PROSTHETIC LIGAMENT RECONSTRUCTION OF THE KNEE

Edited by

MARC J. FRIEDMAN, M.D.

Southern California Orthopedic and Sports
Medicine Group; Clinical Instructor of Orthopedics
University of California, Los Angeles,
Van Nuys, California

RICHARD D. FERKEL, M.D.

Director, Center for Disorders of the Knee,
Southern California Orthopedic and Sports
Medicine Group, Van Nuys, California

1988

W. B. SAUNDERS COMPANY

Harcourt Brace Jovanovich, Inc.

Philadelphia, San Diego, London, Toronto, Montreal, Sydney, Tokyo

W. B. SAUNDERS COMPANY
Harcourt Brace Jovanovich, Inc.

West Washington Square
Philadelphia, PA 19105

Editor: Tracy N. Tucker
Production Manager: Frank Polizzano
Cover Illustrator: Stela Mandel

Prosthetic Ligament Reconstruction of the Knee   ISBN 0-7216-2559-2

Last digit is the print number: 9   8   7   6   5   4   3   2   1

To Donna, Michelle
and the kids
for their love, support and understanding.

PREFACE

Over the past century, a multitude of surgical procedures have been described for stabilization of the "cruciate-deficient knee." Unfortunately, the majority of these techniques have necessitated sacrificing normal structures and involve prolonged recovery periods with variable results. It has become apparent that the ideal cruciate reconstruction would allow for arthroscopic insertion, early range of motion, immediate weightbearing, and no immobilization, and would last a lifetime.

The obvious solution to this problem would be a prosthetic ligament substitute. This book details the current status of prosthetic ligament materials currently being studied in the United States. Although the field is changing quickly, the book should serve to give the reader a solid basis of core information about prosthetic materials. Currently in Europe, numerous other devices are being tested, and some of these will certainly make their way over to the United States as well.

In order to disseminate information to the orthopedic community about these materials, we organized in 1984 a course entitled "Prosthetic Ligament Reconstruction of the Knee." As the field has evolved, so has the course. This book contains many of the ideas discussed over the past four years, and the refinements that have been made to achieve a more ideal prosthetic material.

There have now been over 4000 prosthetic ligament reconstructions performed in the United States, with over 1000 being performed arthroscopically. At numerous centers around the country, these are being critically evaluated by the Food and Drug Administration and by prospective studies with clinical and biomechanical testing. Only with a longer follow-up will we know which, if any, prosthetic materials will withstand the test of time, and achieve the goals that we have set forth for the ideal prosthetic device. The future is exciting for this field, but we feel we must also warn the reader that enthusiasm for this type of surgery must be balanced by good common sense about what is truly best for the patient, based on the patient's age, activity level, and future goals.

MARC J. FRIEDMAN, M.D.
RICHARD D. FERKEL, M.D.

CONTRIBUTORS

E. PETER ABBINK, M.D.
Chief of Orthopedics, Willem Alexander Ziekenhuis, The Netherlands
Clinical Experience in Correction of Chronic Anterior Cruciate Ligament Deficiency with Bovine Xenografts: A 5-Year Study

HAROLD ALEXANDER, PH.D.
Professor, Orthopedic Surgery, New York University Medical School; Director, Department of Bioengineering, Hospital for Joint Diseases/Orthopedic Institute
Preclinical Evaluation of Ligament Reconstruction with an Absorbable Polymer-coated Carbon-fiber Stent (Integraft)*

JAMES R. BAIN, M.S.
Orthopedic Division, W. L. Gore and Associates, Inc., Flagstaff, Arizona
Functional Biomechanics of the Gore-Tex Cruciate-Ligament Prosthesis: Effects of Implant Tensioning

ANDREW B. BERMAN, B.S.M.E.
Orthopedic Division, W. L. Gore and Associates, Inc., Flagstaff, Arizona
Functional Biomechanics of the Gore-Tex Cruciate-Ligament Prosthesis: Effects of Implant Tensioning

WILLIAM C. BRUCHMAN, B.S.M.E.
Orthopedic Division, W. L. Gore and Associates, Inc., Flagstaff, Arizona
Functional Biomechanics of the Gore-Tex Cruciate-Ligament Prosthesis: Effects of Implant Tensioning

ROBERT BURKS, M.D.
Director of Sports Medicine Center of Harper Hospital, Assistant Professor and Athletic Director at Wayne State University, Detroit, Michigan
Anterior Cruciate Ligament Graft Isometry and Tensioning

H. ROYER COLLINS, M.D.
Orthopedic Surgeon, St. Luke's and Thunderbird Samaritan Hospitals; Department of Sports Medicine, St. Luke's, St. Joseph, and John C. Lincoln Hospitals
U.S. Experience with Gore-Tex Reconstruction of the Anterior Cruciate Ligament

DALE M. DANIEL, M.D.

Clinical Associate Professor, Orthopedic Surgery, UCSD; Staff Orthopedic Surgeon, Kaiser Permente Medical Center, San Diego, California

Anterior Cruciate Ligament Graft Isometry and Tensioning; Synthetic Angmentation of Biologic Anterior Cruciate Ligament Substitution; The Marshall/Macintosh Anterior Cruciate Ligament Reconstruction with the Kennedy Ligament Augmentation Device: Report of the United States Clinical Trials

RICHARD D. FERKEL, M.D.

Clinical Instructor of Orthopedic Surgery, UCLA School of Medicine; Chief of Arthroscopic Surgery, Wadsworth V.A.; Director, Center for Disorders of the Knee and Orthopedic Surgeon, Southern California Orthopedic and Sports Medical Group, Van Nuys, California

Biomechanics of the Knee; Instrumented Knee Testing

JANET G. FERL, M.S.

Biomechanical Engineer

FDA Regulation of Prosthetic Ligament Devices

SCOTT P. FISCHER, M.D.

Former Fellow in Athletic Medicine, Southern California Orthopedic and Sports Medical Group; Staff Orthopedic Surgeon, Community Memorial Hospital, Ventura, California

Biomechanics of the Knee; Instrumented Knee Testing

JAMES M. FOX, M.D.

Associate Director, Center for Disorders of the Knee, Southern California Orthopedic and Sports Medical Group, Staff Orthopedic Surgeon, Valley Presbyterian Hospital, Van Nuys, California

Arthroscopic Insertion of the Prosthetic Gorè-Tex Ligament

E. PAUL FRANCE, PH. D.

Research Instructor of Surgery, University of Utah School of Medicine; Salt Lake Knee Research Foundation, University of Utah

The Biomechanics of Anterior Cruciate Allografts

MARC J. FRIEDMAN, M.D.

Assistant Clinical Professor of Orthopedic Surgery, UCLA School of Medicine; Associate Director, Center for Disorders of the Knee and Southern California Orthopedic and Sports Medical Group; Orthopedic Surgeon, Valley Presbyterian Hospital, Van Nuys, California

A Review of Autogenous Intra-Articular Reconstruction of the Anterior Cruciate Ligament

KYOSUKE FUJIKAWA, M.D., M.P.H.

Assistant Professor, Department of Orthopedic Surgery, School of Medicine, Keio University, Tokyo, Japan; Knee Surgery in Chief, Keio University Hospital, Tokyo, Japan

Clinical Study of Anterior Cruciate Ligament Reconstruction with the Leeds-Keio Artificial Ligament

KAREN L. GOLDENTHAL, M.D.

Center for Biologies Evaluation and Research, Food and Drug Administration

FDA Regulation of Prosthetic Ligament Devices

WILLIAM DOUG GURLEY, M.D.
Fellow, Athletic Medicine, Salt Lake Knee and Sports Clinic
Anterior Cruciate Ligament Allografts

CHRISTOPHER D. HARNER, M.D.
Assistant Professor of Orthopedic Surgery, University of Pittsburgh, School of Medicine;
Fellow, Athletic Medicine, Salt Lake Knee and Sports Clinic
The Biomechanics of Anterior Cruciate Allografts

DAVID JENKINS, M.B., CH.B, F.R.C.S., CH.M.
Consultant and Orthopedic Surgery, University Hospital of Wales, Cardiff, Wales, U.K.
Carbon Fiber in Ligament Reinforcement

JOHN C. KENNEDY, M.D., F.R.C.S.(C) *(Deceased)*
Professor, Division of Orthopedics, University of Western Ontario, London, Ontario, Canada
Polypropylene-Braid-Augmented Anterior Cruciate Ligament Reconstruction

ROBERT L. LARSON, M.D.
Orthopedic Consultant, Athletic Department, University of Oregon, Eugene, Oregon; Clinical
Associate Professor of Surgery, Division of Orthopedics and Rehabilitation, School of Medi-
cine, Oregon Health Sciences Center, Portland, Oregon; Staff, Sacred Heart General Hospital,
Eugene, Oregon
*Indications for Prosthetic Ligament Reconstruction; Future of Prosthetic Ligament
Reconstruction*

GARY M. LOSSE, M.D.
*The Marshall/Macintosh Anterior Cruciate Ligament Reconstruction with the Kennedy
Ligament Augmentation Device: Report of the United States Clinical Trials*

WILLIAM C. McMASTER, M.D.
Adjunct Professor, Orthopedics, University of California, Irvine, Irvine, California; Attending
Orthopedist, St. Joseph Hospital, Orange, California; Attending Orthopedist, Children's Hos-
pital, Orange County, Orange, California
*Biomechanics Profile of the ProCol Cruciate Bioprosthesis; Open Anterior Cruciate
Ligament Reconstruction with ProCol Bioprosthesis: Results at 24 Months—U.S. Series*

KEITH L. MARKOLF, PH.D.
Adjunct Professor, Division of Orthopedic Surgery, UCLA
Clinical and Laboratory Studies with the Gore-Tex Ligament at UCLA

NIRMAL K. MISHRA, D.V.M., PH.D.
Chief of Restorative Devices
FDA Regulation of Prosthetic Ligament Devices

ELVERT F. NELSON, M.D.

North Pacific Orthopedic Sports Medical Clinic; Private Practice, Portland, Oregon

Integraft* Anterior Cruciate Ligament Reconstruction: Arthroscopic Technique

JAMES A. NICHOLAS, M.D.

Professor of Orthopedic Surgery, New York Medical College; Director, Department of Orthopedic Surgery, Lenox Hill Hospital, New York, New York; Founding Director, Nicholas Institute of Sports Medicine and Athletic Trauma (NISMAT), Lenox Hill Hospital, New York, New York

Prosthetic Ligament Reconstruction

DONALD NOEL, O.P.A.

North Pacific Orthopedic Sports Medical Clinic

Integraft* Anterior Cruciate Ligament Reconstruction—Arthroscopic Technique

RICHARD D. PARKER, M.D.

Head of Sports Medicine, Mt. Sinai Medical Center, Cleveland, Ohio; Clinical Instructor in Orthopedics/Orthopedic Surgery, Case Western Reserve University, Cleveland, Ohio; Mt. Sinai Medical Center, Cleveland, Ohio; Fellow, Athletic Medicine, Salt Lake Knee and Sports Clinic

Prosthetic Ligament Reconstruction

JOHN R. PARSONS, PH.D.

Associate Professor and Director of Orthopedic Research, University of Medicine and Dentistry New Jersey—New Jersey Medical School; Associate Professor, Graduate Faculty, Biomedical Engineering, Rutgers University, New Brunswick

Preclinical Evaluation of Ligament Reconstruction with an Absorbable Polymer-coated Carbon-fiber Stent (Integraft*)

GARY A. PATTEE, M.D.

Former Fellow in Athletic Medicine, Southern California Orthopedic and Sports Medical Group; Orthopedic Surgeon, Saint John's Hospital and Health Center, Santa Monica, California; Orthopedic Surgeon, Santa Monica Hospital Medical Center, Santa Monica, California

A Review of Autogenous Intra-Articular Reconstruction of the Anterior Cruciate Ligament; Prosthetic Reconstruction of the Anterior Cruciate Ligament: Historical Overview

LONNIE E. PAULOS, M.D.

Clinical Associate Professor, University of Utah School of Medicine; Co-Director, Salt Lake Knee and Sports Clinic

The Biomechanics of Anterior Cruciate Allografts; Anterior Cruciate Ligament Allografts; Prosthetic Ligament Reconstruction

DARRELL A. PENNER, M.D., F.R.C.S.(C)

Orthopedic Surgeon, Colonel Belcher and Holy Cross Hospitals, Calgary, Alberta, Canada

Anterior Cruciate Ligament Graft Isometry and Tensioning

THOMAS D. ROSENBERG, M.D.

Clinical Associate Professor, University of Utah; Salt Lake Knee and Sports Clinic

The Biomechanics of Anterior Cruciate Allografts; Anterior Cruciate Ligament Allografts; Prosthetic Ligament Reconstruction

JAMES H. ROTH, M.D.

Clinical Associate Professor, Division of Orthopedic Surgery, University of Western Ontario, London, Ontario, Canada; Attending Surgeon, Victoria Hospital, London, Ontario, Canada

Polypropylene-Braid–Augmented Anterior Cruciate Ligament Reconstruction

ROY M. RUSCH, M.D.

Senior Clinical Instructor, University of Oregon Medical School; Director, North Pacific Orthopedic Sports Medical Clinic; Active Staff, Portland Adventist Medical Center; Courtesy Staff, Woodland Park Hospital; Courtesy Staff, MT. Hood Medical Center

Integraft* Anterior Cruciate Ligament Reconstruction; Integraft* Anterior Cruciate Ligament Reconstruction: Arthroscopic Technique

BAHAA B. SEEDHOM, B.S.C., PH.D.

Arthritis and Rheumatism Council, Senior Lecturer (Bioengineering) at The Rheumatology and Rehabilitation Research Unit, LEEDS University, Leeds, West Yorkshire, U.K.

The Leeds–Keio Ligament: Biomechanics

STEPHEN J. SNYDER, M.D.

Associate Director, Center for Disorders of the Knee, Southern California Orthopedic and Sports Medical Group; Orthopedic Surgeon, Valley Presbyterian Hospital, Van Nuys, California; Associate Director, Center for Disorders of the Knee, Van Nuys, California; Coordinator for Shoulder Arthroscopy Study Groups, Southern California

Prosthetic Reconstruction of the Anterior Cruciate Ligament: Historical Overview

MARY LOU STONE, R.P.T.

Clinical Specialist and Research Therapist, San Diego, California

The Marshall/Macintosh Anterior Cruciate Ligament Reconstruction with the Kennedy Ligament Augmentation Device: Report of the United States Clinical Trials

SCOTT N. STONEBROOK, B.S.E.

Research Engineer, LDS Hospital, Salt Lake City, Utah

Functional Biomechanics of the Gore-Tex Cruciate-Ligament Prosthesis: Effects of Implant Tensioning

C.L. VAN KAMPEN, PH.D.

Technical Supervisor, Orthopedic Products Division/3M

Synthetic Augmentation of Biologic Anterior Cruciate Ligament Substitution

ANDREW B. WEISS, M.D.

Professor and Chief, University of Medicine and Dentistry of New Jersey—New Jersey Medical School, Section of Orthopedic Surgery; Chief, Orthopedic Surgery, University Hospital, Newark, New Jersey; Attending, Hospital Center at Orange, New Jersey; Attending, Kennedy Memorial Hospital, Saddlebrook, New Jersey; Attending, United Hospitals Medical Center, Newark, New Jersey; Consultant, V.A. Medical Center, East Orange, New Jersey

Preclinical Evaluation of Ligament Reconstruction with an Absorbable Polymer-coated Carbon-fiber Stent (Integraft*)

TERRY L. WHIPPLE, M.D., F.A.C.S.

Assistant Clinical Professor, Medical College of Virginia; President, Orthopedic Research of Virginia; Consultant, Hand and Sports Medicine, University of Virginia; Chief of Orthopedics, Humana Hospital, St. Lukes, Richmond, Virginia; Attending Surgeon, St. Mary's Hospital, Richmond, Virginia

Arthroscopic Anterior Cruciate Ligament Reconstruction with ProCol Xenograft Bioprosthesis

E. PAUL WOODWARD, M.D.

Assistant Clinical Professor of Surgery/Orthopedic School of Medicine, UCSD; Sharp Memorial Hospital; Scruppa Memorial Hospital; Mercy Hospital; Childrens Hospital

The Marshall/Macintosh Anterior Cruciate Ligament Reconstruction with the Kennedy Ligament Augmentation Device: Report of the United States Clinical Trials

CONTENTS

1

PROSTHETIC LIGAMENT RECONSTRUCTION   1
    JAMES A. NICHOLAS, M.D.

2

BIOMECHANICS OF THE KNEE   3
    SCOTT P. FISCHER, M.D., and RICHARD D. FERKEL, M.D.

3

INSTRUMENTED KNEE TESTING   10
    SCOTT P. FISCHER, M.D., and RICHARD D. FERKEL, M.D.

4

ANTERIOR CRUCIATE LIGAMENT GRAFT ISOMETRY AND TENSIONING   17
    DALE M. DANIEL, M.D., DARRELL A. PENNER, M.D., and
    ROBERT BURKS, M.D.

5

A REVIEW OF AUTOGENOUS INTRA-ARTICULAR RECONSTRUCTION
OF THE ANTERIOR CRUCIATE LIGAMENT   22
    GARY A. PATTEE, M.D., and MARC J. FRIEDMAN, M.D.

6

PROSTHETIC RECONSTRUCTION OF THE ANTERIOR CRUCIATE
LIGAMENT: HISTORICAL OVERVIEW   29
    GARY A. PATTEE, M.D., and STEPHEN J. SNYDER, M.D.

7

INDICATIONS FOR PROSTHETIC LIGAMENT RECONSTRUCTION   34
    ROBERT L. LARSON, M.D.

8

CARBON FIBER IN LIGAMENT REINFORCEMENT 39

DAVID JENKINS, M.D.

9

PRECLINICAL EVALUATION OF LIGAMENT RECONSTRUCTION WITH
AN ABSORBABLE POLYMER-COATED CARBON-FIBER STENT
(INTEGRAFT*) 41

HAROLD ALEXANDER, PH.D., JOHN R. PARSONS, PH.D., and
ANDREW B. WEISS, M.D.

10

INTEGRAFT* ANTERIOR CRUCIATE LIGAMENT RECONSTRUCTION 52

ROY M. RUSCH, M.D.

11

INTEGRAFT* ANTERIOR CRUCIATE LIGAMENT RECONSTRUCTION:
ARTHROSCOPIC TECHNIQUE 59

ROY M. RUSCH, M.D., ELVERT F. NELSON, M.D., and DONALD NOEL, O.P.A.

12

SYNTHETIC AUGMENTATION OF BIOLOGIC ANTERIOR CRUCIATE
LIGAMENT SUBSTITUTION 65

DALE M. DANIEL, M.D., and C.L. VAN KAMPEN, PH.D.

13

THE MARSHALL/MACINTOSH ANTERIOR CRUCIATE LIGAMENT
RECONSTRUCTION WITH THE KENNEDY LIGAMENT AUGMENTATION
DEVICE: REPORT OF THE UNITED STATES CLINICAL TRIALS 71

DALE M. DANIEL, M.D., E. PAUL WOODWARD, M.D., GARY M. LOSSE, M.D.,
and MARY LOU STONE, RPT

14

POLYPROPYLENE-BRAID–AUGMENTED ANTERIOR CRUCIATE
LIGAMENT RECONSTRUCTION 79

JAMES H. ROTH, M.D., and JOHN C. KENNEDY, M.D.

15

BIOMECHANICS PROFILE OF THE PROCOL CRUCIATE
BIOPROSTHESIS 89

WILLIAM C. MCMASTER, M.D.

16

OPEN ANTERIOR CRUCIATE LIGAMENT RECONSTRUCTION WITH
PROCOL BIOPROSTHESIS: RESULTS AT 24 MONTHS—U.S. SERIES 95

WILLIAM C. MCMASTER, M.D.

17

CLINICAL EXPERIENCE IN CORRECTION OF CHRONIC ANTERIOR
CRUCIATE LIGAMENT DEFICIENCY WITH BOVINE XENOGRAFTS: A 5-
YEAR STUDY   101
  E. PETER ABBINK, M.D.

18

ARTHROSCOPIC ANTERIOR CRUCIATE LIGAMENT RECONSTRUCTION
WITH PROCOL XENOGRAFT BIOPROSTHESIS   112
  TERRY L. WHIPPLE, M.D.

19

THE LEEDS–KEIO LIGAMENT: BIOMECHANICS   118
  BAHAA B. SEEDHAM, B.SC., PH.D.

20

CLINICAL STUDY OF ANTERIOR CRUCIATE LIGAMENT
RECONSTRUCTION WITH THE LEEDS–KEIO ARTIFICIAL LIGAMENT   132
  KYOSUKE FUJIKAWA, M.D., M.P.H.

21

FUNCTIONAL BIOMECHANICS OF THE GORE-TEX CRUCIATE-
LIGAMENT PROSTHESIS: EFFECTS OF IMPLANT TENSIONING   140
  SCOTT N. STONEBROOK, B.S.E., ANDREW B. BERMAN, B.S.M.E.,
  WILLIAM C. BRUCHMAN, B.S.M.E., and JAMES R. BAIN, M.S.

22

CLINICAL AND LABORATORY STUDIES WITH THE GORE-TEX
LIGAMENT AT UCLA   149
  KEITH L. MARKOLF, PH.D.

23

U.S. EXPERIENCE WITH GORE-TEX RECONSTRUCTION OF THE
ANTERIOR CRUCIATE LIGAMENT   156
  H. ROYER COLLINS, M.D.

24

ARTHROSCOPIC INSERTION OF THE PROSTHETIC GORE-TEX
LIGAMENT   165
  JAMES M. FOX, M.D.

25

THE BIOMECHANICS OF ANTERIOR CRUCIATE ALLOGRAFTS   180
  E. PAUL FRANCE, PH.D., LONNIE E. PAULOS, M.D.,
  THOMAS D. ROSENBERG, M.D., and CHRISTOPHER D. HARNER, M.D.

26

ANTERIOR CRUCIATE LIGAMENT ALLOGRAFTS   186
LONNIE E. PAULOS, M.D., THOMAS D. ROSENBERG, M.D., and
WILLIAM DOUG GURLEY, M.D.

27

ALLOGRAFT ANTERIOR CRUCIATE LIGAMENT RECONSTRUCTION: AN
ARTHROSCOPICALLY GUIDED TECHNIQUE   193
THOMAS D. ROSENBERG, M.D., LONNIE E. PAULOS, M.D., and
RICHARD D. PARKER, M.D.

28

FDA REGULATION OF PROSTHETIC LIGAMENT DEVICES   202
JANET G. FERL, M.S., KAREN L. GOLDENTHAL, M.D., and
NIRMAL K. MISHRA, D.V.M., PH.D.

29

FUTURE OF PROSTHETIC LIGAMENT RECONSTRUCTION   209
ROBERT L. LARSON, M.D.

INDEX   213

1

PROSTHETIC LIGAMENT RECONSTRUCTION

JAMES A. NICHOLAS, M.D.

INTRODUCTION

For the past four decades, I am fortunate to have been intimately associated with the frustrating problem of the torn anterior cruciate ligament, and its resultant patterns of instability. I am delighted to write an introduction to this book detailing the important new developments concerning the synthetic approach.

First, as to historical credit, World War I and polio spurred interest in attempts to repair surgically and reconstruct anterior cruciate instability using fascial iliotibial strips passed through drill holes in the femur and tibia, with some remarkable results. Hey Groves (1917) and Alwyn Smith (1918) were the first to try to make new anterior cruciate ligaments; over the following years, all types of procedures have not solved this dilemma satisfactorily, and synthetics are another approach.

In 1986 we are still trying to do this. Whereas extra-articular procedures, and the intra-articular operations of the 1950s to the 1970s, reported 60 to 70 per cent satisfactory results, present-day combined intra-articular and extra-articular techniques have reached the 90 per cent level. So we have gained 19 per cent good to excellent results in three decades. There has been no breakthrough in this period. ''How-to'' techniques abound. Advocates of nonrepair, exercise, bracing, and menisci preservation by repair are quite vocal, as opposed to those who believe in repair–reconstruction with acute anterior cruciate tears.

So what is the reason for this diversity? Obviously, the problem is a common one. In the past three weeks, as I have written this, my professional football team has had five different combinations of instability as a result of acute anterior cruciate ligament tears (in a squad of 45). It is extremely important for a surgeon to have a broad perception of instability, and he or she should understand the classification, clinical patterns, and the unpredictable nature of instability. Surgeons should recognize that not all such knees end up on the same road. Some stabilize without reconstruction and repair with slight arthritis, and function for decades without much difficulty, permitting skiing, but not deceleration from heavy jumping, such as in basketball. Individuals who have loose joints, as well as those with floppy heart valves, have a different pattern of function than those with inherently tight knees, be it topography, contracture, or actual differences in collagen tensile strength.

No surgeon should ever forget these facts when making a careful clinical diagnosis, abetted by arthroscopy, anesthesia, and, if necessary, arthrography (for capsular, blind-spot meniscal integrity) in planning treatment. All surgeons interested in this subject must know the literature since 1918, and the current prodigious debate that goes on, and be prepared to modify their own bias. Rehabilitation is always important, whatever will be used to stabilize the knee. The strain on the anterior cruciate ligament will increase by rotation, and in flex-

1

ion beyond 60 degrees, the hamstrings, as well as the medial–lateral adductor/abductor hip–knee components, must be made as strong as possible to counteract excessive knee extension/rotation activity. One of the most important tests of knee stability in performance is the ability to hop and jump forward. Without strong hip flexors, hamstrings, calves, abductors, and adductors, buckling of the knee will occur, or be enhanced at lower forces.

On the subject of other knee tests for instability, such as the pivot shift and Lachman and drawer signs, their presence will point to an anterior cruciate deficiency. However, and I emphasize this, retraining a knee to normal ability to balance body weight is also a function of proprioceptive stability, something that Michael Freeman has emphasized so well in his studies of the unstable ankle. After knees are injured or operated on, a number of balancing-performance moves, such as deceleration or inside–out–inside cuts, require 12 to 15 months of training in proprioception, with strong musculature before the knee can be safely stressed. This is important in any rehabilitation program for these knees. Prosthetic ligaments alone cannot provide this essential proprioceptive component when nerves supplying the anterior cruciate and capsular complexes are disrupted; the nerves must be intact again to carry proprioceptive balance with phasic muscle contraction in sports movements and gait, with higher loads of force.

There are many other unsolved problems to keep in mind. Does a new ligament or synthetic repair, as is reported in autografts with collagen in.

Are the best results correlated to a loss of movement in tibial rotation with decreased end points? Does this cause a greater load on the knee, producing arthritis? Can machines measure dynamic as opposed to static laxity, in vivo?

Is arthroscopic reconstruction ignoring the secondary stabilizers, which are likely to produce greater damage (by ignoring the posterolateral and medial capsular corners)? Are not allografts, if autogenicity can be blocked, more likely to simulate the normal cruciate twisting collagenous structure? Or do synthetics have this capability?

When are extra-articular procedures indicated? Do we test knees as carefully now with the arthroscope available, as we did in the 1960s, when examinations emphasized careful four-quadrant evaluation of the knee clinically and, if necessary, under anesthesia using dye?

Finally, do synthetics have the capability of functioning as viable ligaments, which can resist repeated tensile stresses? My experience with polyethylene ligaments in 1973 to 1975 was dismal when a knee recovered its motion; all broke when flexion was recovered to 90 degrees, and the instability problem was then worse, because the synthetics had to be removed.

With all this, it is an exciting future for a difficult challenge. The authors of this book deserve our thanks for their courage and interest in furthering what our grandfather pioneers first attempted.

2

BIOMECHANICS OF THE KNEE

SCOTT P. FISCHER, M.D.
RICHARD D. FERKEL, M.D.

The knee is the largest and possibly the most complex joint in the human body. It allows rotation about two axes. It restrains rotation about a third axis and controls translation in all three planes. The knee bears loads that frequently exceed the body's weight by two to three times, and its location between the body's two longest lever arms makes it especially prone to injury. Because it lacks any great amount of bony stability, it depends upon a complex arrangement of ligaments, menisci, and musculotendinous units to maintain normal alignment and stability.

When excessive load or stress is applied to the lower extremity, it is not unusual for the result to be a ligamentous or meniscal injury to the knee. Damage to these structures may compromise the stability of the knee and allow abnormal motion with altered biomechanics. This change in knee function may ultimately express itself as a functional instability, as secondary degeneration of the joint, or as both. Our goal in treatment is to control this instability and arrest secondary degenerative changes. To accomplish this, it is necessary first to have a clear understanding of the anatomy, kinematics, and biomechanics of the knee.

It is outside the scope of this book to present a treatise on these topics comparable to that of Müller [17] or Nordin and Frankel [18]. Our purpose in this chapter is to review terms and concepts pertinent to the discussion in the following chapters.

ANATOMY AND KINEMATICS

Knee flexion and extension comprises a complex series of motions occurring between the femur and the tibia. Far from being a simple hinge-type joint, rolling, sliding, and axial rotation occur simultaneously during different portions of the knee's normal range of motion. Comparison of the weight-bearing surfaces of the femoral and tibial condyles reveals the femoral surface to be significantly longer than that of the tibia. If one plots the serial contact points between the femur and the tibia throughout the full range of flexion, it is apparent that the distance between successive points is greater on the femur than on the tibia (Fig. 2–1). This reflects the combination of rolling and sliding that is present during flexion of the knee. In early flexion, the ratio of rolling to sliding is approximately 1:2, whereas late in flexion it approaches 1:4 [17].

In addition to this combination of rolling and sliding, axial rotation also occurs between the femur and the tibia, especially as the knee nears extension. Examination of the femoral–tibial joint reveals its division into slightly different medial and lateral compartments. The two femoral condyles are asymmetric in shape with the medial femoral condyle (MFC) longer and narrower than the lateral femoral condyle (LFC). During the final 15 degrees of terminal extension, the LFC is

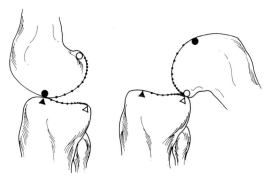

Figure 2–1. The distance between serial femoral–tibial contact points is greater on the femur than on the tibia, reflecting the necessary combination of sliding and rolling during flexion. (Adapted from Müller [17].)

blocked from further sliding by engagement of the anterolateral tibial plateau in the terminal sulcus of the LFC. At this point in extension, there is remaining weight-bearing surface anteriorly and centrally on the longer MFC. Therefore additional medial compartment extension is possible and occurs by further MFC sliding until full knee extension is accomplished. Because the lateral compartment does not participate in this additional sliding, the tibia must automatically rotate externally approximately 15 degrees to allow this medial compartment motion to occur. It is this combination of extension and automatic axial rotation that is frequently referred to as the "screw-home mechanism."

The tibial plateaus are also asymmetric. The medial surface is concave and larger compared to the lateral surface, which is relatively convex. Interposition of the menisci in each compartment improves the adaptation of the tibial and femoral surfaces. This increases the surface area for load transmission through the joint, and thereby decreases joint surface stress. The menisci also have been shown to contribute to knee-joint stability in the anterior cruciate deficient knee [1, 14]. The lateral meniscus is more loosely attached to the tibia than the medial meniscus, allowing greater anterior–posterior excursion of this meniscus with flexion and extension. Rising up from the tibial plateau between the medial and lateral compartments are the anteromedial and posterolateral tibial spines, which may provide stability against medial–lateral translation [9].

Inspection of the contour of the femoral condyles in the sagittal plane reveals that they have a changing radius of curvature from anterior to posterior, giving them a cam-shaped appearance. This varying radius of curvature produces a change in position of the center of rotation (for flexion–extension) as the knee passes through its range of

motion. One must therefore speak of an "instant center" of rotation for the knee over a defined arc of flexion [5, 6, 17, 22].

If a line is drawn joining this instant center of rotation to the joint-surface contact point, the velocity vector for the motion between the weight-bearing surfaces of the joint is defined as the perpendicular to this line. In a normal joint, this vector is tangential to the femoral surface, and parallel to the tibial surface, so that pure sliding occurs without joint-surface compression or distraction (Fig. 2–2). When there is internal derangement of the knee, such as with cruciate ligament insufficiency or meniscal tears, the instant center of rotation may change to an abnormal position [5, 6]. If this occurs, the joint-surface velocity vector may not be tangential to the joint surfaces, but may produce articular surface compression or distraction with flexion and extension (Fig. 2–2). This may in part explain the accelerated and abnormal joint-surface wear associated with these conditions. An attempt to restore more normal knee kinematics and biomechanics should therefore be a significant concern to the clinician.

The anterior cruciate ligament (ACL) and the posterior cruciate ligament (PCL) are the two major intra-articular ligaments of the knee. Located in the intercondylar region between the medial and lateral compartments, they are responsible for controlling and guiding the knee through most of its range of motion. The ACL is comprised of a multitude of fibers of varying lengths, which twist upon each other as the knee flexes. Fibers inserting

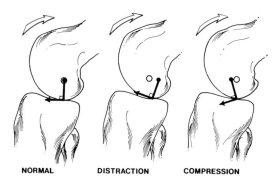

NORMAL   DISTRACTION   COMPRESSION

Figure 2–2. The joint-surface velocity vector of the femur during flexion is perpendicular to a line connecting the joint-surface contact point and the instant center of rotation (solid circle). In a normal knee, this velocity vectory is parallel to the corresponding portion of the tibial articular surface, representing joint sliding with further flexion. In a knee with ligamentous or meniscal injury, the instant center of rotation shifts location in the femur. This results in an altered femoral-surface velocity vector, producing articular distraction or compression with further knee flexion. (Adapted from Frankel VH, Nordin M. Biomechanics of the musculoskeletal system, Philadelphia: Lea and Febiger, 1980.)

more anteriorly and medially on the tibia, originate most posteriorly and proximally on the LFC in the intercondylar notch [7]. These fibers tend to remain taut through most of the knee's range of motion. The fibers of the ACL that insert more posteriorly on the tibia tend to be taut in extension, but become lax as the knee flexes. The ACL has been reported to be approximately 38 mm in length and 11 mm in width [7]. Its average strength has been determined to be approximately 1730 N in young individuals [2, 19], and it contributes 86 per cent of the knee's stability to anterior tibial translation. In addition, it contributes to stabilization against varus and valgus displacement in the knee [11] and against anterolateral tibial rotation [8].

The PCL is comprised of a large anterior portion, which comprises the bulk of the ligament, and a smaller oblique posterior portion. Its average length and width have been measured as approximately 38 mm and 13 mm, respectively [7]. It inserts into a depression in the tibia that is inferior to the articular surface and posterior to the intercondylar area. It originates on the lateral aspect of the medial femoral condyle, posterior in the intercondylar notch [7]. The PCL contributes 95 per cent of the knee's stability to posterior tibial translation when flexed to 90 degrees [2]. It also contributes to knee stability against varus–valgus rotation [8, 11] and posterolateral tibial rotation [8].

During flexion and extension, the ACL and PCL function together to control the tibia as it moves on the femur. The interaction between these ligaments and joint surfaces has been modeled by Menschik (in Müller [17]) with the ''crossed four-bar linkage.'' In this model, the ACL and PCL are represented by rigid bars of proportionate length, with fixed femoral attachments. At their tibial insertions they are connected to a mobile tibial bar. When passed through a range of motion, this ''tibial surface'' is seen to produce a series of tangent lines, which together accurately reproduce the contour of the posterior portion of the femoral condyle (Fig. 2–3).

The point at which the ACL and PCL cross is coincident with the instant center of rotation for that arc of motion. In the normal knee, a line joining the femoral attachments of the ACL and PCL is found to be at a 40-degree angle to the long axis of the femur (Fig. 2–3). When a crossed four-bar linkage is constructed in this fashion, a normal range of motion of approximately −5 degrees to 145 degrees is allowed. If the ACL and PCL femoral attachments are altered, such that the line between them is at less than a 40-degree angle to the longitudinal axis of the femur, full extension is restricted [17]. Similarly, if there is greater than a 40-degree angle, hyperextension is allowed. If the

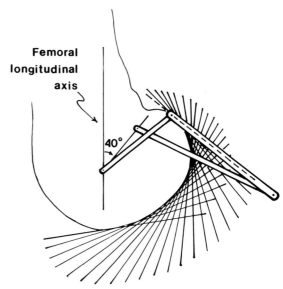

Figure 2–3. The crossed four-bar linkage model. When passed through a range of motion, the tibial surface traces a series of tangent lines reproducing the contour of the posterior portion of the femoral condyle. (Adapted from Müller [17].)

femoral attachment site of the ACL is moved anteriorly in the intercondylar notch, ligament laxity will be present early in knee flexion. As further flexion occurs, the ligament will become taut and restrict full flexion [17] (Fig. 2–4). Under these circumstances, attempts to achieve a full range of motion will be unsuccessful until the ligament with the improper length and attachment site is ruptured. Such improper ligament placement also alters the site at which the ligaments cross, reflecting a change in location of the instant center of rotation (possibly resulting in abnormal joint-surface velocity vectors).

The ideal and actual attachment sites for the extra-articular collateral stabilizers of the knee

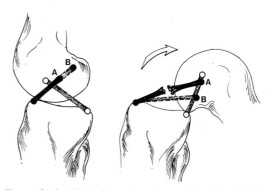

Figure 2–4. If the femoral attachment site of the ACL is moved anteriorly (A) in the intercondylar notch from its normal position (B), it will either restrict full flexion or it will rupture. (Adapted from Müller [17].)

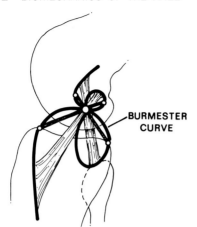

Figure 2—5. The isometric attachment sites for lines that cross the knee lie along the Burmester curve and pass through the instant center of rotation (large open circle). Note that the cruciate and collateral ligament insertions lie upon the curve and intersect at the center of rotation. (Adapted from Müller [17].)

have been determined to lie along a complex line described by two third-order curves developed by Burmester in 1888 [see 17]. The Burmester curve determines points of isometry between the "cammed" femoral side of the joint, and the "flat" tibial side of the joint (Fig. 2–5). The cruciate ligaments as well as the medial and lateral collateral ligament fibers passing from the tibial to the femoral portion of the curve are found to cross at the instant center of rotation. Fibers that lie outside the curve are either lax for a portion of the joint's range of motion, or attach to a musculotendinous unit capable of tensioning those fibers through the range of motion (such as the semimembranosus). The curve also provides the rationale for the asymmetry between the femoral and tibial attachment sites of the collateral ligaments present not only in the human knee, but in essentially all tetrapod species [see 4].

BIOMECHANICS

In subsequent chapters, various biomechanical properties of the normal ACL and proposed prosthetic replacements will be discussed. Many terms that must be understood to avoid later confusion commonly arise in these discussions. Several of these terms and their definitions are listed in Table 2–1. When specific structures are biomechanically tested to determine how much elongation occurs with an applied force, a load-deformation curve (Graph 2–1) is generated for that structure. This type of curve is dependent upon the structural properties of the specimen. A stress–strain curve is similar to a load-deformation curve; however, its charted values are derived numbers (refer to Table 2–1). A stress–strain curve is not dependent upon a specimen's physical dimensions and therefore is more of a measure of the specimen's material properties.

Stiffness and strength are parameters used to describe specific properties of prosthetic ligaments for purposes of comparison with the expected demands to which they will be subjected. Because it is a viscoelastic structure, the rate at which a ligament is loaded will have dramatic effects upon its ultimate strength and stiffness, as demonstrated in Graph 2–2 [13]. The ACL is routinely exposed to loads that vary from 70 N while ascending stairs, to 210 N with level walking. ACL loads increase to 485 N descending an incline and 630 N while jogging [3]. The strength of the ACL in young persons has been measured to be 1730 N ($\pm$ 270 N) [19]. This appears to leave significant reserve for ACL protection with routine activities, however, loads with aggressive athletic activities are as yet unmeasured and are certain to be significantly greater. For this reason, selection of the ideal strength of an ACL graft will depend not only upon

TABLE 2–1. DEFINITIONS

Load	Applied force (Newtons)
Deformation	Amount object stretches or elongates (millimeters)
Stress	Amount of load divided by area over which it is applied (megapascals)
Strain	Deformation divided by the initial length (per cent)
Stiffness	Amount of applied load necessary to produce a given deformation (Newtons per millimeter)
Ultimate Strength	Measure of how much load a structure can bear prior to failure (also maximum load)
Load-deformation curve	A graph of the relationship between the load applied to an object and its resulting change in dimension. (Depends upon the structural properties of the specimen)
Stress–strain curve	A graph of the relationship between the stress applied to a material and its resulting strain. (Similar to load-deformation curve, but does not depend upon specimen physical dimensions; measurement of material properties)
Creep	Progressive material deformation over time under a constant load
Viscoelasticity	A time-related material property that allows creep to occur, or that results in a relaxation of internal stress when deformation is constant

GRAPH 2–1.

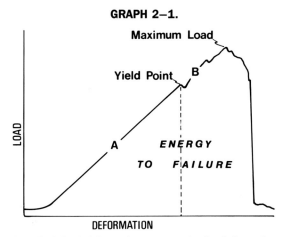

A typical load-deformation curve; elastic deformation (A) occurs up to the yield point, after which plastic deformation (B) occurs. Energy to failure is to the area beneath the entire curve.

GRAPH 2–2.

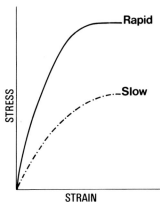

Viscoelastic properties of ligaments result in different amounts of ligament strain for an equal amount of stress, depending upon the rate of loading. There is increased ligament stiffness (the slope of the curve) and energy absorbed (area under the curve) with rapid loading.

the range of loads to which it will be routinely subjected after implantation, but also upon the margin of safety desired to protect the graft during uncontrolled and athletic activities. This concept of reserve strength or "safety zones" in ligament substitution as described by Noyes et al. [19] is important when considering material and structural properties for prosthetic ACL grafts. Table 2–2 compares these biomechanical properties for several of the prosthetic ligaments under current investigation. At this time, however, the desired combination of properties such as strength, maximum stress, stiffness, and ultimate strain have not

been adequately defined experimentally for prosthetic ACL replacements or augmentation devices.

BIOMECHANICS OF THE ACL-DEFICIENT KNEE

The ACL is the "primary anterior stabilizer" in the knee, contributing 86 per cent of the resistance to anterior displacement forces [2]. As noted in Chapter 3, the anterior laxity of an uninjured knee (in 30 degrees of flexion) is approximately 5 mm, with 2 mm or less difference between the right and

TABLE 2–2.   COMPARISON OF ACL PROSTHETIC LIGAMENTS

	Normal ACL	Gortex	Xenotech	LAD	Stryker	Leeds-Keio	Integraft
Animal model	Human (16–26 yr)	Sheep	Dog	Goat	Dog	Pig	Dog
Fixation	Bone	Bone	Bone	Soft tissue	Bone	Bone	Soft tissue
Type of prosthesis		Permanent	Permanent	Stent	Stent	Ingrowth	Ingrowth
Material		PTFE	Bovine tendon	Polypropylene braid	Dacron fabric	Dacron mesh	Coated carbon
Ultimate tensile strength (N)	1730	>4448	3000–4000	1730 (8 mm) 1500 (6 mm)	3110	2000	425 per tow
Stiffness (N/mm)	182	322	53	56 N/mm (8 mm) 15 cm long 61 N/mm (6 mm) 15 cm long	39	>182	33 × 10⁶ psi*
Ultimate strain (%)	60	9	10	22 (8 mm) 22 (6 mm)	18	35	1

*Cannot be stated in N/mm; material used as composite, and stiffness will change with method of insertion.

left knee in 95 per cent of normal individuals. With isolated ACL deficiency, mean anterior instability becomes approximately 10 mm with an injured versus normal knee difference averaging 5 mm [21]. Anterior stiffness in extension is similarly reduced to 30 per cent of normal with ACL sectioning [16]. With loss of the ACL, other "secondary stabilizers" contribute whatever residual anterior stability is present [see 12]. The hamstring musculotendinous units may function as effective dynamic stabilizers when the knee is flexed; however, as the knee approaches extension, they function at an increasing biomechanical disadvantage for controlling anterior translation. Similarly, other secondary restraints, such as the medial collateral ligament (MCL), function more effectively when the knee is flexed because of their fiber orientation. Butler et al. [2] found equal contributions to anterior stability in the ACL-deficient knee (at 90 degrees of flexion) by the MCL, lateral collateral ligament, medial and lateral capsule, and the iliotibial band. The medial meniscus also makes a contribution to anterior stability in the ACL-deficient knee [1, 14, 20]. While medial meniscectomy does not produce significantly increased anterior instability in an otherwise normal knee, medial meniscectomy in the ACL-deficient knee produces an additional anterior laxity of approximately 5 mm when measured at 20 to 30 degrees of flexion (Graph 2–3). Under static conditions, weight-bearing loads have been shown to have a significant stabilizing effect on anterior instability [10], decreasing it by up to 66 per cent. Under dynamic conditions (such as running and pivoting), weight-bearing loads may be expected to have a variable effect on knee stability, depending upon the degree of knee flexion and rotation.

Rotatory instability has also been studied under weight-bearing conditions. Here, the ACL has been determined to be the primary stabilizer against anterolateral rotatory instability (ALRI) [15]. Lipke et al. report [15] that secondary stability against ALRI in the ACL-deficient knee, is provided by the posterolateral complex and the lateral collateral ligament. (Sectioning of these structures in the ACL-intact knee, however, does not produce any increase in ALRI.) This study suggested that the axial center of rotation shifts medially within the knee when the ACL is absent. With this change in rotational axis, alteration in the kinematics and biomechanics of knee motion must be expected. When coupled with the change in instant center of rotation for flexion–extension that accompanies ACL insufficiency, the potential for degenerative changes in the knee with anterior instability and ALRI is readily appreciated.

Upon consideration of the abnormal knee kinematics and biomechanics resulting from ACL insufficiency, the potential benefits of ACL reconstruction beyond the restoration of stability become apparent. It remains to be shown, however, that ACL reconstruction is capable of restoring to normal the altered biomechanics of an ACL-deficient knee, and that this reconstructive surgery has a protective effect on the knee with regard to future degenerative changes.

REFERENCES

1. Bargar WL, Moreland JR, et al. In vivo stability testing of post meniscectomy knees. Clin Orthop 1980; 150:247–252
2. Butler DL, Noyes FR, Grood ES. Ligamentous restraints to anterior-posterior drawer in the human knee. J Bone Joint Surg (Am) 1980; 62:259–270.
3. Chen EH, Black J. Materials design analysis of the prosthetic anterior cruciate ligament. J Biomed Mater Res 1980; 14:567–586.
4. Dye SF. An evolutionary perspective of the knee. J Bone Joint Surg (Am), 1987; G9:976–983.
5. Frankel VH, Burstein AH, Brooks DB. Biomechanics of internal derangement of the knee. J Bone Joint Surg (Am) 1971; 53:945–962.
6. Gerber C, Matter P. Biomechanical analysis of the knee after rupture of the anterior cruciate ligament and its primary repair—an instant-center analysis of function. J Bone Joint Surg (Br) 1983; 65:391–399.
7. Girgis FG, Marshall JL, Al Monajem ARS. The cruciate ligaments of the knee joint: anatomical, functional and experimental analysis. Clin Orthop 1975; 106:216–231.
8. Gollehon DL, Torzilli PA, Warren RF. The role of the posterolateral and cruciate ligaments in the stability of the human knee. J Bone Joint Surg (Am) 1987; 69:233–242.
9. Graf B. Biomechanics of the anterior cruciate ligament. In: Jackson DW, Drez D, eds. The anterior cruciate deficient knee. St. Louis: Mosby, 1987:55–71.
10. Hsieh HH, Walker PS. Stabilizing mechanisms of the

GRAPH 2–3.

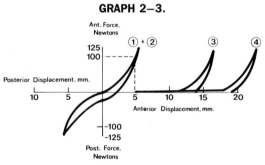

Displacement of the tibia on the femur at 30 degrees of flexion. Curves are numbered as follows: ① = normal knee, ② = status post medial meniscectomy, ③ = status post division of ACL, ④ = status post division of ACL and medial meniscectomy. (Adapted from Levy et al. [14].)

Ant. denotes anterior and Post. posterior.

loaded and unloaded knee joint. J Bone Joint Surg (Am) 1976; 58:87–93.

11. Inoue M, et al. Treatment of the medial collateral ligament injury: the importance of the anterior cruciate ligament on the varus-valgus knee laxity. Am J Sports Med 1987; 15:15–21.

12. Insall JN. Chronic instability of the knee. In: Insall JN, ed. Surgery of the knee. New York: Churchill Livingstone, 1984: 303.

13. Jobe CM. Special properties of living tissue that affect the shoulder in athletes. Clin Sports Med 1983; 2:271–280.

14. Levy IM, Torzilli PA, Warren RF. The effect of medial meniscectomy on anterior-posterior motion of the knee. J Bone Joint Surg (Am) 1982; 64:883–888.

15. Lipke JM, Janecki CJ, et al. The role of incompetence of the anterior cruciate and lateral ligaments in anterolateral and anteromedial instability. J Bone Joint Surg (Am) 1981; 63:954–960.

16. Markolf KL, Mensch JS, Amstutz HC. Stiffness and laxity of the knee—the contributions of the supporting structures. J Bone Joint Surg (Am) 1976; 58:583–593.

17. Müller W. The knee: form, function and ligament reconstruction. New York: Springer-Verlag, 1983.

18. Nordin M, Frankel VH. Biomechanics of the knee. In: Frankel VH, Nordin M, ed. Biomechanics of the musculoskeletal system. Philadelphia: Lea and Febiger, 1980: 113–148.

19. Noyes FR, Butler DL, et al. Biomechanical analysis of human ligament grafts used in knee ligament repairs and reconstruction. J Bone Joint Surg (Am) 1984; 66:344–352.

20. Noyes FR, DeLucas JL, Torvik PJ. Biomechanics of anterior cruciate ligament failure: an analysis of strain-rate sensitivity and mechanisms of failure in primates. J Bone Joint Surg (Am) 1974; 56:236–253.

21. Sherman OH, Markolf KL, Ferkel RD. Measurements of anterior laxity in normal and anterior cruciate absent knees with two instrumented test devices. Clin Orthop 1987; 215:156–161.

22. Tamea CD, Henning, CE. Pathomechanics of the pivot shift maneuver—an instant center analysis. Am J Sports Med 1981; 9:31–37.

3

INSTRUMENTED KNEE TESTING

SCOTT P. FISCHER, M.D.
RICHARD D. FERKEL, M.D.

"Determination of the nature of the injury and its degree remains the most important factor in successful treatment of injured knee ligaments."

D. O'Donoghue, 1973

The importance of the anterior cruciate ligament (ACL) is unquestioned, and its function in normal knee kinematics has been described. Injury to the ACL, with subsequent laxity, is known to contribute to the clinical syndrome of the "unstable knee" with its rotatory instability and susceptibility to further injury. In this context we define laxity as a static "looseness" of the ACL, while instability refers to a functional "looseness" of the knee during activity.

ACL laxity can be determined by the Lachman and anterior drawer tests, while instability can be elicited by the pivot shift or other similar clinical tests. These maneuvers have been shown to have excellent qualitative correlation with ACL dysfunction [6, 9, 12, 20, 29, 32, 33, 34]. However, attempts to quantify these tests are subject to variation in examiner execution and perception [7, 14]. Results of clinical examination can be influenced by the skill of the examiner, variability among multiple examinations, and a variable definition of laxity among examiners. The common 1 + , 2 + , or 3 + notations of laxity and instability are imprecise and therefore inadequate when making patient comparisons for the evaluation of various reconstructive procedures and protocols. Several investigators have developed techniques to

quantitate more accurately the measurement of knee-joint laxity in a reproducible manner.

In the laboratory *in vitro* setting, isolated cadaveric knee-joint specimens can be rigidly mounted on an examination apparatus, and tibial–femoral displacements resulting from applied forces can be measured accurately. Laboratory testing apparatuses employing load cells, potentiometers, goniometers, and force transducers are used to provide measurements and observations that are objective and reproducible. Studies using these techniques have furthered our understanding of the contribution to normal knee stability by the menisci, the cruciate ligaments, and the capsular structures [4, 5, 8, 11, 18, 19, 21, 22, 25, 27, 36]. They have also defined the destabilizing result produced by the sacrifice of these structures individually and in combination. However, such *in vitro* studies can provide only a partial representation of the normal *in vivo* function of these structures. As additional clinical studies are performed, it is imperative that the degree of objectivity and accuracy obtained in the clinical evaluation of these patients be similar to that accomplished in the laboratory setting.

The goal for use of a clinical knee-testing device should be to provide objective and reproducible

10

measurements that quantify laxity in the injured and uninjured knee. Such data is necessary to improve diagnostic accuracy for knee-ligament injuries, and to evaluate and compare results from different treatment protocols.

Several investigators have developed objective techniques to measure anterior–posterior knee laxity clinically. These various techniques can be grouped into three different methods: *(1)* those utilizing measurements on stress radiographs, *(2)* those with the application of a mechanical device to the knee, providing direct measurement of tibial–femoral displacement, and *(3)* those with remote sensors measuring tibial–femoral motion.

Radiographic techniques for evaluation of knee stability were first employed by Kirchmeyer in 1920 [17]. He used stress radiographs to evaluate medial–lateral instability as well as the anterior drawer sign. This technique was refined by later authors [2, 15, 26,]

Quellet [28] reported the use of a device that applied a constant anterior force to the proximal tibia with a system of ropes and weights. Through measurements on lateral stress radiographs, he determined the normal anterior laxity at 90 degrees of flexion to be approximately 5 mm. Two years later, Kennedy and Fowler [16] evaluated sagittal-plane mobility of the knee at 90 degrees of flexion with a clinical stress machine. The patient was seated in a device that held the thigh immobile while an anteriorly directed, measured force was applied to the proximal tibia by a pneumatic load actuator. Lateral stress radiographs were compared to nonstress radiographs to determine relative displacements of the joint surfaces. Templates overlaid on the x-rays and vernier calipers allowed the displacements to be measured to the nearest 0.1 mm (Fig. 3–1). With this technique, they also determined normal anterior mobility at 90 degrees (with an unspecified stress) to be 5.0 mm. Similar measurements in patients with injured ACLs showed increased mobility (6.0 to 20.0 mm).

In 1976, Jacobsen [13] refined the technique of Kennedy and Fowler (Fig. 3–2), and he demonstrated the presence of tibial rotation with the anterior drawer. He determined a difference in anterior drawer between the right and left knees of more than 3.1 mm to be abnormal. More recently, Torzilli et al. [35] observed that "large errors in measurement of laxity were found to exist if rotational motions were not accounted for." They applied a spring tension device to the proximal tibia in an unconstrained testing apparatus, and then measured anterior drawer displacement at 90 degrees of flexion on lateral x-rays. He corrected for rotation of the tibia and femur by a series of additional measurements on the radiographs. His results were

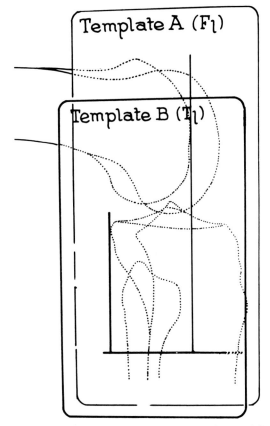

Figure 3–1. Stress radiograph template overlays used by Kennedy and Fowler to determine anterior knee laxity. (With permission, from Kennedy and Fowler [16].)

similar to those previously described, however, several additional x-rays were required for this technique.

There are inherent limitations using these radiographic techniques of laxity measurement. Adjustments for the magnification factor must be made, precise identification of landmarks on serial films may be difficult, and rotational discrepancies must be eliminated. There is the additional limitation of determining displacement at only one load (rather than over the entire range of load). Finally, these studies measured anterior tibial displacement at 90 degrees of flexion, rather than at the preferred 20 degrees.

A second approach to clinical knee-laxity measurement has been the development of mechanical devices that attach directly to the leg. These measure tibial–femoral displacement (laxity) via change in relative position of bony landmarks about the knee during the application of a measured load. Markolf and associates [23] were the first investigators to use an instrumented clinical testing apparatus to quantify knee laxity in human

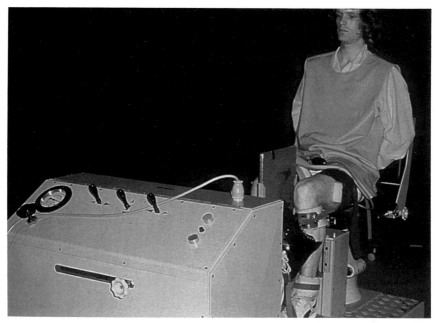

Figure 3–2. Hydraulic clinical testing device used to apply measured anterior drawer force to the tibia for stress radiographs. (Courtesy of K. Jacobsen.)

subjects. Their ''UCLA apparatus'' was a modification of a device previously used [25] to measure laxity and stiffness of knee ligaments in cadaver specimens accurately. For human testing, the femur was immobilized by grasping the thigh in a padded clamping device. The foot was immobilized and anterior–posterior forces were applied to

GRAPH 3–1.

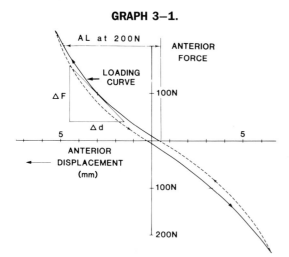

Typical load-displacement curve for anterior laxity in a normal knee. Anterior laxity is the displacement of the tibia as 200 N of anterior force is applied to the proximal tibia. Anterior stiffness is the slope of the curve (F/d = FORCE/displacement) at an applied force of 100 N.

the proximal tibia with an instrumented force handle. Displacement was measured by a potentiometer. This device produced a continuous recording of load versus displacement (Graph 3–1), allowing the determination of stiffness as well as laxity for sagittal-plane knee displacement. Current studies utilize a portable version of the device (Fig. 3–3). A study of 49 uninjured subjects documented that maximum anterior–posterior laxity occurred at 20 degrees of flexion. Average anterior–posterior laxity at 20 degrees and 90 degrees was determined to be 5.5 mm and 4.8 mm, respectively, under a 200-N load. They also found a 25 to 50 per cent decrease in laxity when the patient tensed the muscles crossing the knee. In another study [1], the UCLA apparatus demonstrated no measurable change in laxity of postmeniscectomy knees unless a cruciate ligament injury was also present.

With this device, it has been shown that anterior laxity in ACL-deficient knees is also best measured at 20 degrees of flexion [24]. The injured versus normal knee anterior laxity was determined to be 2.3 times greater at 20 degrees of flexion than at 90 degrees (tested at 200 N of force). Similarly, the difference in stiffness is 2.7 times greater at 20 degrees than at 90 degrees (tested at 100 N of force). The mean anterior laxity (at 20 degrees of flexion) for ACL-deficient knees is approximately 10 mm, with a mean injured–normal difference of 5 mm. Injured–normal differences of 2 mm or less

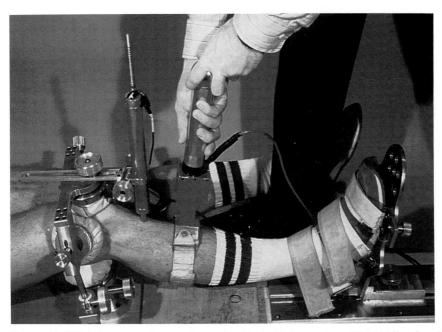

Figure 3–3. The portable UCLA instrumented knee-testing device. The distal femur is immobilized while a force handle applies anterior load to the tibia. Continuous displacement is measured at the tibial tubercle by the transducer. (Courtesy of K. Markolf.)

are present in 95 per cent of patients with normal knees (Graph 3–2).

In the late 1970s and early 1980s, Malcom and Daniel developed a portable and self-contained instrumented knee-testing machine (KT-1000) (Fig. 3–4) [5]. This knee arthrometer is applied along the anterior tibial crest, and monitors relative motion between the tibia and the patella which is

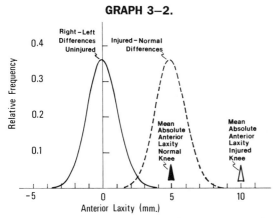

GRAPH 3–2.

A representation of the right–left differences in anterior knee laxity for normal and ACL-injured patient populations. Note that there is a low frequency of overlap between the two patient groups. Also shown is the mean laxity for normal and ACL-injured knees.

held immobilized against the femoral condyles. Tibial–femoral displacement is measured as anterior–posterior forces are applied to the proximal tibia with a force handle. Daniel et al. [5] have reported the results of testing 338 uninjured and 89 ACL-deficient subjects with this device. With the knee at 20 degrees of flexion, the mean anterior displacement at 89 N for the uninjured subjects was 5.7 mm. Persons with ACL disruptions had a mean displacement of 13.0 mm. Right-to-left variation in anterior displacement was less than 2.0 mm for 92 per cent of the normal subjects, and more than 2.0 mm for 96 per cent of those with ACL disruptions. Changes in anterior stiffness were similar to those previously reported by Markolf et al. [24] (55 per cent change comparing injured to normal knee).

Recently, Sherman et al. [30] compared the UCLA device to the KT-1000. In examining 48 normal and 19 ACL-deficient patients, the UCLA device gave consistently lower absolute displacement readings than the KT-1000 at the same displacement force (89 N). However, when the recommended displacement force of 200 N was used for the UCLA machine, similar displacements were observed. These discrepancies were attributed to difference in device design, highlighting the importance of the proper use of these devices as recommended by their developers. Each apparatus, when used as recommended, was 90 to 95 per

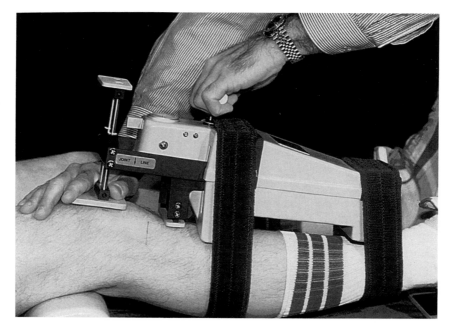

Figure 3–4. The Medmetric KT-1000 knee arthrometer being used to measure anterior knee laxity.

cent accurate in correctly classifying ACL-deficient knees as being outside the normal range of anterior displacement and having abnormal side-to-side difference.

The Stryker knee-laxity tester (Fig. 3–5) was recently used by Boniface et al. [3] to evaluate 123 normal and 30 ACL-deficient patients. They reported an injured–normal knee difference of 2 mm (anterior displacement) to be significant for an ACL injury (88 per cent accuracy). Shino et al. [31] reported preliminary results with an apparatus similar in design to these previous devices. In a

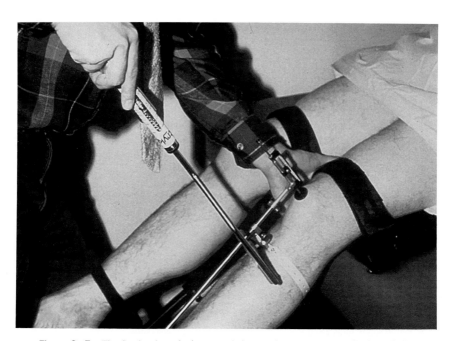

Figure 3–5. The Stryker knee-laxity tester being used to measure anterior knee laxity.

study of 30 normal and 73 ACL-injured patients, his findings were comparable to those previously cited.

In 1984, Johnson and associates [14] reported on a series of patients more than five years post ACL reconstruction with a patellar tendon graft. They developed a clinical apparatus that used rotary potentiometers to measure tibial–femoral displacement via a system of small cables and pulleys. They concluded that "the laxity-measuring device was better able to resolve the laxity in both the Lachman and the anterior drawer tests than the clinical examination." With their device, the mean anterior laxity at 20 degrees of flexion for normal knees was 4.8 mm. The clinical result of the reconstructed knee was correlated with the injured-versus-normal-knee difference in anterior laxity. Those reconstructions with a good or excellent result had a mean laxity difference of 2.5 mm, while those with fair or poor results had a mean laxity difference of 3.9 mm.

The third type of knee-testing device is that represented by the Genucom knee-analysis system. A six-degrees-of-freedom force platform dynamometer measures forces and moments manually applied to the knee. Tibial–femoral displacements are concurrently measured by an electrogoniometer through an instrumented linkage attached to the proximal tibia. Early trials with this system seem to indicate good reproducibility for knee-motion analysis in all three planes simultaneously [10]. Studies using this device to evaluate and compare the differences in anterior laxity for normal and injured knees are as yet unpublished. Similar models are currently being developed by other investigators.

This overview of investigational and clinical knee-testing devices serves to highlight their usefulness in assessment of anterior knee laxity. While each has slightly different normal ranges for injured and uninjured knees, each has given consistent and reproducible data when properly used. Use of these devices to provide objective measurement of anterior knee laxity and injured–normal knee laxity difference is preferable to data reported with more qualitative measurements of laxity (such as 1 + , 2 + , 3 + laxity). Future use of these devices in clinical research projects should provide objective and reproducible means to quantify and monitor changes in knee laxity and stiffness. This type of data should provide a basis for the meaningful comparison of results from different treatment protocols and different treatment centers. This will become critical as one tries to evaluate the effectiveness of prosthetic ligaments in reconstructive surgery of the knee.

REFERENCES

1. Bargar WL, Moreland JR, et al. In vivo stability testing of post-meniscectomy knees. Clin Orthop 1980; 150:247–252.
2. Bohler J. Rontgenollogishe Darstellung von Kreuzbandverletzungen. Chirung 1943; 16:136.
3. Boniface RJ, Fu FH, Ilkhanipour K. Objective anterior cruciate ligament testing. Orthopedics 1986; 9:391–393.
4. Butler DL, Noyes FR, Grood ES. Ligamentous restraints to anterior-posterior drawer in the human knee. J Bone Joint Surg (Am) 1980; 62:259–270.
5. Daniel DM, Malcom LL, et al. Instrumented measurement of anterior laxity of the knee. J Bone Joint Surg (Am) 1985; 67:720–726.
6. DeHaven KE. Diagnosis of acute knee injuries with hemarthrosis. Am J Sports Med 1980; 8:9–14.
7. Ferkel RD, Markolf E, et al. Treatment of the anterior cruciate ligament—absent knee with associated meniscal tears. Clin Orthop 1987; 222:117–126.
8. Fukubayashi T, Torzilli PA, et al. An in vitro biomechanical evaluation of anterior-posterior motion of the knee. J Bone Joint Surg (Am) 1982; 64:248–264.
9. Galway HR, MacIntosh DL. The lateral pivot shift: a symptom and sign of anterior cruciate ligament insufficiency. Clin Orthop 1980; 147:45–50.
10. Highgenboten CL, Jackson A. The reliability of the genucom knee analysis system. (Unpublished.)
11. Hsieh HH, Walker PS. Stabilizing mechanisms of the loaded and unloaded knee joint. J Bone Joint Surg (Am) 1976; 58:87–93.
12. Hughston JC, Andrews JR, Cross MJ, et al. Classification of knee ligament instabilities. Part I. J Bone Joint Surg (Am) 1976; 58:159–172.
13. Jacobsen K. Stress radiographical measurement of the anteroposterior, medial and lateral stability of the knee joint. Acta Orthop Scand 1976; 47:335–344.
14. Johnson RJ, Eriksson E, et al. Five to ten year follow-up evaluation after reconstruction of the anterior cruciate ligament. Clin Orthop 1984; 183:122–140.
15. Jonasch E. Zerreissung des ausseren und inneren Knieseitenbandes. Mschr Unfallheilk Beiheft 1958; 59:21.
16. Kennedy J, Fowler PJ. Medial and anterior stability of the knee: an anatomical and clinical study using stress machines. J Bone Joint Surg (Am) 1971; 53:1257–1270.
17. Kirchmeyer L. Das Rontgenbild als diagnostisches Hilfsmittel bei Zerreissungen der Kniegelenksbander. Forschr Roentgenstr 1920; 27:425.
18. Levy IM, Torzilli PA, Warren RF. The effect of medial meniscectomy on anterior-posterior motion of the knee. J Bone Joint Surg (Am) 1982; 64:883–888.
19. Lipke JM, Janecki CJ, et al. The role of incompetence of the anterior cruciate and lateral ligaments in anterolateral and anteromedial instability. J Bone Joint Surg (Am) 1981; 63:954–960.
20. Losse RE, Johnson TR, Southwick WD. Anterior subluxation of the lateral tibial plateau: a diagnostic test and operative repair. J Bone Joint Surg (Am) 1978; 60:1015–1030.
21. Mains DB, Andrews JG, Stonecipher T. Medial and anterior-posterior ligament stability of the human knee measured with a stress apparatus. Am Sports Med 1977; 5:144–153.
22. Markolf KL, Bargar WL, et al. The role of joint load in knee stability. J Bone Joint Surg (Am) 1981; 63:570–585.

23. Markolf KL, Graff-Radford A, Amstutz HC. In vivo knee stability, a quantitative assessment using an instrumented testing apparatus. J Bone Joint Surg (Am) 1978; 60:664–674.

24. Markolf KL, Kochan A, Amstutz HD. Measurements of knee stiffness and laxity in patients with documented absence of the anterior cruciate ligament. J Bone Joint Surg (Am) 1984; 66:242–253.

25. Markolf KL, Mensch JS, Amstutz HC. Stiffness and laxity of the knee—the contributions of the supporting structures. J Bone Joint Surg (Am) 1976; 58:583–593.

26. Palmer I. On the injuries to the ligaments of the knee joint, a clinical study. Acta Chir Scand [Suppl] 1938; 53:78.

27. Piziali RL, Seering WP, et al. The function of the primary ligaments of the knee in anterior-posterior and medial-lateral motions. Biomechanics 1980; 13:777–784.

28. Quellet R, Levesque HP, Laurin CA. The ligamentous stability of the knee: an experimental investigation. Can Med Assoc J 1969; 100:45–50.

29. Rosenberg TD, Rasmussen GL. The function of the anterior cruciate ligament during anterior drawer and Lachman's testing: an in vivo analysis on normal knees. Am J Sports Med 1984; 12:318–322.

30. Sherman OH, Markolf KL, Ferkel RD. Measurements of anterior laxity in normal and anterior cruciate absent knees with two instrumented test devices. Clin Orthop 1987; 215:156–161.

31. Shino K, Hirose H, et al. In vivo knee stability measurement using a clinical knee testing apparatus on normal and anterior cruciate deficient knees. (Unpublished.)

32. Slocum DB, James SL, Larson RL, et al. Clinical test for anterolateral rotatory instability of the knee. Clin Orthop 1976; 118:63–69.

33. Torg SS, Conrad W, Kalen V. Clinical diagnosis of anterior cruciate ligament instability in the athlete. Am J Sports Med 1976; 4:84–92.

34. Torsten J, Bo A, Peterson L, et al. Clinical diagnosis of ruptures of ACL: a comparison study of the Lachman test and the anterior drawer sign. Am J Sports Med 1982; 10:100–102.

35. Torzilli PA, Greenberg RL, Insall J. An in vivo biomechanical evaluation of anterior-posterior motion of the knee. J Bone Joint Surg (Am) 1981; 63:960–968.

36. Wang CJ, Walker PS. Rotatory laxity of the human knee joint. J Bone Joint Surg (Am) 1974; 56:161–170.

4

ANTERIOR CRUCIATE LIGAMENT GRAFT ISOMETRY AND TENSIONING

DALE M. DANIEL, M.D.
DARRELL A. PENNER, M.D.
ROBERT T. BURKS, M.D.

There is an intimate relationship between the geometry of the cruciate ligaments and the shapes of the articular surfaces of the tibial–femoral joint. The relationship of these structures in the sagittal plane has been modeled as a four-bar linkage as shown in Figure 4–1. The cruciate ligaments are represented as straight-line tension-bearing elements of constant length and the bone ends and their articular surfaces are taken to be rigid. There is much to support this model. It nicely predicts the sliding and rolling motion of the knee joint during flexion and extension [6, 8, 9]. When forces are added to represent tendons, the mechanical calculations of muscle–ligament interaction are found to be in close agreement with observations on cadaveric human knee joints [O'Connor JJ: personal communication]. The premise of the model is that the distance between the cruciate ligaments' origins and insertions remain at constant length throughout knee flexion and extension.

Numerous authors have performed cadaveric studies to document the distance between the origin and insertion of the anterior cruciate ligament (ACL) during passive knee motion. Wang et al. [13] used a radiographic technique with metal markers to measure the distance between the "neutral points" of the cruciate ligaments' attachment sites. They recorded the distance between the ACL

attachment-site markers increased 10 per cent (3 mm) between 0 and 120 degrees of flexion. Crowninshield et al. [4] measured length and used an analytical model to calculate length changes for the anterior and posterior fibers of each of the cruciate ligaments. Their model predicted the anterior fibers of the anterior cruciate ligament to be longest in the position of flexion and the posterior fibers to be longest in extension. Presumably there would be some intermediate fiber that remained at constant length.

Arms et al. [1] placed a strain transducer on the anteromedial fibers of the ACL. The cadaver was placed on an autopsy table with the knee hanging freely over the end of the table. Passive ACL strain tests were performed by lowering the leg while grasping the toes. This revealed a decrease in ACL strain as the knee was flexed to 40 degrees and then returned to the initial strain level with the knee at 90 degrees. Active knee motion was investigated by pulling through the quadriceps tendon to control knee motion. This resulted in an increased strain in the ACL from 0 to 40 degrees of knee motion and then similar strains as were seen in the passive tests with further knee flexion. An increased strain indicates that the ligament is lengthening. This study documents the interaction between the quadriceps and the anterior cruciate

17

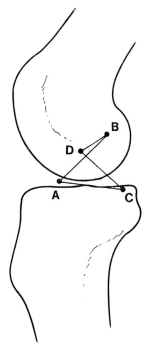

Figure 4—1. Cruciate four-bar linkage. AB denotes the anterior cruciate ligament, CD the posterior cruciate ligament, AC the tibial link, and DB the femoral link.

ligament and reveals that the measurements of ligament lengths will vary depending on the joint load.

Other investigators have replaced the cruciate ligament with a heavy thread [11], a 6-mm polypropylene braid [12], or a steel cable [7] to document the change in distance between origin and insertion sites as the knee is passed through a range of motion. Odensten and Gillquist [11] joined different points on the tibia shelf and on the lateral femoral condyle by a nonelastic thread, 1 mm in diameter, that was pulled through drill holes at different points in the tibia and femur. The thread was fixed to the femur but free to move in the hole through the tibia. The distance between the central points of the insertion areas on the tibia and on the lateral femoral condyle did not change throughout the whole range of knee motion (0 to 135 degrees) as determined by excursion of the thread. Reported studies on attachment-site isometry are presented in Table 4–1. An attachment site in the geographic center of the normal ligament attachment is referred to as the neutral position.

Conditions that result in no change in the distance between the ligament graft-attachment sites as the knee is passed through a range of motion are referred to as isometric graft placement. A nonisometric placement results in a change in distance between the tibial and femoral insertion sites. We have used the convention of describing

TABLE 4–1. THE CHANGE IN LENGTH BETWEEN THE TIBIAL AND FEMORAL ANTERIOR CRUCIATE LIGAMENT GRAFT SITES WITH KNEE MOTION

Author	Range of Motion	Orientation*		Specimen Number	Mean Length Change[†]
		Tibia	*Femur*		
Odensten [11][‡]	0 to 135	N	N	10	0
Hoogland [7][§]	0 to 130			4	−3 mm
Odensten	0 to 135	N	P	10	−10 mm
Hoogland	0 to 130			4	−8 mm
Penner [12][¶]	0 to 90			17	−4.5 mm
Odensten	0 to 135	N	A	10	+7 mm
Hoogland	0 to 130			4	+10 mm
Penner	0 to 90			8	+5.7 mm
Odensten	0 to 135	A	N	10	+5 mm
Hoogland	0 to 130			4	+3 mm
Odensten	0 to 135			10	−9 mm
Hoogland	0 to 130			4	−4 mm

*N denotes insertion neutral position (geographic center of the normal ligament attachment; P denotes posterior position, estimated to be 10 to 15 mm posterior to the neutral position; and A denotes anterior position, estimated to be 10 to 15 mm anterior to the neutral position. In Hoogland's study the anterior data reported here was measured with the cable passed over the front of the tibia.

[†]Positive (+) denotes that the attachment-site distance increases with knee flexion, and negative (−) that the attachment-site distance decreases with knee flexion.

[‡]Odensten did not apply a load to the measuring thread.

[§]Hoogland applied a 5-kg load to the measuring thread.

[¶]Penner maintained constant tension on the tibial end of the polypropylene braid with a load cell.

an increase in the distance between insertion sites with knee flexion as a positive length change and a decrease in insertion-site distance with knee flexion as a negative length change. Movement of either tibial or femoral insertion sites from the central area of normal ACL insertion results in a nonisometric condition.

Let us first consider the condition of moving the femoral site of attachment while maintaining the tibial site in the neutral position. Posterior movement of the femoral attachment site results in a negative nonisometric graft orientation (graft insertion site distance decreases with knee flexion). Placing the graft in the over-the-top position resulted in a negative nonisometric orientation in all specimens reported [7, 11, 12]. Anterior placement of the femoral attachment site resulted in a positive nonisometric orientation (increasing length with knee flexion (Table 4–1).

The effect of movement of the tibial insertion site when the femur was in the neutral position resulted in a less consistent effect (Table 4–1). However, both Penner [12] and Hoogland [7] reported that if the femoral placement was in the over-the-top position, anterior movement of the tibial hole decreased the negative length change with knee flexion and posterior placement of the tibial hole increased the negative length change. The surgeon must be aware, however, that anterior placement of the tibial hole may result in graft impingement on the anterior portal of the intercondylar notch with knee extension resulting in possible graft abrasion and graft failure. If an anterior placement of the tibial hole is used, ostectomy of the femur may be necessary to prevent graft impingement.

Penner [12] evaluated the surgical technique of modifying the over-the-top orientation by making an estimated 5-mm posterior bone trough, thus bringing the femoral graft closer to the neutral site. The modified over-the-top position produced a mean 1.4-mm decrease in attachment-site distance when the knee was ranged from 0 to 90 degrees (7 specimens studied).

CLINICAL EVALUATION OF ISOMETRY

The object of ligament repair and reconstruction is to reestablish the ligament guidance system and normal joint kinematics. There is an intimate relationship between the geometry of the ligaments and the articular surface contours. The distance between the neutral points of the anterior cruciate attachments are isometric to passive knee motion. As the ligaments are viscoelastic structures, they will lengthen when loaded. Surgical reconstruction consists of placing a cord of tissue or synthetic material through the knee to reconstruct the complex anterior cruciate ligament. It is likely that to simulate best the complex normal ligament, the replacement structure should be placed along the neutral axis of the normal ligament, which we believe is isometric with passive motion. The measurement of graft isometry allows the surgeon to evaluate the graft replacement.

Clinically, we strive to place ligament grafts in an isometric position and routinely document the graft placement isometry. Our current practice in ACL reconstruction is to evaluate the distance change between origin and insertion with knee flexion from 0 to 90 degrees. It would be optimal to evaluate isometry through the full range of flexion as attachment-site distance changes from 0 to 135 degrees of flexion may be as much as twice the distance change measured from 0 to 90 degrees. However, we find that surgical positioning, the thigh tourniquet, and surgical draping prevent unobstructive full motion. We have rated as a satisfactory placement an attachment-site distance change from 0 to 90 degrees of not greater than 2 mm. A 2-mm increase in graft length is less than a 10 per cent change in length in a 30-mm distance between attachment sites and should not result in tissue injury [5, 10]. Our surgical technique using the MEDmetric Tension/Isometer (TI) is as follows:

1. Place a 3- or 4-mm pilot hole in the femur and in the tibia in the assumed isometric locations. In selecting the initial pilot holes it should be remembered that pilot holes placed too far posteriorly on the femur or anteriorly on the tibia are easily modified. The surgeon may not be able to modify successfully pilot holes placed too far anteriorly on the femur or posteriorly on the tibia.
2. Pass a braided wire of heavy suture through the pilot holes.
3. Clamp the suture with a hemostat as it exits the femoral hole laterally.
4. Pass the suture exiting from the tibial hole through the TI suture nose.
5. Adjust the TI to apply a 4-lb load and cycle the knee from 0 to 90 degrees of flexion five times. With the knee in 0 degrees of flexion readjust the load to 4 lb and read the linear scale. Flex the knee to 90 degrees, adjust the tension knob to apply a 4-lb load, and read the linear scale (Fig. 4–2).
6. If the linear scale change when the knee is ranged from 0 to 90 degrees is not satisfactory, one or both pilot holes should be replaced and the measurement repeated.

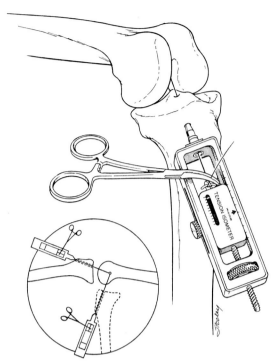

Figure 4—2. The tension on the suture passed through the pilot holes is kept constant as the knee is passed through a range of motion. The length change between the graft attachment sites is measured (Medmetric Tension/Isometer).

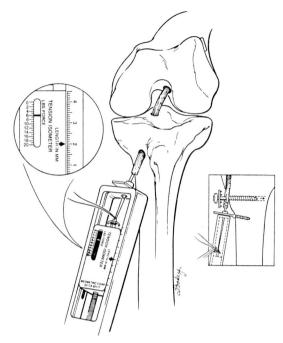

Figure 4—3. A measured load is applied with the Medmetric Tension/Isometer. The instrument is stabilized on the tibia with a skeletal fixation plate.

7. With a cylindrical size template, determine the smallest hole through which the ligament graft will pass. Place guide wires in the selected pilot holes and enlarge the holes with a cannulated reamer 1 mm larger than the graft size. Do not make the holes any larger than necessary. A snug fit of the graft in the holes results in good consistency between the suture isometry and the implanted-graft isometry.

8. Pass the graft and secure the femoral end. Secure a suture passed through the tibial end of the graft to the TI, which is skeletally stabilized either with an extension nose or the skeletal fixation plate (Figure 4–3). Apply a 4-lb load to the graft and cycle the knee from 0 to 90 degrees of flexion five times. With the knee in 0 degrees of flexion adjust the tension knob to apply a 4-lb load and read the linear scale. Flex the knee to 90 degrees, adjust the tension knob to 4 lb and read the linear scale. Note the length change and record it in the surgical record. We have found that the length change of the graft seldom varies more than 1 mm from the length change measured with the pilot holes, provided that the graft fills the bone tunnel.

When the over-the-top orientation is used, the tibial hole is placed as far anteriorly as possible without resulting in graft impingement on the anterior portal of the intercondylar notch with knee extension. A trough is made posteriorly where the graft exits the intercondylar notch to bring the over-the-top position nearer the femoral neutral point. A curved osteotome and a rat-tailed rasp with the teeth removed from the convex side—to prevent injury to the posterior cruciate ligament—are instruments useful in making the trough. The trough is deepened until the isometry is satisfactory (no greater than a 2-mm length change with the knee ranged from 0 to 90 degrees of flexion).

GRAFT TENSIONING

Reports of ACL reconstruction procedures usually include a statement about tensioning the graft to achieve normal joint laxity. At the time of graft tensioning there is a direct relation between ligament tension and joint laxity [2]. There are, however, other factors that will effect the relation between ligament tension and joint laxity: ligament stiffness, ligament length, displacement load, and stress relaxation. Loaded grafts will deform with time. It is unlikely that the tension applied at the time of graft fixation will exist at the time of wound closure and the tension will undoubtedly diminish in the postoperative period. Synthetic grafts are less likely to deform than collagen grafts. Care should be taken, especially with synthetic grafts, not to apply graft tension that will eliminate normal joint laxity.

If the graft is isometrically oriented, ligament tension will remain constant as the knee is passed through a range of motion. However, if the graft is not oriented isometrically, with knee motion an increasing distance between fixation sites will result in an increase in graft tension, while decreasing distance between fixation sites will result in a decrease in graft tension [12]. An example of the relation between graft tension and knee range of motion with the ligament in a nonisometric orientation (+9 mm) with an implanted 6-mm polypropylene braid (3M Kennedy LAD) is presented in Graph 4–1. When an increasing distance between fixation sites occurs with knee flexion, if the graft is tensioned and fixed with the knee in extension, knee flexion will be limited or result in ligament deformity and possible disruption. If the graft is nonisometric, the graft should be tensioned and fixed at the angle of flexion at which the distance between the fixation sites is maximal.

Our clinical procedure is to first skeletally fix the femoral end of the graft. If the orientation is satisfactory, we then tension the tibial end of the graft with the knee in 30 degrees of flexion with the MEDmetric Tension/Isometer (TI). The linear scale on the TI is then locked so the tibial end of the graft cannot move. The knee is then passed through a full range of motion five times and the joint laxity is manually evaluated. If the laxity is judged to be satisfactory (similar to the subject's normal knee) the graft is fixed to the tibia. If the

laxity is not judged to be satisfactory, the graft is retensioned at a new load. Tension levels we have used in surgery have ranged from 1 to 15 lbs. The graft load is recorded in the operative record. Under anesthesia, prior to surgery and after wound closure, we measure the anterior–posterior knee laxity with an arthrometer in the normal and injured knee to document preoperative pathologic knee laxity and the postrepair knee laxity. Our present goal in anterior cruciate ligament surgery is to establish anterior laxity in the operated knee to within 2 mm of the normal knee.

The measurement of graft isometry, ligament tensioning, and the postrepair measurement of knee laxity with an arthrometer will allow the surgeon to correlate the relations between these variables. Documenting these values in the operative notes will allow for the later correlation with the clinical outcome. A nonisometric orientation will result in tension changes in the graft with knee motion. If an early passive-motion program is utilized the graft will be at risk of rupturing [3]. If an early motion is not used and the joint is immobilized in a position to relieve tension on the graft, the healed graft may prevent normal motion.

REFERENCES

1. Arms SW, et al. The biomechanics of anterior cruciate ligament rehabilitation and reconstruction. Am J Sports Med 1984; 12(1):8.
2. Burks RT, Daniel DM. Anterior cruciate graft preload and knee stability. Orthop Trans 1984; 8:52.
3. Burks RT, Daniel DM, et al. The effect of continuous passive motion on anterior cruciate ligament reconstruction stability. Am J Sports Med 1984; 23(4):323.
4. Crowninshield R, Pope MH, Johnson RJ. An analytical model of the knee. J Biomechanics 1976; 9:397.
5. Frank C, et al. Medial collateral ligament healing: a multidisciplinary assessment in rabbits. Am J Sports Med 1983; 11(6):379.
6. Goodfellow J, O'Connor J. The mechanics of the knee and prosthesis design. J Bone Joint Surg (Br) 1978; 60:358.
7. Hoogland T, Hillen B. Intra-articular reconstruction of the anterior cruciate ligament. Clin Orthop 1984; 185:197.
8. Kapandji IA. The physiology of the joints. Vol. 2. Lower limb. London: Churchill Livingstone, 1970, 120.
9. Mueller W. The knee. New York: Springer-Verlag, 1982; 8.
10. Noyes FR, Keller CS, et al. Advances in the understanding of knee ligament injury, repair and rehabilitation. Med Sci Sports Medicine and Science in Sports and Exercise 1984; 16(5):427.
11. Odensten M, Gillquist J. Functional anatomy in anterior cruciate ligament surgery. J Bone Joint Surg (Am) 1985; 67:257.
12. Penner DA, Daniel DM, Wood P, Mishra D. An in vitro study of anterior cruciate ligament graft orientation and isometry. Presented at the Annual Meeting of the American Orthopedics and Sports Medicine Society, July, 1986.
13. Wang C, Walker PS. The effects of flexion and rotation on the length patterns of the ligaments of the knee. J Biomechics 1973; 6:587.

GRAPH 4–1.

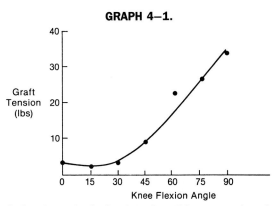

Cadaveric study. Graft orientation: tibia = neutral position, femur = anterior position. With fixation of the proximal end of the graft to the femur and fixation of the distal end to a load cell, the tension in the graft was measured as the knee was ranged from 0 degrees to 90 degrees. (When the attachment to the load cell was adjusted to keep the tension constant, there was a 9-mm increase in distance between the attachment sites between 0 and 90 degrees of flexion.)

5

A REVIEW OF AUTOGENOUS INTRA-ARTICULAR RECONSTRUCTION OF THE ANTERIOR CRUCIATE LIGAMENT

GARY A. PATTEE, M.D.
MARC J. FRIEDMAN, M.D.

The anterior cruciate ligament is an important structure within the human knee and loss of its functions often leads to significant disability [16, 17, 26, 43, 44]. Numerous methods of intra-articular reconstruction of the anterior cruciate ligament (ACL) have been reported using iliotibial band, semitendinosus and gracilis tendons, patellar tendon, and meniscus. Comparisons among various studies of anterior cruciate ligament reconstruction are difficult due to differences in surgical technique, lack of uniform evaluation systems, and small numbers of patients. Success rates of 80 to 90 per cent have been reported with relatively short follow-up [10, 15, 35] but satisfactory results seem to diminish over time [28]. Thus length of follow-up becomes a critical factor when evaluating various methods of stabilizing the ACL-deficient knee.

In general, the indications for ACL reconstruction include functional disability in patients unwilling to alter their life styles, symptomatic instability with activities of daily living, and failure of a rehabilitation program [43]. The risks of meniscal injury and accelerated development of degenerative arthritis must also be considered [17, 44]. Relative contraindications to such procedures include degenerative joint disease, failure of patients to comply with preoperative and postoperative rehabilitation programs, a sedentary life style, and relatively mild instability [26, 27].

Kennedy et al. stated in 1980 that no completely satisfactory transfer exists for ACL reconstruction [34] and Noyes et al. [42] viewed the long-term success of biologic grafts for cruciate reconstruction with pessimism. Autogenous substitutes for the anterior cruciate ligament have been shown to undergo a process of necrosis during revascularization in the early postoperative period [9, 34], predisposing them to failure. Kennedy et al. demonstrated that the normal semitendinosus tendon of the rabbit fails at 10 kg, but after being transplanted intra-articularly, fails at only 4 to 5 kg [34]. At one year after ACL reconstruction in rhesus monkeys, the patellar tendon graft has been shown to have 81 per cent of its original tensile strength and only 52 per cent of the strength of the normal anterior cruciate ligament [9].

Numerous biomechanical studies have been performed on the various substitutes used in ACL reconstruction (Table 5–1) [33, 34, 42]. Noyes et al. determined that the central 14 mm of a bone–patellar tendon–bone preparation has approximately 168 per cent of the strength of the normal anterior cruciate ligament [42]. In reviewing this data, one should keep in mind the fact that Kennedy used specimens from older cadavers and that the harvested tissues were not necessarily of equal dimensions.

In 1905, Wilhelm Roux [49] stated that "an organ will adapt itself structurally to an alteration, quantitative or qualitative in function." Autoge-

**TABLE 5–1. RELATIVE STRENGTHS OF ANTERIOR
CRUCIATE LIGAMENT SUBSTITUTES
(listed as per cent of "normal" ligament strength).***

	Noyes et al. [42]	Kennedy et al. [33, 34]
Anterior cruciate ligament	100% (1730 N)†	100% (626 N)‡
Bone–PT–bone		
Medial third	—	64%
Medial 14 mm	159%	—
Central 14 mm	168%	—
Semitendinosus	70%	104%
Gracilis	49%	75%
Fascia lata (proximal)	36% (16-mm strip)	109% (unknown width)
Iliotibial band (distal)	44% (18-mm strip)	176% (unknown width)
Q–PR–PT	—	13%
Medial	21%	—
Central	15%	—
Lateral	14%	—
Medial meniscus	—	84%
Lateral meniscus	—	100%

*Q denotes quadriceps, PR patellar retinaculum, and PT patellar tendon. Note the difference in ''normal'' anterior cruciate ligament strengths. The fact that Noyes et al. [42] used younger specimens than Kennedy et al. [33, 34] and that strain rates differed may help account for this discrepancy.
†Strain rate = 100% per second.
‡Strain rate = 50 cm per minute.

nous tissue when placed in the synovial fluid environment and acted upon by appropriate biomechanical forces may undergo morphologic changes over time and take on the histologic appearance of the normal anterior cruciate ligament [3, 4]. In the rabbit model, it has been shown that when the patellar tendon is placed in the environment and anatomic position of the normal anterior cruciate ligament, the cell morphology and Type III collagen content change to that of the normal anterior cruciate ligament by 30 weeks [3].

Revascularization of the patellar tendon graft in the dog has been shown to occur by six weeks with contributions from the fat pad, the tibial stump of the anterior cruciate ligament, and the posterior synovial tissues. It would therefore appear that the patellar tendon graft is essentially an avascular free graft and that preservation of the fat pad and synovium optimize revascularization and viability of the graft [4]. The inferior medial and lateral geniculate arteries have been shown to be important to the vascular supply of the patellar tendon [10, 47] and attempts have been made to preserve the vasculature to the medial third of the tendon, producing a vascularized graft. However, the importance of using a vascularized graft has not been determined at this time [47].

It has been stated that failure to place the ACL substitute at the exact point of anatomic attachment of the normal ligament on the distal femur may make the difference between success and failure of the reconstructive procedure [21]. Hoogland and Hillen [24] have demonstrated a variety of length changes of reconstructed anterior cruciate ligaments, depending on the placement of the tibial and femoral tunnels through which the graft is routed. They recommend a posterosuperior tunnel through the femoral condyle to produce minimal changes in length of the graft with flexion and extension.

INTRA-ARTICULAR AUTOGENOUS SUBSTITUTES FOR THE ANTERIOR CRUCIATE LIGAMENT

Iliotibial Band

In 1917, Hey Groves [22] reported the use of a proximally based strip of iliotibial band that was passed through drill holes in the lateral femoral condyle and proximal tibia to substitute for the original anterior cruciate ligament. Although no follow-up was available, one patient reported to have undergone this procedure was able to walk without a limp and return to work.

In 1918, Smith described the use of a distally based strip of iliotibial band [53], and in 1920, Hey Groves modified his earlier procedure, also using a distally based graft to replace the anterior cruciate ligament. The terminal portion of the graft was used to reinforce the medial collateral ligament [23]. Fourteen patients were reported on, but with short follow-up because of their military status. Four patients were able to return to active service, four patients noted some benefit from the surgery, and four patients had no benefit. Two patients were in the immediate postoperative period at the time of the report and were not included.

In 1963, O'Donoghue modified Hey Groves' procedure, using a thickened distal portion of the iliotibial band routed from distal to proximal, leaving better-quality tissue within the knee joint [45]. Twenty-nine patients were followed for slightly less than three years with 27 reporting subjective improvement. Twenty-three of the 29 patients had 0 to 1+ instability as compared with the uninjured knee.

Bertoia et al. [5] also used a distally based strip of iliotibial band, but routed it in an over-the-top fashion and through the intercondylar notch to be secured through a hole in the tibia. Thirty-four patients were followed for a minimum of two years with 23 per cent excellent and 68 per cent good combined objective and subjective results. Eighty-eight per cent had a positive anterior drawer sign at follow-up but 91 per cent were converted to a negative pivot shift.

Zarins and Rowe [58] described the combined use of a distally based strip of iliotibial band and distally based semitendinosus tendon transfer. They reported 100 patients at a follow-up of 3 to $7\frac{1}{2}$ years with the anterior drawer sign eliminated or reduced to 1+ in 80 per cent. Ninety-one per cent of the patients had a 0 to 1+ pivot shift and 90 per cent noted functional stability. The best results were reported in patients who were operated on within two years of their injury, prior to the development of associated lesions.

Nicholas and Minkoff [41] described an iliotibial band pullthrough, using a three-quarter inch proximally based strip of iliotibial band as a dynamic reconstruction of the anterior cruciate ligament. A bone block from Gerdy's tubercle was left attached distally, brought through the posterior capsule and attached to the anteromedial tibial margin with a screw. Thirteen of 15 patients were noted to be markedly improved with a change in the preoperative anterior drawer of 3+ to 1+ in the postoperative period. They cautioned against taking more than one third of the iliotibial band due to problems with varus instability.

In 1981, Insall et al. [25] reported the use of a "tubed" graft consisting of the anterior two thirds of the iliotibial band and the lateral portion of the patellar retinaculum with a bone block from Gerdy's tubercule. This proximally based graft was brought through the intercondylar notch and fixed to a point just medial to the tibial tubercule with a cancellous screw and washer. Twenty-four patients were reported with 88 per cent improved stability at a follow-up of two to four years.

Scott and Schosheim [52] modified the technique of Insall et al. [25] to maintain attachment of the iliotibial band to the lateral intermuscular septum by limiting posterior dissection to the proximal pole of the patella. The graft was placed in the tightest possible position on the tibia and secured with a cancellous screw. Sixty-two patients were reported with a follow-up of 24 to 55 months. Subjective results were 64 per cent excellent and 29 per cent good while five patients had a positive Lachman test and four patients had a positive pivot-shift test.

Scott et al. [51] reported further follow-up on 111 knees in 1985 and noted 95 per cent excellent and good results with 94 per cent of the patients having a negative pivot shift and 81 per cent having a negative Lachman test. The proximally based graft is felt to be an advantage, in that it is not dependent on revascularization.

Pes Tendons

In 1975, Cho [11] described a distally based semitendinosus tendon transfer in which the graft was brought through drill holes in the tibia and femur and sutured to the iliotibial band. Maintaining an intact tendon sheath was thought to prevent necrosis and degeneration of the graft by maintaining vascularity. Of five patients with a follow-up of 21.4 months, no subjective instability was noted, although two of the patients each had a positive anterior drawer sign. Using a similar procedure, Lipscomb et al. [36] reported an 11-month follow-up of 78 patients. Seventy-two of the patients were reported to be subjectively more stable and satisfied with their surgery and 86 per cent had 0 to 1+ anterior or anteromedial rotatory instability.

In 1980, Puddu [48] described a procedure in which a proximally based semitendinosus tendon was routed through tibial and femoral drill holes and sutured to the iliotibial band. This technique was combined with an extra-articular augmentation. Twelve patients were reported on, with an average follow-up of eight months, all of whom were noted to have less than a 1+ anterior drawer sign.

Zaricznyj reported on 22 patients who underwent ACL reconstruction with an average follow-up of 5.4 years [57]. In 5 patients, the fifth-toe extensor tendon was used as the cruciate substitute, and 17 underwent reconstruction with the semitendinosus tendon. Although a significant number of patients had a 0 to 1+ anterior drawer sign at follow-up, Zaricznyj later recommended double-looping the semitendinosus tendon for added strength. Gomes and Marczyk also used a double loop of semitendinosus tendon in 26 patients, with a follow-up of three years [20]. Twenty of the patients also underwent posteromedial capsular reefing. Bone plugs were used to secure the double loop of semitendinosus tendon within the bone tunnels both proximally and distally. Twenty-four patients were satisfied with the procedure and were able to return to their previous levels of athletic activity. One patient had a positive Lachman test and none of the patients had a positive pivot shift.

DuToit [13] stated that a ligament substitute with intact proprioceptors gives greater awareness of tension than a denervated free graft. He reported on a dynamic transfer using a proximally based gracilis tendon routed through the posterior capsule and intercondylar notch of the knee and secured to the tibia through a drill hole anterior to the normal ACL attachment. It was hoped that reflex muscle tone would preserve tension and prevent stretching of the graft. No objective data were presented, but improved subjective stability was noted in all 12 patients.

Thompson et al. [54] also used the gracilis tendon as a dynamic stabilizer of the ACL-deficient knee in eight patients. All but one were able to return to their preoperative activity level, although objectively all of the patients still had a positive anterior drawer sign and evidence of rotatory instability.

Lipscomb et al. [35] described a combined transfer of the semitendinosus and gracilis tendons, which were left attached distally and passed through drill holes in the tibia and femur. The authors reported 284 total cases in 1981, which included 88 patients with a semitendinosus transfer alone, 97 patients with combined semitendinosus and gracilis transfers, and 99 patients with a lateral extra-articular reconstruction in addition to the pes tendon transfer. Overall, 84 per cent good results were noted at a follow-up of five years.

The combined use of the gracilis and semitendinosus tendon was also reported by Moyer et al. in 1986 [40]. The tendons were left attached distally, and brought through tibial and femoral tunnels, and stapled to the lateral femoral condyle. Thirty-one patients were reported, half of whom underwent arthroscopic reconstruction. No long-term results were reported but the patients who underwent arthroscopic reconstruction were noted to have less pain, shorter hospitalizations, and fewer complaints of patellofemoral pain.

Patellar Tendon

Portions of the extensor mechanism have been used as a substitute for the anterior cruciate ligament [1, 2, 7, 8, 10, 19, 28, 29, 30, 31, 32]. Complications resulting from use of the patellar tendon have rarely been reported, but include fracture of the patella [39] and rupture of the remaining portion of the tendon, presumably due to a reduction in the mass of the structure or interruption of its vascular supply [6].

In the 1930s, Campbell reconstructed the anterior cruciate ligament using the medial border of the quadriceps tendon, joint capsule, and patellar tendon, which were routed through tibial and femoral drill holes in a distal-to-proximal direction. He reported on nine patients, all of whom were noted to have excellent results, many being able to return to their previous level of athletic activity [7, 8].

In 1963, Jones described using the central third of the patellar tendon as an ACL substitute [29]. In addition to the patellar tendon, the graft consisted of a triangular block of bone from the superficial half of the patella and a strip of quadriceps tendon taken to one inch above the superior pole of the patella. This structure was left attached distally and brought into the joint through a notch beneath the fat pad. The graft was then pulled through a tunnel in the lateral femoral condyle and secured with sutures to the periosteum of the distal femur. The defect in the patellar tendon was routinely closed. Initially, 11 patients were followed for two years and although no subjective instability was noted, 4 patients had to give up sports activities. In 1970, Jones modified the original procedure to include the use of a 2.4-mm Kirschner wire passed percutaneously across the femoral condyle to lock the graft in the femoral tunnel [30]. Forty-six patients who underwent the modified procedure were reported on, with a minimum follow-up of two years [31]. Twenty-nine of the 46 patients had a positive anterior drawer sign, although most were able to return to sports activities with little restriction.

Alm and Gillquist [2] studied 164 patients who underwent reconstruction of the anterior cruciate ligament using the medial third of the patellar ligament, which was taken from the superior pole of the patella to the tibial tubercle, where it was left attached. This graft was brought up through a hole in the tibia and secured at the original sight of insertion of anterior cruciate ligament, with sutures brought out through drill holes in the lateral femoral condyle. One hundred thirty-one of the cases were followed for two years and eight patients were noted to have sustained further injuries. Of the remaining 123 patients, 66 per cent were able to resume competitive sports activities, although the majority still had a slightly increased anterior drawer sign.

Eriksson [15] described four modifications of the Jones procedure [29] and felt that the best results were obtained by taking a block of bone from the distal two thirds of the medial patella and anchoring this portion of the graft to the lateral femoral condyle with sutures placed through drill holes. He also stressed the importance of anchoring the ligament substitute at the normal ACL insertion site on the femur and tensioning the graft when securing the sutures. Seventy-two cases were evaluated at one year and 80 per cent were noted to have stable knees with no anterior drawer sign.

In 1979, Marshall et al. described the use of a cruciate ligament substitute consisting of the central portion of the quadriceps tendon, the prepatellar tissue and the central portion of the patellar tendon measuring 1 cm in width [38]. This graft was left attached to the tibial tubercle distally and brought through a proximal tibial drill hole and through the intercondylar notch in an over-the-top fashion. They also emphasized suturing the synovium and fat pad to the graft for enhanced revascularization. Forty patients were followed for an average of 22 months and 18 were able to return to sports. All of the patients had a positive anterior drawer sign and 22 of the 40 patients had a positive pivot shift but no giving way. Clinical results were rated using the Hospital for Special Surgery scoring system [37] and were noted to change from a preoperative value of 28 to a postoperative value of 39.1.

Paulos et al. [47] reported the use of a vascularized patellar tendon graft consisting of the medial third of the patellar tendon, preserving the blood supply from the inferior medial geniculate artery. Thirty-five patients were followed for a minimum of two years with ''encouraging results,'' although the authors noted some problems in gaining extension and with intercondylar calcification.

Clancy et al. [10] also reported on the use of a vascularized graft consisting of the central one third of the patellar ligament with a laterally based vascular fat-pad pedicle, supplied by the lateral inferior geniculate artery. The graft was detached with bone blocks from the patella and tibial tubercle, each measuring 4 mm in depth, 10 mm in width, and 25 mm in length. This vascularized structure was rotated 180 degrees and secured within the bone tunnels with buttons. The authors also emphasized precise placement of the tibial and femoral tunnels for isometric positioning of the substitute. Clinical results were reported on 50 patients who were followed for an average of thirty-three months. None of the patients had postoperative instability and 46 were able to return to sports activities consisting of acceleration, deceleration, and cutting maneuvers. The pivot shift was absent in 41 patients and the Lachman test was negative or only trace positive in 20 patients, while the remaining 30 had only a mildly positive Lachman

sign with a firm end point. Overall, combined subjective and objective results were excellent in 30 patients and good in 17.

In a long-term follow-up study of 88 patients undergoing reconstruction of the anterior cruciate ligament with the medial third of the patellar ligament, Johnson et al. [28] reported 71 per cent satisfactory results. Objective measurement of the Lachman test revealed 6.8 mm of anterior translation on the reconstructed side, as compared with 4.8 mm on the uninjured side. No evidence of anterolateral rotatory instability could be demonstrated in 56 of 80 patients.

Forty patients were followed for an average of 3.1 years by Fried et al. [19] after undergoing a Jones procedure [29] combined with an extra-articular iliotibial band transfer [14]. Twenty-four of the 40 patients were noted to have good or excellent results and 8 were able to return fully to sports activities. Twenty-nine of the patients had a 0 or 1+ Lachman test and only six patients had a pivot shift. The time interval from injury to reconstruction averaged 2.7 years and the authors noted a high incidence of arthritic changes and meniscal tears.

Paterson and Trickey [46], using a modification of the Jones procedure [29], followed 40 patients for an average of 2.7 years. The patellar ligament was taken as a free graft, secured in the tibial drill hole with a wedge of bone, and placed over the top of the lateral femoral condyle. Subjectively, 72.5 per cent good results were reported.

Meniscus

Walsh reported use of the meniscus in reconstruction of the anterior cruciate ligament in 1972 [56]. Thirteen cases were studied, all with unsatisfactory results. Seven patients were noted to be significantly worse and five required re-exploration for symptoms of intercondylar meniscal dislocation. Collins et al. [12] studied the histology of the meniscus when used as a substitute for the anterior cruciate ligament in dogs. The grafts were noted to become vascularized and to undergo morphologic changes in response to the new functional demands and intra-articular environment.

Tillberg [55] reported the use of meniscal substitution of the cruciate ligament in 45 patients followed from 1 to 31 years. This study included four posterior cruciate ligament reconstructions. Forty-four of the 45 patients subjectively reported feeling more stable, and 31 knees demonstrated less than a 2-mm difference in anterior translation, as compared with the normal side. Twenty-two of the 45 patients had some intermittent instability of the knee on stair climbing or on uneven ground and all were able to return to work, two requiring a lighter occupation. Twenty-seven of the patients were able to participate in sports.

Ferkel et al. [18] reported 84 per cent excellent or good objective results in 100 patients undergoing meniscal substitution of the anterior cruciate ligament, with an average follow-up of 42 months. Five per cent of the patients had a positive pivot shift. The reconstructed knees demonstrated an average of 2.1 mm greater laxity than the uninjured side at 200 N of force.

Recently, the functional deficit often resulting from the ACL-deficient knee has become better defined and indications for operative intervention outlined. However, the biomechanical and histologic properties of the various autogenous substitutes for the anterior cruciate ligament fail to duplicate those of the normal structure adequately, and the large number of studies presenting clinical results following reconstruction are difficult to compare.

This overview of autogenous ACL reconstruction helps to demonstrate the need for consistent evaluation and adequately long follow-up in an attempt to find the "ideal" procedure for reconstruction of the anterior cruciate ligament.

REFERENCES

1. Alm A. Survival of part of patellar tendon transposed for reconstruction of anterior cruciate ligament. Acta Chir Scand 1973; 139:443–447.
2. Alm A, Gillquist J. Reconstruction of the anterior cruciate ligament by using the medial third of the patellar ligament. Acta Chir Scand 1974; 140:289–296.
3. Amiel D, Kleiner JB, Roux RD, Harwood FL, Akeson WH. The phenomenon of "ligamentization": anterior cruciate ligament reconstruction with autogenous patellar tendon. J Orthop Res 1986; 4:162–172.
4. Arnoczky SP, Tarvin GB, Marshall JL. Anterior cruciate ligament replacement using patellar tendon. J Bone Joint Surg (Am) 1982; 64:217–224.
5. Bertoia JT, Urovitz EP, Richards RR, Gross AE. Anterior cruciate reconstruction using the MacIntosh lateral-substitution over-the-top repair. J Bone Joint Surg (Am) 1985; 67:1183–1187.
6. Bonamo JJ, Krinick RM, Sporn AA. Rupture of the patellar ligament after use of its central third for anterior cruciate reconstruction. J Bone Joint Surg (Am) 66:1294–1297.
7. Campbell WC. Repair of the ligaments of the knee. Surg Gynecol Obstet 1936; 62:964–968.
8. Campbell WC. Reconstruction of the ligaments of the knee. Am J Surg 1939; 43:473–480.
9. Clancy WG, Narechania RG, Rosenberg TD, Gmeiner JG, Wisnefske DD, Lange TA. Anterior and posterior cruciate ligament reconstruction in Rhesus monkeys. J Bone Joint Surg (Am) 1981; 63:1270–1284.
10. Clancy WG, Nelson DA, Reider B, Narechania RG. Anterior cruciate ligament reconstruction using one-third of the patellar ligament, augmented by extra-articular tendon transfers. J Bone Joint Surg (Am) 1982; 64:352–359.
11. Cho KO. Reconstruction of the anterior cruciate ligament by semitendinosus tenodesis. J Bone and Joint Surg (Am) 1975; 57:608–612.
12. Collins HR, Hughston JC, DeHaven KE, Bergfeld JA, Evarts CM. The meniscus as a cruciate ligament substitute. Am J Sports Med 1974; 2:11–21.
13. DuToit GT. Knee joint cruciate ligament substitution: the Lindemann (Heidelberg) operation. S Afr J Surg 1967; 5:25–30.
14. Ellison AE. Distal iliotibial band transfer for anterolateral rotatory instability of the knee. J Bone Joint Surg (Am) 1979; 61:330–337.
15. Eriksson E. Reconstruction of the anterior cruciate ligament. Orthop Clin North Am 1976; 7:167–179.
16. Feagin JA, Abbott HG, Rokous JR. The isolated tear of the anterior cruciate ligament. J Bone Joint Surg (Am) 1972; 54:1340–1341.
17. Feagin JA, Curl WW. Isolated tear of the anterior cruciate ligament: 5 year follow-up study. Am J Sports Med 1976; 4:95–100.
18. Ferkel RD, Goodfellow D, Markolf K, et al. The ACL deficient knee: substitute or follow along? Orthop Trans 1984; 8:257.
19. Fried JA, Bergfeld JA, Weiker G, Andrish JT. Anterior cruciate ligament reconstruction using the Jones–Ellison procedure. J Bone Joint Surg (Am) 1985; 67:1029–1033.
20. Gomes JLE, Marczyk LRS. Anterior cruciate ligament reconstruction with a loop or double thickness of semitendinosus tendon. Am J Sports Med 1984; 12:199–203.
21. Hewson GF. Drill guides for improving accuracy in anterior cruciate ligament repair and reconstruction. Clin Orthop 1983; 172:119–124.
22. Hey Groves EW. Operation for the repair of the crucial ligaments. Lancet 1917; 2:674–675.
23. Hey Groves EW. The crucial ligaments of the knee joint: their function, rupture, and operative treatment of the same. Br J Surg 1920; 7:505–515.
24. Hoogland T, Hillen B. Intra-articular reconstruction of the anterior cruciate ligament: an experimental study of the length changes in different ligament reconstructions. Clin Orthop 1984; 185:197–202.
25. Insall J, Joseph DM, Aglietti P, Campbell R Jr. Bone block iliotibial band transfer for anterior cruciate insufficiency. J Bone Joint Surg (Am) 1981; 63:560–569.
26. Johnson RJ. The anterior cruciate: a dilemma in sports medicine. Int J Sports Med 1982; 3:71–79.
27. Johnson RJ. Natural history of anterior cruciate ligament injuries. Presented at the American Academy of Orthopaedic Surgeons Winter Sports Injuries—1986, Snowmass, Colorado, March 13, 1986.
28. Johnson RJ, Eriksson E, Haagmark T, Pope MH. Five- to ten-year follow-up evaluation after reconstruction of the anterior cruciate ligament. Clin Orthop 1984; 183:122–140.
29. Jones KG. Reconstruction of the anterior cruciate ligament: a technique using the central one-third of the patellar ligament. J Bone Joint Surg (Am) 1963; 45:925–932.
30. Jones KG. Reconstruction of the anterior cruciate ligament using the central one-third of the patellar ligament. J Bone Joint Surg (Am) 1970; 52:838–839.
31. Jones KG. Reconstruction of the anterior cruciate ligament using the central one-third of the patellar ligament: a follow-up report. J Bone Joint Surg (Am) 1970; 52:1302–1308.
32. Jones KG. Results of use of the central one-third of the patellar ligament to compensate for anterior cruciate ligament deficiency. Clin Orthop 1980; 147:39–44.

33. Kennedy JC. Chronic ligamentous instability of the knee joint. In: Straub LR, Wilson PD Jr, (eds.) Clinical trends in orthopaedics. New York: Thieme-Stratton, 1982:224–236.

34. Kennedy JC, Roth JH, Mendenhall HV, Sanford JB. Intra-articular replacement in the anterior cruciate ligament-deficient knee. Am J Sports Med 1980; 8:1–8.

35. Lipscomb AB, Johnston RK, Snyder RB. The technique of cruciate ligament reconstruction. Am J Sports Med 1981; 9:77–81.

36. Lipscomb AB, Johnston RK, Snyder RB, Brothers JC. Secondary reconstruction of the anterior cruciate ligament in athletes by using the semitendinosus tendon. Am J Sports Med 1979; 7:81–84.

37. Marshall JL, Fetto JF, Botero PM. Knee ligament injuries: a standardized evaluation method. Clin Orthop 1977; 123:115–129.

38. Marshall JL, Warren RF, Wickiewicz TL, Fetto JF. Reconstruction of a functioning anterior cruciate ligament. Orthop Rev 1979; 6:49–55.

39. McCarroll JR. Fracture of the patella during a golf swing following reconstruction of the anterior cruciate ligament. Am J Sports Med 1983; 11:26–27.

40. Moyer RA, Betz RR, Iaquinto J, Marchetto P, Alburger PD, Clancy M. Arthroscopic anterior cruciate ligament reconstruction using the semitendinosus and gracilis tendons: preliminary report. Contemp Orthop 1986; 12:17–22.

41. Nicholas JA, Minkoff J. Iliotibial band transfer through the intercondylar notch for combined anterior instability (ITPT procedure). Am J Sports Med 1978; 6:341–353.

42. Noyes FR, Butler DL, Grood ES, Zernicke RF, Hefzy MS. Biomechanical analysis of human ligament grafts used in knee-ligament repairs and reconstructions. J Bone Joint Surg (Am) 1984; 66:344–352.

43. Noyes FR, Matthews DS, Mooar PA, Grood ES. The symptomatic anterior cruciate-deficient knee. Part II: The results of rehabilitation, activity modification, and counseling on functional disability. J Bone Joint Surg (Am) 1983; 65:163–174.

44. Noyes FR, Mooar PA, Matthews DS, Butler DL. The symptomatic anterior cruciate-deficient knee. Part I: The long-term functional disability in athletically active individuals. J Bone Joint Surg (Am) 1983; 65:154–162.

45. O'Donoghue DH. A method for replacement of the anterior cruciate ligament of the knee. J Bone Joint Surg (Am) 1963; 45:905–924.

46. Paterson FWN, Trickey EL. Anterior cruciate ligament reconstruction using part of the patellar tendon as a free graft. J Bone Joint Surg (Br) 1986; 68:453–457.

47. Paulos LE, Butler DL, Noyes FR, Grood ES. Intra-articular cruciate reconstruction. II: Replacement with vascularized patellar tendon. Clin Orthop 1983; 172:78–84.

48. Puddu G. Method for reconstruction of the anterior cruciate ligament using the semitendinosus tendon. Am J Sports Med 1980; 8:402–404.

49. Roux W. Die Entwicklungsmechanic. Leipzig: 1905.

50. Rovere GD, Adair DM. Anterior cruciate-deficient knees: a review of the literature. Am J Sports Med 1983; 11:412–419.

51. Scott WN, Ferriter P, Marino M. Intra-articular transfer of the iliotibial tract. J Bone Joint Surg (Am) 1985; 67:532–538.

52. Scott WN, Schosheim PM. Intra-articular transfer of the iliotibial muscle-tendon unit. Clin Orthop 1983; 172:97–101.

53. Smith A. The diagnosis and treatment of injuries of the crucial ligaments. Br J Surg 1918; 6:176–189.

54. Thompson SK, Calver R, Monk CJE. Anterior cruciate ligament repair for rotatory instability: the Lindemann dynamic muscle-transfer procedure. J Bone Joint Surg (Am) 1978; 60:917–920.

55. Tillberg, B. The late repair of torn cruciate ligaments using the menisci. J Bone Joint Surg (Br) 1977; 59:15–19.

56. Walsh JJ Jr. Meniscal reconstruction of the anterior cruciate ligament. Clin Orthop 1972; 89:171–177.

57. Zaricznyj B. Reconstruction of the anterior cruciate ligament using free tendon graft. Am J Sports Med 1983; 11:164–176.

58. Zarins B, Rowe CR. Combined anterior cruciate ligament reconstruction using semitendinosus tendon and iliotibial tract. J Bone Joint Surg (Am) 1986; 68:160–177.

6

PROSTHETIC RECONSTRUCTION OF THE ANTERIOR CRUCIATE LIGAMENT: Historical Overview

GARY A. PATTEE, M.D.
STEPHEN J. SNYDER, M.D.

Corner was perhaps the first to describe prosthetic reconstruction of the anterior cruciate ligament [11]. In 1914, he used a loop of silver wire to replace the torn anterior cruciate ligament in a football player. Several years later, Smith used multiple silk sutures pulled through channels in the tibia and femur to reconstruct a torn anterior cruciate ligament, although a severe inflammatory reaction necessitated removal of the sutures after 11 weeks [34].

Although von Mironova [38] began using Lavsan, a form of polyester, for human anterior cruciate ligament reconstruction almost 30 years ago, most of the modern research on prosthetic cruciate ligament reconstruction began with investigations in animals. Because anterior cruciate ligament tears are relatively common in dogs, veterinarians have provided much of the early experience in prosthetic ligament reconstruction [7, 12, 17, 21, 27, 32]. In 1960, Emery and Rostrup [12] described the use of an 8-mm tube of Teflon to replace the anterior cruciate ligament in nine dogs. They reported only a slight increase in anterior–posterior laxity and minimal joint reaction at six months, but noted fraying of the Teflon in the region of entrance into the femoral tunnel. In the same year, Johnson [21] reported excellent results using No. 4 braided nylon suture anchored by vi-

tallium screws to replace the anterior cruciate ligament in 20 dogs. Butler [7] implanted Teflon mesh into the knees of 15 dogs and cats to replace the anterior cruciate ligament and reported good results, with little or no tissue reaction.

In 1969, Gupta and Brinker [17] used braided Dacron cord coated with silicone rubber as an anterior cruciate ligament prosthesis in the dog. The rubber coating was intended to protect the Dacron from the synovial fluid environment, but 7 of 10 prostheses fragmented after two to four months. The failures were believed to be due to loosening of the silicone coating and exposure of the Dacron to the intra-articular environment. Andrish and Woods [3] used a 4-mm woven Dacron graft to augment reconstruction of the anterior cruciate ligament using the central third of the patellar tendon. All of the tendon grafts that were augmented had failed by three months, while all of the non-augmented reconstructions remained intact. This was believed to be due to the stress-shielding effect of the Dacron graft, leading to resorption of the autogenous tissue.

In 1973, the FDA approved implantation of the Proplast (Vitek, Inc.) prosthetic anterior cruciate ligament [40]. This prosthesis was intended to be used as a stint, or temporary internal splint, augmenting medial and lateral extra-articular procedures by providing stability until healing took place [19]. The implant consists of a core of polyaramid fiber and fluorinated ethylene propylene polymer, and a coating of a porous low-modulus composite of polytetrafluoroethylene and vitreous carbon fiber. In biomechanical studies, the prosthesis failed at a force of 158 kg with 23.6 per cent elongation. James et al. [19] reported implantation of the prosthesis as a salvage procedure in 15 patients with disabling chronic knee instability due to anterior cruciate ligament deficiency. They reported only 50 per cent satisfactory results, although the anterior drawer was eliminated in 10 patients. Stint breakage occurred in 8 of the 15 patients, most failures occurring within one year, and six implants requiring removal.

Rubin and Marshall [29] reported the use of a Hydron sponge–Dacron prosthesis in six beagle dogs to replace the anterior cruciate ligament. Hydron is a polyhydroxyethyl methacrylate compound, noted to be extremely biocompatible and was used in a porous cylindrical sponge form, reinforced longitudinally with loosely knitted Dacron fabric. The dogs were studied at 8 to 15 months postoperatively, and bony fixation within the tibial and femoral tunnels was noted to be slightly retarded compared with the fixation of bare Dacron prostheses. The Hydron sponge appeared to disintegrate, exposing the Dacron to the synovial fluid environment. In the same year, Rubin et al. [30] compared the use of loosely knitted Dacron mesh to tightly woven Dacron tape in two groups of dogs and noted tissue ingrowth in the mesh but not in the tape prostheses. Most joints in which the implants remained intact were free of arthritis, while changes typical of the anterior cruciate ligament–deficient knee development in every knee in which the implant failed.

The use of a polyethylene prosthetic anterior cruciate ligament was reported by Kennedy in 1975 [22] and in 1976, Grood and Noyes [16] reported the results of biomechanical testing of a Hercules 1900 medical-grade ultra-high-molecular-weight polyethylene prosthesis. This device measures 6.35 mm in diameter and 178 mm in length, with a 35- to 40-mm central section with a diameter of 4.76 mm. This was known as the Polyflex ligament (Richards Manufacturing Company). Fixation was accomplished with a threaded nut augmented with polymethylmethacrylate cement. Ultimate tensile stress at failure was 6000 psi and occurred at elongations from 350 to 450 per cent. The mode of failure was pull-out of the threaded portion of the implant following elongation. After cyclic loading at 250 N (250,000 cycles), elongation of 7.6 mm resulted, which

showed only a 40 per cent recovery after 1000 sec. Overall, the margin of safety of the implant was felt to be low in terms of its ability to resist expected in vivo forces without sustaining permanent deformation. Chen and Black [9] also concluded, after biomechanical evaluation, that the Polyflex ligament was unsatisfactory for anterior cruciate ligament replacement. In a clinical study of 38 patients with an average follow-up of 12 to 18 months after implantation of the Polyflex ligament, 30 patients had pain, 7 had instability, 16 had greater than 5 mm of anterior displacement, and 6 implants had broken [14]. In another study, 52 per cent of 29 patients had undergone revision or removal of the prostheses within one year of implantation [13].

Kennedy [23] began implanting a prosthetic device in 1979 to augment autogenous tissue used in reconstruction of the anterior cruciate ligament. This was a 6-mm, flat, diamond-braided polypropylene ligament augmentation device (LAD), which was developed in conjunction with the 3M Company. Kennedy believed that autogenous tissue used in anterior cruciate reconstruction was subject to stretch and rupture in the early postoperative period and that immobilization and subsequent collagen breakdown placed the graft in jeopardy. The LAD was developed to supplement the biologic graft during this critical period of remodeling.

Biomechanical testing of the LAD revealed a tensile load failure of 140 kg and excellent creep resistance when subjected to over one million load cycles [23]. Extensive animal studies have shown a significant increase in strength of the autogenous tissue with ingrowth of collagen throughout the host tissue [24]. Using the MacIntosh procedure for anterior cruciate ligament reconstruction in young swine, the nonaugmented prepatellar tissue failed at an average load of 22.5 kg. With augmentation using the braided polypropylene device, the average load to failure was 29.5 kg immediately postoperatively and increased to 49.5 kg 44 days after surgery [24].

In 1983, Kennedy [23] reported the clinical use of the LAD in 110 human knees, with encouraging results. The LAD was sutured from the insertion of the patellar tendon, through the prepatellar tissue and into a section of the rectus femoris. The augmented graft is then passed through the knee joint and over the top of the lateral femoral condyle, where it is secured with a staple. The increased tensile strength of the composite graft allows appropriate intraoperative tensioning, and since the synthetic device is secured to bone only at one end, the effects of stress shielding are minimized [26].

As ingrowth and recollagenization strengthens the autogenous graft, the LAD is protected from creep and fatigue failure. Roth [28] reported significantly improved results in 45 patients using the LAD at an average of 50 months of follow-up, when compared with a similar group of patients with nonaugmented grafts.

In 1978, Jenkins [20] was the first to report the use of flexible carbon fiber to replace the anterior cruciate ligament. The implant consists of 40,000 individual strands of carbon fiber tow. The carbon matrix is thought to act as a temporary scaffold, inducing the ingrowth of fibroblastic tissue, and may encourage the orientation of new collagen in the direction of the original ligament. Jenkins originally implanted the devices in sheep and at three to eight months noted initial covering of the implant with synovium and eventual envelopment of the carbon with what appeared to be a new ligament. However, with fragmentation of the fibers, particles of carbon were noted to migrate to regional lymph nodes. In 1983, Rushton et al. [31] reported on 39 patients who underwent anterior cruciate reconstruction with carbon fiber and a lateral extra-articular augmentation. Ten patients required arthroscopic examination at an average of 16.9 mo for persistent pain and mild effusion. They were unable to demonstrate ingrowth of organized fibroblastic tissue, but only a thin fibrous covering over the carbon-fiber implant. Also noted was the presence of carbon fiber within the joint, which possibly contributed to persistent effusions and synovial thickening.

To reduce carbon-particle migration and improve handling properties, carbon fiber implants have been coated with polylactic acid polymer [2]. Theoretically, the copolymer is resorbed shortly after implantation and the carbon undergoes gradual mechanical degradation over a long period of time. Stress is initially taken up by the prosthesis and gradually transferred to the newly formed collagen. In April 1981, clinical testing of the carbon–polylactic acid composite ligament prosthesis was begun in a multicenter study [39]. The prosthesis is woven through a strip of distally detached iliotibial band, passed through the posterior capsule of the knee, and passed through a tibial tunnel. Fixation to the tibia is accomplished with a carbon–polylactic acid fastener. Clinical improvement was reported in most patients who underwent anterior cruciate ligament reconstruction as a salvage procedure using the prosthesis [39]. However, Strum and Larson [35] used the polylactic acid–coated carbon implant (Hexcel Medical) to augment anterior cruciate ligament reconstructions utilizing the central third of the patellar tendon or a double loop

of semitendinosus tendon. They found no apparent benefit at one year when compared to a similar group of patients undergoing the same reconstruction without augmentation.

The xenograft (Xenotech Laboratories, Irvine, Calif.) is a bovine extensor tendon with a bifurcation at one end. Treatment with glutaraldehyde protects the collagen bundles from proteolytic action by cross-linking lysine radicals on adjacent proteoglycan molecules. This treatment produces an implant that does not undergo remodeling and is thus considered a permanent prosthesis [25]. The tensile strength of the implant is over 3000 N and animal studies have demonstrated host tissue ingrowth, strong biologic fixation within bone tunnels, and no evidence of resorption of the graft [25].

Clinical trials using the bovine xenograft began in The Netherlands in January 1981 [1]. Of the first 50 patients undergoing implantation of the xenograft for anterior cruciate insufficiency, only 52 per cent had good or excellent functional results. This was thought to be at least partially due to fraying or rupture of the graft secondary to impingement on the femoral notch or at the entrance to the bone tunnels. A second series of 89 patients had 92 per cent good and excellent functional results after modification of the surgical technique, using a wide notchplasty, chamfering the bone tunnel entrance sites, and further correcting rotational instability with a lateral extra-articular procedure [1]. Successful results have been reported in the United States, but at the present time, no long-term clinical experience is available [40].

Tremblay et al. [37] feel that prosthetic ligament implants fail due to inadequate functional, physiologic, and biomechanical characteristics necessary to replace the normal anterior cruciate ligament. They devised a prosthesis consisting of a hollow cylindrical Silastic core around which is woven a polytetrafluoroethylene-impregnated Dacron suture with a predetermined weave angle. By varying the weave angle of the nonelastic fiber, the strength and elastic characteristics of the implant can be altered to match those of the normal anterior cruciate ligament. At the present time, no clinical data on this device have been reported.

Cabaud et al. [8] reported the use of a braided polyglycolic acid ligament (Dexon, Davis and Geck) to augment anterior cruciate ligament repair in dogs. The implant provided sufficient protection to allow healing of the cruciate repair and was almost completely resorbed by five weeks. The results are encouraging, but no further work with this implant has been reported.

The Leeds–Keio prosthetic ligament is made of

pure polyester in an open-weave structure with both tubular and flat sections [15, 33]. The maximum tensile load is approximately 2000 N and the stiffness of the ligament is comparable to that of the normal anterior cruciate ligament [28]. It is anchored to both the femur and the tibia with bone plugs, allowing bone ingrowth, which strengthens the fixation of the ligament. No autogenous tissue is sacrificed in using the prosthesis for anterior cruciate reconstruction, and the implant is thought to act as a scaffold for natural tissue ingrowth [15]. Since February 1982, more than 220 Leeds–Keio artificial ligaments have been used for anterior cruciate reconstruction, with very satisfactory results reported, although the follow-up period is less than five years [15].

The Gore-Tex graft is an expanded polytetrafluoroethylene (PTFE) prosthesis that was originally developed as a single-filament device and later replaced with a multifilament design [5]. The structure consists of PTFE nodules interconnected with strong fibrils of the same substance. This porous structure allows host tissue ingrowth, although the device is intended for use as a permanent prosthesis, independent of host tissue for strength. The prosthesis is secured to cortical bone with self-tapping screws inserted through loops at each end of the implant. Mechanical testing revealed an average ultimate tensile strength of 4830 N with a mean elongation of 8.9 per cent. After cyclical loading, no reduction in tensile strength was noted. The device was initially tested in 17 sheep and no instability was noted at one year [6]. Biomechanical testing following implantation revealed maximum fixation strength due to tissue ingrowth at 218 days.

Investigational use of the Gore-Tex graft in humans began in October 1982, with implantation using a modified over-the-top procedure [4]. Over 160 patients have be followed for two or more years postoperatively and encouraging functional results have been reported. Eighteen devices have failed, presumably due to impingement against sharp bone edges, including the anterior and posterior intercondylar notches and the posterior femoral and tibial intra-articular bone tunnels. The impingement is thought to cause strand failure by "cold flow" and possibly by abrasion. In another series, marked improvement in activities of daily living was noted in patients followed for more than two years, with 3.1 per cent of the grafts requiring removal due to failure or infection [10].

The Stryker Meadox ligament graft is a composite of four Dacron tapes surrounded by a woven Dacron velour sleeve [18, 36]. It is intended to be used as an augmentation device with the iliotibial band in anterior cruciate reconstruction and in animal studies has demonstrated significant bone and fibrous tissue ingrowth [36]. Biomechanical testing of the ligament reveals a tensile strength of 2670 N, with an average ultimate elongation of 18 per cent. In canine studies, little instability was noted using the over-the-top intra-articular procedure with iliotibial band augmentation, and there was only a slight loss of strength at one year. Further investigations in dogs are in progress [18].

Since Edred Corner used a wire loop over 70 years ago, numerous attempts have been made to find a prosthetic device with the appropriate characteristics and longevity to substitute for the anterior cruciate ligament. Whether to be used as permanent prostheses, as supporting structures for the host tissues, or as scaffolds to allow eventual biologic replacement with collagenous tissue, many of the devices have been removed from clinical use, while others await further investigation.

REFERENCES

1. Abbink EP. Surgical technique for correction of chronic anterior cruciate ligament deficiency with bovine xenografts. Presented at the Third Annual Symposium on Prosthetic Ligament Reconstruction of the Knee, Scottsdale, Arizona, April, 1986.
2. Alexander H, Parsons JR, Smith G, Fong R, Mylod A, Weiss AB. Anterior cruciate ligament replacement with filamentous carbon. Trans Orthop Res Soc 1982; 7:45.
3. Andrish JT, Woods LD. Dacron augmentation in anterior cruciate ligament reconstruction in dogs. Clin Orthop 1984; 183:298–302.
4. Bolton CW. Three years of clinical experience with the Gore-Tex cruciate ligament prosthesis: what we have learned. Presented at the Third Annual Symposium on Prosthetic Ligament Reconstruction of the Knee, Scottsdale, Arizona, April, 1986.
5. Bolton W, Bruchman B. Mechanical and biological properties of the Gore-Tex expanded polytetrafluoroethylene (PTFE) prosthetic ligament. Aktuel Prob Chir Orthop 1983; 26:40–51.
6. Bolton CW, Bruchman WC. The Gore-Tex expanded polytetrafluoroethylene prosthetic ligament. Clin Orthop 1985; 196:202–213.
7. Butler HC. Teflon as a prosthetic ligament in repair of ruptured anterior cruciate ligaments. Am J Vet Res 1964; 25:55–60.
8. Cabaud HE, Feagin JA, Rodkey WG. Acute anterior cruciate ligament injury and repair reinforced with a biodegradable intraarticular ligament. Am J Sports Med 1982; 10(5):259–265.
9. Chen EH, Black J. Materials design analysis of the prosthetic anterior cruciate ligament. J Biomed Mater Res 1980; 14:567–586.
10. Collins HR. The Gore-Tex artificial anterior cruciate ligament results. Presented at the Third Annual Symposium on Prosthetic Ligament Reconstruction of the Knee, Scottsdale, Arizona, April, 1986.
11. Corner EM. Notes of a case illustrative of an artificial anterior crucial ligament, demonstrating the action of that ligament. Proc R Soc Med 1914; 7:120–121.

12. Emery MA, Rostrup O. Repair of the anterior cruciate ligament with 8 mm. tube Teflon in dogs. Can J Surg 1960; 4:111–115.
13. FDA Orthopaedic Device Classification Panel. Initial survey of Richards Polyflex cruciate ligament prosthesis. Transcript, Washington, D.C., November, 1978.
14. Fox J. Report on the clinical results of Polyflex (TM) ligament replacement. Prepared for the FDA Orthopaedic Panel, April 15, 1977. Presentation to the panel April 15, 1977.
15. Fujikawa K. Clinical study of the Leeds–Keio artificial ligament. Presented at the Third Annual Symposium on Prosthetic Ligament Reconstruction of the Knee, Scottsdale, Arizona, April, 1986.
16. Grood ES, Noyes FR. Cruciate ligament prosthesis: strength, creep, and fatigue properties. J Bone Joint Surg (Am) 1976; 58:1083–1088.
17. Gupta BN, Brinker WO. Anterior cruciate ligament prosthesis in the dog. J Am Vet Med Assoc 1969; 154(9):1057–1061.
18. Hoffman H. Development and evaluation of a synthetic ligament prosthesis. Presented at the Third Annual Symposium on Prosthetic Ligament Reconstruction of the Knee, Scottsdale, Arizona, April, 1986.
19. James SL, Woods GW, Homsy CA, Prewitt JM, Slocum DB. Cruciate ligament stents in reconstruction of the unstable knee. Clin Orthop 1979; 143:90–96.
20. Jenkins DHR. The repair of cruciate ligaments with flexible carbon-fibre. J Bone Joint Surg (Br) 1978; 60:520–522.
21. Johnson FL. Use of braided nylon as a prosthetic anterior cruciate ligament of the dog. J Am Vet Med Assoc 1960; 137(11):646–647.
22. Kennedy JC. Experience with polypropylene ligament. Presented at the Canadian Orthopaedic Association Meeting, Ottawa, Canada, June, 1975.
23. Idem. Application of prosthetics to anterior cruciate ligament reconstruction and repair. Clin Orthop 1983; 172:125–128.
24. Kennedy JC, Roth JH, Mendenhall HV. Intraarticular replacement in the anterior cruciate ligament-deficient knee. Am J Sports Med 1980; 8:1–8.
25. McMaster WC. A histologic assessment of canine anterior cruciate substitution with bovine xenograft. Clin Orthop 1985; 196:196–201.
26. McPherson GK, Mendenhall HV, Gibbons DF, et al. Experimental mechanical and histologic evaluation of the Kennedy ligament augmentation device. Clin Orthop 1985; 196:186–195.
27. Meyers JF, Grana WA, Lesker PA. Reconstruction of the anterior cruciate ligament in the dog. Am J Sports Med 1979; 7(2):85–90.
28. Roth JH. Polypropylene braid augmented and nonaugmented intraarticular anterior cruciate ligament reconstruction. Presented at the Third Annual Symposium on Prosthetic Ligament Reconstruction of the Knee, Scottsdale, Arizona, April, 1986.
29. Rubin RM, Marshall JL. Porous hydrophilic polymer: good and bad news in the orthopedic application of cruciate ligament substitution. J Biomed Mater Res 1975; 9:375–380.
30. Rubin RM, Marshall JL, Wang J. Prevention of knee instability. Clin Orthop 1975; 113:212–236.
31. Rushton N, Dandy DJ, Naylor CPE. The clinical arthroscopic and histological findings after replacement of the anterior cruciate ligament with carbon-fibre. J Bone Joint Surg (Br) 1983; 65:308–309.
32. Saidi K, Beauchamp P, Laurin CA. Prosthetic replacement of the anterior cruciate ligament in dogs. Can J Surg 1976; 19:547–549.
33. Seedhom BB. The Leeds–Keio ligament: concepts and mechanical aspects of the device. Presented at the Third Annual Symposium on Prosthetic Ligament Reconstruction of the Knee, Scottsdale, Arizona, April, 1986.
34. Smith A. The diagnosis and treatment of injuries of the crucial ligaments. Br J Surg 1918; 6:176–189.
35. Strum GM, Larson RL. Clinical experience and early results of carbon fiber augmentation of anterior cruciate reconstruction of the knee. Clin Orthop 1985; 196:124–138.
36. Technical Report: Stryker Corporation, Kalamazoo, Michigan January, 1983.
37. Tremblay GR, Laurin CA, Drovin G. The challenge of prosthetic cruciate ligament replacement. Clin Orthop 1980; 147:88–92.
38. von Mironova SS. Spatresultate der Rekonstruktion des Bandapparates des Kniegelenks mit Lawsan, Zentralbl Chir 1978; 103:432.
39. Weiss AB, Blazina ME, Goldstein AR, Alexander H. Ligament replacement with an absorbable copolymer carbon fiber scaffold—early clinical experience. Clin Orthop 1985; 196:77–85.
40. Whipple TL. The role of exogenous materials in arthroscopic management of cruciate-deficient knees. In: McGinty JB, ed. Techniques in orthopaedics: arthroscopic surgery update. Baltimore: University Park Press, 1985: Vol 5, 139–154.

7

INDICATIONS FOR PROSTHETIC LIGAMENT RECONSTRUCTION

ROBERT L. LARSON, M.D.

INTRODUCTION

The anterior cruciate ligament, which we as orthopedists have held in such respect and which has commanded our attention for so many years, has been a challenge to our surgical ingenuity and skill since 1917 when Hey Groves [3] first attempted its reconstruction. Even then one of Hey Groves' contemporaries, Alwyn Smith, [2] tried silk as an artificial replacement and failed.

We are still looking for a replacement that will act as a true prosthesis, recognizing the rigid specifications of elasticity, tensile strength, creep, and multi-axial function that it must meet. Our objectives have broadened. We are now investigating synthetic materials that will augment autogenous tissue or other biologic tissue. Such synthetics are used to increase the tensile strength of deficient tissue, to act as a scaffold for collagen growth, and to provide a stent to protect biologic tissue while it regains a blood supply and develops tensile strength. Some synthetics will provide all of the above benefits and possibly stimulate collagen production. The collagen produced must be of the physiologic type that provides normal alignment, normal linkage, and adequate tensile strength.

Many of the properties of a normal anterior cruciate ligament are difficult if not impossible to reduplicate synthetically. Normal ligaments have proprioceptive nerve endings, which respond to the musculoligamentous reflex. This reflex causes the muscles around the knee to contract when the ligaments are placed under tension. The anterior cruciate ligament has a viscoelasticity that allows it to elongate to 25 per cent of its normal length before plastic deformation occurs. In normal use of flexion and extension the anterior cruciate goes through 14 per cent elongation and returns to its resting length without producing any permanent elongation. (Elongation of synthetic materials after repetitive stretches is called "cyclic creep" and is expressed as percentage of increased length.) Living tissue can respond to minimal tears or injury with healing, while synthetic material produces fatigue failure. Finally, the anterior cruciate ligament has a broad attachment site, which allows the twisted fibers to provide a multi-axial function, producing some tension in different parts of the ligament in all degrees of flexion, extension, and rotation.

A need exists to provide some enhancement of our present methods of autogenous replacement of the anterior cruciate ligament. The protection necessary for autogenous tissue to develop revascularization, collagen maturation, and tensile strength produces changes in muscle, bone, and cartilage, some of which may be irreversible. These changes include loss of bone mass and decreased strength due to prolonged immobilization, surface deterioration of articular cartilage due to altered chondrocyte metabolism, and breakdown of cells and contractile proteins of muscle tissue.

Recent surgical techniques, which emphasize isometric placement of attachment sites and more secure fixation, has stimulated interest in earlier motion and quicker rehabilitation. Still, autogenous tissue undergoes considerable reduction in its tensile strength when placed in the avascular cavern of the intra-articular notch and bathed in the unrelenting phagocytic action of the synovial fluid. Therefore the goal is to find materials and methods that allow rehabilitation to be completed not in months or years but in days or weeks.

To achieve this goal, we need to consider two factors. These are function and longevity. Function depends on attachment points, tension, and compliance. Attachment should allow normal motion without laxity or limitation of normal range of motion. Proper tension is necessary to guide the knee through its physiologic arc without abnormal stress to the supporting ligaments. It may be as detrimental to make a ligament too tight as it is to make it too loose. An attempt should be made to mimic the normal laxity of the uninjured knee. Compliance is the property that allows the ligament to return to its normal length and strength after the stretching or tension that occurs with cyclic use.

Longevity is influenced by fixation strength at attachment sites, by the tensile strength of the material being used, and by the fatigue properties of the material being used. Biologic tissues have a better potential for withstanding fatigue failure because of healing qualities that may be required after excess stretch produces minor tears or wear that may occur at areas of concentration of load.

TYPES AND CATEGORIES OF SYNTHETIC LIGAMENTS

Artificial substances are used with different objectives, with different indications, and in various configurations to enhance or substitute for the anterior cruciate ligament.

SCAFFOLDS. Scaffolds provide a latticework for ingrowing tissue, which ensures its proper orientation, supports the ingrowth of tissue, and increases its tensile strength, and possibly induces collagen ingrowth. It may be designed to be biodegradeable, removable, or a permanent composite of the reconstructed anterior cruciate ligament. Carbon filament fibers have been proposed as a substance that, when implanted into the autogenous tissue, would add tensile strength and induce and align collagen ingrowth. Because of its biodegradeable property it would allow gradual transference of stress to the autogenous tissue as degradation occurs.

Permanent scaffolds include the Stryker–Meadox ligament, which is made of Dacron–Velour; the Leeds–Keio, made of a loose Dacron weave; the ligament augmentation device (LAD), made of polypropylene; and allografts of biologic tissue. The bovine xenograft, though originally proposed as a degrading scaffold, has been found to have long-lasting properties that make it fall into the classification of a permanent prosthesis.

Scaffolding for augmentation of autogenous tissue would be indicated in patients who have had previously failed or stretched tissue. Its use would be indicated to enhance the strength of autogenous tissue when such tissue requires increased tensile or fixation strength. Scaffolding would be proper in persons with hyperelastic tissue, which suggests a tendency for autogenous tissue to stretch. It may be indicated for the augmentation of acute repair to the anterior cruciate ligament, both as a scaffolding and for increased tensile strength.

The use of a synthetic material must eventually allow the autogenous tissue to assume the load of joint stress so that the autogenous tissue will develop the necessary collagen maturation and tensile strength.

STENTS. Stents protect the implanted tissue from excessive stress while the autogenous tissue is going through the period of degradation, revascularization, and collagen maturation that produces a functional ligament. This parallels, to some extent, the function of scaffolds. The stents, however, will eventually break or need to be removed so that the autogenous tissue can assume the function of stabilizing the joint. Until this occurs, the tissue is stress-protected and therefore does not develop tensile strength.

PROSTHESES. Prostheses are designed to be a permanent replacement for the anterior cruciate ligament. No autogenous tissue is used to reconstruct the anterior cruciate ligament and no ingrowth that will materially alter the function of the prosthesis used is expected. One of the first materials to be used for prosthetic replacement of the anterior cruciate ligament was Proplast, a composite of a polyaramid fiber, Teflon, tetrafluorethylene, and vitreous carbon. As a true prosthesis it was found to be too stiff and to break from fatigue failure at an average of 13.2 months after its implantation. Its use was then changed to a stent to maturing extra-articular repairs. When breakage did occur in the latter instances, an increase of the anterior drawer test was evident. Satisfactory results were present in only 50 per cent in a review of 46 cases by Kellam et al. [5]

The Gore-Tex ligament has received FDA approval for use in a previously failed anterior ligament reconstruction. It can be inserted using arthroscopic control, but requires incisions over the anterior tibia and distal lateral femoral area for the screw fixation necessary.

Xenograft, Pro-Tek (polyethylene terephthalate), and other synthetic materials and configurations are being investigated for use as true prostheses.

The indication for the use of a true prosthesis is for people in whom multiple reconstructive procedures have failed to produce a stable joint. As with any newer procedure or device the indications may change as improvement and knowledge of its efficiency is accumulated. The patient with degenerative joint disease in whom early motion is necessary to prevent further changes would also seem to be a candidate for such a device. An older individual with less activity potential or a person who economically cannot afford the time required for protection of an autogenous reconstruction and is willing to reduce his or her activity level would benefit from a procedure that would allow early function with reduced morbidity. The long-time wear potential, the effects on the joint's articular surfaces, and possibly other unknown factors need be determined before more-widespread indications can be proposed. In my opinion, the use of such prostheses in an athlete to provide a quicker return to a sport is not an indication for their use.

ILLUSTRATIVE CASES

The following cases are examples of the use of synthetic materials in the investigational trials of these devices by the author.

CARBON FILAMENT (HEXCEL). This was used in a series of patients intramedulating the carbon filament in autogenous tissue used for the reconstruction of the anterior cruciate ligament. The middle third of the patellar tendon or the semitendinosus tendon double-looped was used as the autogenous material.

CASE 1

A woman aged 20 years had sustained a ligament and meniscal injury four years prior to the present surgery. A medial meniscectomy and pes anserine transfer had been done, but the patient continued to have problems with instability. Findings included a Lachman score of 2+ and a positive pivot shift test of 2+. Early degenerative changes were evident on x-ray. A middle third of patellar tendon augmented with carbon filament and an iliotibial band tenodesis was done. Follow-up three years after her last surgery revealed a minimal Lachman score, no pivot shift, and a side-to-side arthrometer difference of 3 mm. Some discomfort with overuse of the knee was present with vigorous activity.

CASE 2

An 18-year-old male football player sustained an anterior cruciate ligament tear three weeks prior to being examined. Clinical findings revealed positive Lachman and pivot shift tests. A double-looped semitendinosus tendon augmented with carbon filament was used to reconstruct the anterior cruciate ligament, and an iliotibial-band tenodesis was done. A three-year follow-up revealed no instability and no complaints relative to the injured knee. He returned to playing football for a major university.

CASE 3

A 25-year-old man who had had multiple previous procedures, including an intra-articular patellar tendon replacement of the anterior cruciate ligament (Jones technique), continued to have global instability. A procedure was performed that consisted of tightening the previous intra-articular reconstruction and augmenting it with carbon filament. Then a semitendinosus tendon was augmented with carbon filament and placed through the posterior capsule, exiting through the tibial drill hole (Lindemann technique). An extra-articular reconstruction medially, also using carbon filament as an augmentation, was used to stabilize the knee. Further deterioration of both symptoms and function required repeat medial- and lateral-ligament—complex reconstructions, removal of the previous anterior cruciate reconstructions, a high tibial osteotomy, and placement of a permanent anterior cruciate prosthesis (Gore-Tex).

Comment. Ten cases of carbon-filament—augmented reconstructions were compared with a similar group done in a like manner without augmentation. Comparison of the two groups after one year showed essentially no difference on two different rating scales. [6] Though the carbon fiber seems to have considerable tensile strength to longitudinal stress, its fragility to any bending or shear stress makes it somewhat difficult to handle during its implantation. No evidence of intolerance to the foreign substance in the tissues was noted.

LIGAMENT AUGMENTATION DEVICE (LAD–POLYPROPYLENE). The LAD was used in a series of Marshall–Macintosh procedures to augment the deficiency of the tensile strength of the prepatellar tissue used in this type of reconstruction.

CASE 1

A 31-year-old woman injured her knee in 1979, at which time an acute repair of the anterior cruciate ligament, posterior cruciate ligament, and the medial collateral ligament was done. Fifteen months post surgery a second injury occurred. When seen in 1985, the patient had a 2+ valgus instability at 30 degrees of flexion, a 3+ Lachman score, a 3+ pivot shift test, and a side-to-side arthrometer difference of 8 mm. A patellar tendon/

LAD reconstruction for the anterior cruciate ligament, an iliotibial tenodesis, and a medial collateral ligament reconstruction using the semitendinosus tendon were carried out. Follow-up at 14 months showed a 1+ Lachman score with no pivot shift.

CASE 2

A 19-year-old male sustained a skiing injury in 1980. In 1982, an arthroscopic debridement of stumps of an old anterior cruciate ligament was done. A re-injury occurred in 1983. An evaluation in February 1984 showed a 2+ Lachman score and a 2+ anterior drawer sign, but no pivot shift could be elicited without anesthesia. A 15-mm side-to-side difference by arthrometer testing was demonstrated. Surgical reconstruction of the anterior cruciate ligament, using the middle third of the patellar tendon with an LAD augmentation and an iliotibial-band tenodesis, was carried out in June 1984. At follow-up at 26 months, the patient had no Lachman score, no pivot shift, no anterior drawer laxity, and no side-to-side difference on arthrometer testing.

CASE 3.

A man 28 years of age sustained an anterior cruciate tear in 1980, which was repaired acutely. When seen in 1985, he had a 2+ Lachman score, a 2+ pivot shift, and a side-to-side difference of 9 mm on arthrometer testing. Anterior cruciate reconstruction using the medial third of the patellar tendon and an iliotibial-band tenodesis was done. At a one-year re-evaluation the patient had no Lachman score, no pivot shift, and a side-to-side difference of 2 mm on arthrometer testing.

Comment. All patients in this group were required to have a side-to-side difference of more than 3 mm by arthrometer testing for the Lachman test and a positive pivot shift to qualify for this investigation. A review of the results at a 24-month follow-up of 75 patients in a study in the United States showed an improvement in the Lachman test from 2+ preoperatively to less than 0.05+ postoperatively. The pivot shift, which was present in 100 per cent of patients preoperatively, improved to 82 per cent having no pivot shift postoperatively. The side-to-side difference was reduced from 6.21 mm to 1.47 mm at the two-year follow-up. Augmentation of other tissues, such as the middle third of the patellar tendon with bone-to-bone fixation and the semitendinosus tendon, are not being done as a Phase II extension of this study. The LAD as an augmentation for the patellar tendon reconstruction done in the manner of Marshall–Macintosh (as in the above cases) has been approved by the FDA advisory panel.

GORE-TEX LIGAMENT. The Gore-Tex ligament has been used as a true prosthesis. It can be placed arthroscopically, and because of its firm fixation by screw fixation early mobilization is possible.

CASE 1

A 31-year-old man had an acute repair of an anterior cruciate ligament tear in 1975. In 1977, reconstruction was performed using the semitendinosus tendon in the manner of Lindemann for the anterior cruciate ligament, with a reconstruction of the posterior oblique ligament and the medial collateral ligament and a medial meniscectomy. In 1984, the patient was having problems with instability, even with the use of a brace. Examination showed a 3+ Lachman score, a 3+ anterior drawer sign, and a positive pivot shift, which was difficult to elicit because of guarding by the patient. A Gore-Tex prosthesis was inserted. At follow-up 16 months after surgery, the patient had no Lachman score, a 2+ anterior drawer sign, and no pivot shift. Side-to-side difference on arthrometer testing was 2 mm. The patient continued to have some discomfort with use, but felt the knee was considerably improved since surgery. He had considerable quadriceps atrophy and had a 46 per cent quadriceps strength deficit with Cybex testing. He returned to work supervising brick laying six weeks after surgery.

CASE 2

A 26-year-old man sustained a rupture of the anterior cruciate ligament in 1974. An acute repair and two anterior cruciate reconstructions were done between the time of injury and 1981. When seen in 1983, the patient had a 2+ Lachman score, a 2+ anterior drawer sign, and a 1+ pivot shift. In November 1983 a Gore-Tex prosthetic ligament was implanted and an iliotibial-band tenodesis was done. In February 1985 the patient had increased laxity over that immediately after surgery, and an arthroscopic evaluation was carried out. The ligament was relaxed, and 50 to 75 per cent of its fibers were seen to be disrupted. A tightening of the prosthesis was carried out by advancing the proximal screw. In January 1986, the patient complained of marked discomfort and giving way. A 1+ Lachman score, a 1+ anterior drawer sign, and a 1+ pivot shift was present. Re-implantation of a new Gore-Tex ligament prosthesis was recommended.

CASE 3

A 29-year-old woman sustained an anterior cruciate ligament injury to her right knee in 1984. An arthroscopic debridement of the anterior cruciate ligament and a lateral meniscectomy were done one month after injury. A previous medial meniscectomy had been done in 1975. The patient also had marked instability, with a 3+ pivot shift on her left knee. The right knee showed a 2+ Lachman score, a 3+ pivot shift, and degenerative changes.

It was necessary for her to use a cane and she was unable to work as a nurse. A Gore-Tex anterior cruciate prosthesis was implanted along with a tenodesis of the iliotibial band on the right. Six months after her Gore-Tex ligament implantation, an anterior cruciate ligament reconstruction was done on the left knee, using the patellar tendon augmented with an LAD and an iliotibial-band tenodesis. At follow-up, two years post Gore-Tex and 18 months post LAD, the patient had no instability on clinical testing and no symptoms apparent in her right knee. Her left knee showed a 1+ Lachman score and a 1+ pivot shift but was asymptomatic. She had returned to working full-time as a nurse.

Comment. This replacement has provided satisfactory results in 83 per cent of patients on a rating scale at two years. [1] Subjective patient evaluation shows 87 per cent satisfactory results. However, it is useful to compare this figure with a study by Jensen et al., [4] which showed on computer analysis that 92 per cent of 205 patients who had had autogenous tissue anterior cruciate reconstruction felt their knee was improved after having had surgery. A comparison of patients with Gore-Tex ligaments with a series of patients who had Proplast stents, showed that at one year the Proplast group had 52 per cent satisfactory results and the Gore-Tex group had 80 per cent satisfactory results.

CONTRAINDICATIONS

The use of synthetic material for augmentation or as a true prosthesis is not a panacea for all ligament problems that beset the knee. Patients with poor muscular support, such as a patient with residuals of poliomyelitis are not suitable candidates for reconstructive surgery to stabilize the knee. Muscular support is essential for ligament protection whether it be autogenous or artificial.

Patients with marked degenerative joint disease should be carefully evaluated to determine whether the patient's disability is from instability or the pain of the degenerated joint. Instability may enhance the pain problem, and justification for use of a prosthetic ligament may be present. However, stabilization will not resolve the problem of the degenerated joint, which may continue to cause discomfort with use. In our study of 30 patients with failed knees operated on more than once, in whom a Gore-Tex prosthesis was used, though stability as judged by the Lachman test was improved in 87 per cent, pain at least of a mild degree persisted in 70 per cent of the patients at the one year follow-up. The pain seemed to correlate with the articular changes documented intraoperatively. [1]

Finally, unrealistic expectations are a contraindication for possibly any surgery. This is particularly true with the use of synthetic materials. The notion that 100 per cent satisfactory results are possible with artificial substances, and that their use will absolve the surgeon from the careful surgical techniques that have been developed over the years for cruciate surgery, is a notion that is not only false but will delay the proper investigation and development of newer materials.

SUMMARY

The duplication of the function of the anterior cruciate ligament is one of the most demanding of the clinical applications of synthetic implants. The lack of standard methods for evaluating the biomechanical properties of artificial materials as well as our inability to test biomechanically in vivo our autogenous/synthetic implants, and the difficulty in comparing clinical results because of the subjective interpretation of the patient's history and clinical tests for instability, adds to the problems in assessing the true value of synthetic materials for augmentation of autogenous tissue. Their benefit may be the reduction in time of protective mobilization and a shortened period before return to function. The true prostheses have benefits that are evident in the salvaged knee. The wear properties and the knee's tolerance to their long-time use will determine their ultimate benefit.

REFERENCES

1. Ahlfeld SK, Larson RL, Collins HR. Anterior cruciate reconstruction on the chronically unstable knee using expanded polytetrafluoroethylene (PTFE) prosthetic ligament. Am J Sports Med, 1987; 15:326.
2. Alwyn Smith S. The diagnosis and treatment of injuries to the crucial ligaments. Br J Surg 1918; 6:176.
3. Hey Groves EW. Operation for repair of the crucial ligaments. Lancet 1917; 674:675.
4. Jensen JE, Slocum DB, Larson RL, James SL, Singer KM. Reconstruction procedures for anterior cruciate ligament insufficiency: a computer analysis of clinical results. Am J Sports Med 1983; 11:240.
5. Kellam JF, Larson RL, James SL, Slocum DB, Homsey CA, Woods GW. Proplastic cruciate stents in reconstruction of the unstable knee. Presented at the American Academy of Orthopedic Surgeons 50th Annual Meeting, Anaheim, Calif., 1983.
6. Strum GM, Larson RL. Clinical experience and early results of carbon fiber augmentation of anterior cruciate reconstruction of the knee. Clin Orthop 1985; 196:124:138.

8

CARBON FIBER IN LIGAMENT REINFORCEMENT

DAVID JENKINS, M.B., Ch.B., F.R.C.S., Ch.M

Starting with early experiments on rabbits and sheep, we were able to demonstrate in 1971 that an organized fibroblastic response could be produced in the presence of filamentous carbon fiber. Initial experiments on sheep were performed in which the Achilles tendon was excised and replaced, using a double strand of carbon. This led to an anatomical structure similar to the original being formed. Microscopical examination of samples taken from the newly induced Achilles tendon indicated that there was a very low foreign-body response to the presence of the carbon fiber, but a massive and organized fibroblastic response with new collagen laid down along the lines formed by the individual carbon-fiber filaments.

Our initial use of this material in humans was in 1973, and since that time I have personally placed over 700 carbon implants in humans. The longest follow-up is 13 years. My colleagues and I have found that this material is useful in a number of different applications.

In the acromioclavicular separation, commonly seen in rugby players, it can be used as an alternative to the Bosworth Screw. The technique is to drill a hole through the distal end of the clavicle, and then loop carbon through the hole and under the coracoid, in such a way that the coracoclavicular ligament is reinforced with this material. I normally fix the carbon with a double-drill-hole technique, so this is held in place by friction and finally supported with histo-acryl glue. It has a great advantage in this particular position in that no second operation for removal of an implant is required.

We have similarly used the material to stabilize the distal radial ulnar joints. It has been used around the MP and DIP joints of the hand with less success. The main problem in that position is that the material is superficial and can occasionally erode through the skin. It is therefore not recommended for use in the small joints of the hand.

Carbon-fiber ligaments have been used to stabilize grossly unstable shoulders, normally associated with poliomyelitis. The carbon acts as a capsular plication agent.

The main use of carbon-fiber has been in and around the knee. To date there are over 500 implants in and around the human knee. We have managed to show that it is excellent in the extra-articular situation. That is, when it is used to reinforce the medial or lateral collateral ligaments the results are nearly always good. In the knee we have had less-satisfactory results. In the initial series, the carbon was placed in the knee to replace either the anterior or posterior cruciate ligament, or both. No attempt was made to cover the carbon. We found that considerable carbon staining of the synovium occurred. This led us, in the past 250 internal knee implants, to bury the carbon in the stump of the ligament that has been repaired or reconstituted. This way we have seen no evidence of carbon staining. As an added advantage, we have found that there is less breakage of the carbon in the knee when it is buried in the cruciate stump. The technique used is usually to replace the anterior cruciate first by passing it through a suitable drill hole on the medial aspect of the posterior part of the lateral condyle of the innercondylar notch. This approximates to the midpoint of origin of the anterior cruciate ligament. The carbon is then passed through the stump of the anterior cruciate ligament, to enter the bone at the appropriate point on the tibia, and is then passed through the tibia to come out on the anterior surface. Then, if the collateral ligaments are to be reinforced or replaced, the carbon is turned through a series of drill holes, to match the appropriate origins and insertions of the collateral ligaments. Finally, after skin closure, the leg is immobilized in plaster. The position is normally held at 30 degrees. The plaster cast remains on for six weeks. Following removal, exercises and sports are avoided. Certainly, quadriceps and hamstring drills are considered appropriate, however. At three months after the cast is removed, the patient is encouraged to start gentle jogging, and sports are allowed at eight months.

The other use for carbon fiber around the knee has been to reinforce, and at times replace, either the quadriceps mechanism or the patellar tendon. We have done this in nine patients. The technique is to drill through the patella (or where the patella is missing), through the tibia, and then pass the carbon up into the quadriceps mechanism, rather in the manner of a Bunnel suture. The leg is immobilized in plaster for six weeks, but on this occasion the knee is fully extended.

Lastly, we have found carbon fiber to be a satisfactory material for use around the ankle, particularly in lateral collateral ligament strain. Over 60 such implants have been performed. It is not appropriate to use carbon when there is arthritis present in the ankle. That will simply produce a stable, but still painful, joint. However, it is appropriate to use it for the chronically unstable ankle. The technique is to pass the carbon through a drill hole in the fibula, and then along grooves in the fibular to pass externally to the peroneal tendons; then it is passed through double drill holes in the oscalcis or the talus. Again, the limb is immobilized in plaster, with the foot in a neutral position. The cast remains on for six weeks.

We have considerable enthusiasm for the use of this material in the extra-articular situation, and guarded optimism about its use in the intra-articular placement. There have been no major complications. There is certainly no evidence of carcinogenicity or similar problems. As stated above, this material has been in place in human beings for 13 years and more. There have been occasional breakages and occasional infections, which have led to removal of the carbon, but there has been no single major complication. For this reason we think we can strongly recommend this material for general use.

Around the world there are now 20,000 carbon-fiber implants, and again there have been no reported serious complications following carbon-fiber implantation.

9

PRECLINICAL EVALUATION OF LIGAMENT RECONSTRUCTION WITH AN ABSORBABLE POLYMER-COATED CARBON-FIBER STENT (INTEGRAFT*)

HAROLD ALEXANDER, Ph.D.
JOHN R. PARSONS, Ph.D.
ANDREW B. WEISS, M.D.

INTRODUCTION

Two avenues of research have dominated efforts to replace ligaments. The first is aimed toward the development of an adequately designed, permanent prosthetic replacement. Such a replacement must be constructed of a biocompatible material and it must have sufficient mechanical strength, with some promise of surviving the millions of fatigue cycles associated with normal ligament use.

The second concept utilizes a scaffold replacement approach that encourages the ingrowth of new collagenous tissue. This technique provides only temporary mechanical integrity until the new tissue can assume the mechanical function. Working along these lines, we have found composites of filamentous carbon fiber and absorbable polymers to be useful for this purpose. Ribbonlike composite structures have been utilized in the repair and replacement of ligaments. When used in this way, the composite acts as a scaffold upon which new collagenous tissue can grow.

There may be no other material in the history of orthopedic implants to have been surrounded with such controversy as is carbon fiber. The earliest use of carbon fiber for ligament repair dates to the work of Jenkins et al. [20, 21] in Wales, and Wolter et al. [45] in West Germany in the late 1970s. Since that time, at least 112 papers have been published on this subject. A review of those publications reveals that 87 have reported positively on its use, 13 have published negative reports, and 12 have reported both positive and negative findings.

There are many explanations for the seemingly obvious contradictions on this subject in the literature. However, the overriding explanation is the differences in the materials and devices used by the various investigators. The original work of Jenkins and that of other investigators in the United Kingdom was performed with an extremely brittle fiber that had been coated with a toxic epoxy. Although every effort was made to remove the epoxy, complete removal is impossible. Therefore the negative reports of Dandy et al., [15] Amis et al, [4] and Forster et al. [17] are directly attributable to the use of this uncoated, brittle, potentially toxic

*Integraft is a trademark of Osteonics Biomaterials, Livermore, California.

implant material within the synovial joint. Investigators in West Germany [13, 26–28] have used a woven structure of a different carbon fiber that also had been epoxy-coated. They also tried pyrolytic-carbon coating to improve the tissue response [45]. The fragmentation of the coating resulted in a worse response. They then obtained fiber that had never been epoxy-coated and coated their implant with collagen. This produced a transient foreign-body response, but produced superior long-term results.

Investigators in South Africa have used yet another carbon fiber in a twisted form coated with animal collagen [39, 40]. This material has also been shown to elicit a foreign-body response but provides for adequate tissue ingrowth. Recently, a French group has developed yet another implant of carbon fibers covered with a polyglycolic acid–polylactic acid polymer film [9]. We have drawn upon the successes and the failures of many of these other investigators to produce a carbon-fiber–based ligament repair and reconstruction material that clinical trials have now shown to be a useful addition to the armamentarium of the knee surgeon.

Even though these various carbon-fiber–based implants have some significant differences, a common feature of all has been the demonstration that filamentous carbon implants act as scaffolds for the development of new fibrous tissue. Carbon fiber succeeds as a scaffolding material for a number of reasons. It provides mechanical strength on implantation, allowing early return of function. The material is extremely compatible, permitting the ingrowth of new, aligned fibrous tissue. Finally, the carbon fiber bundles may mechanically degrade as the new tissue matures, allowing for the gradual transfer of load to the regrown tissue structure.

Forster et al. [16] and Jenkins et al. [20, 21] used spun carbon-fiber tows as replacement anterior cruciate ligaments and medial collateral ligaments in sheep. They have since used this raw, uncoated carbon in humans for various ligament reconstructions, [22] including the cruciate ligaments of the knee. Similarly, Wolter et al., [45] Claes et al., [13] and Kinzl et al. [24] used thick braided tows of carbon to replace medial collateral ligaments in sheep and extra-articular knee and ankle ligaments in humans [11]. In the work of these groups, as well as in that reported by Dandy et al. [15] and Rushton et al. [37] for replacing anterior cruciate ligaments, raw carbon fiber was found to partially fragment during and immediately after the operative procedure. This permitted carbon to migrate from the implant site before the new fibrous tissue could encapsulate it. Carbon fragments were found in the lymph nodes of the animals and they are most likely in the nodes of the humans into whom the uncoated carbon was implanted. Although not shown to be detrimental in any way, spread of carbon-fiber fragments to nearby lymph nodes is clearly undesirable.

We report here a program of research in which the problem of the mechanical degradation of the brittle filamentous carbon during its implantation and during the early phases of tissue growth was addressed. This premature mechanical degradation, and the resulting migration of carbon fragments from the implant site, was largely eliminated by utilizing a coating of polylactic acid polymer (PLA) or a copolymer of lactic acid and ε-caprolactone (copolymer). The coated implant has greatly improved handling characteristics when compared with raw carbon fiber. After implantation, the polymer slowly degrades, exposing the fibers to the fibroblast cells. The implant, in a ribbonlike configuration, was used in a variety of animal models. In these studies, the implant material was successful as a scaffold for the development of new soft tissue. The implants allowed early resumption of activity and eventual growth of new structures histologically and mechanically similar to the natural structures.

LIGAMENT REPLACEMENT MATERIAL

Absorbable polymer–filamentous carbon tissue scaffolding ribbons are produced by coating uniaxial filamentous carbon with either PLA or copolymer. The individual carbon-fiber tows typically contain 10,000 fibers, 6 to 10 μm in diameter. The fibers are prepared by pyrolizing a polyacrylonitrile (PAN) fiber tow in an inert atmosphere at approximately 3,000°C. The resulting material is almost pure elemental carbon with mechanical strength and rigidity greater than steel. It has a modulus of over 200 GPa and an ultimate tensile strength of approximately 2.5 GPa.

The polylactic acid polymer is produced from L(−) lactide. This cyclic diester, the lactide of lactic acid, polymerizes by an ionic ring-opening addition mechanism to a high polymer, which can be cast into films, spun into fibers, or extruded into rods similar to the industrial polyesters, such as Dacron. It is a thermoplastic, but can be dissolved readily in a number of solvents. Poly ε-caprolactone alone is similar in character. However, the copolymer of lactic acid and ε-caprolactone is, interestingly, elastomeric in nature. As such, it is tough and flexible.

Fabrication of fiber-coated tows is accomplished by first preparing PLA or copolymer solution. The fibers are coated with the polymer by dipping in solution or spraying. For attachment to soft tissues, suture needles are attached to the ends of the fiber tows. The device is then sterilized by gamma irradiation.

The biocompatibility of carbon fiber, polylactic acid, and polycaprolactone has previously been demonstrated. Finely divided carbon particles have been shown to be well tolerated; they do not cause formation of foreign-body giant cells in the synovial lining of joints, nor do they produce cytotoxic effects [19]. Studies of tissue tolerance of carbon materials by Christel et al. [12] have also indicated that carbon materials are well accepted by connective tissues. Filamentous carbon has been used as a component of implants currently in use in human beings, and studies in rabbits and mice indicate good short- and long-term biocompatibility of this material. The question of foreign-body or physically induced carcinogenicity was addressed in studies using carbon-fiber connective-tissue implants, conducted by Tayton et al. [42] and Claes (personal communication). We also performed a study using 205 Sprague-Dawley rats. The long-term effects of carbon fiber resident in the bone, soft tissue, and vital organs were ascertained. The study lasted for two years, the approximate lifespan of a rat. Gross examination at autopsy and microhistology of organs were largely unremarkable. Tumors were found in both control and experimental animals with similar occurrence rates. The various lesions observed were consistent with the tumor types seen commonly in aging rats. To date, all three research groups have found no abnormal tumor formation attributable to carbon fiber.

The short- and long-term response to polylactic acid has been studied by Cutright et al., [14] Brady et al., [10] and Kulkarni et al [25]. Polylactic acid has been found to be a biocompatible material that elicits little immunologic response, probably because of the absence of peptide linkages. It biodegrades by undergoing hydrolytic de-esterification to lactic acid, a normal metabolic intermediate. The compatibility of poly ϵ-caprolactone has been studied by a number of researchers [33, 36]. The polymer and its degradation product, hydroxycaproic acid, are compatible. Biologic response to and degradation of lactic and caprolactone copolymers have been investigated by Schindler et al [38].

PRECLINICAL EVALUATION

This is a new device produced from new materials without extensive clinical experience. Conse-

TABLE 9–1.
LABORATORY TESTING

Implant mechanical properties
Cell culture–cell-fiber interactions
Carbon-fiber ash weight analysis
Polymer-ash weight analysis
Trace element analysis
Sterilization polymer degradation
Needle attachment strength
Pyrogenicity
Tissue culture cytotoxicity
Quantitative Ames test
Extract cell transformation
Direct contact cell transformation

quently, extensive in vitro and in vivo biocompatibility and bench testing were necessary.

In Vitro Testing

The laboratory testing performed over the eight years during which this device was developed are presented in Table 9–1. The details of much of this in vitro evaluation are beyond the scope of this chapter. However, the cell culture–cell-fiber interactions results are presented to provide an understanding of the basis of the scaffold nature of the device.

Ricci et al. [35] isolated rat tendon fibroblasts from the hind feet of 14-day-old Sprague-Dawley rats. The tendon explants were placed on carbon, Dacron, polyethylene, and Nylon fibers in Dulbecco's modified Eagle's medium containing 10 per cent fetal-calf serum and 1 per cent penicillin–streptomycin. After five to seven days in culture, the cells were fixed and examined by scanning electron microscopy. The orientation of the cells grown on different substrates was controlled by the surface characteristics of the substrate. On smooth substrates, such as the polymer fibers, the cells oriented randomly. On small (7 to 15 μm) striated fibers, such as the carbon fibers used in the ligament implant, the cells aligned parallel to the longitudinal surface striations. Also, cells grown on the striated surfaces lacked the ruffling membrane common to cells grown on smooth surfaces.

Figure 9–1 is a scanning electron micrograph demonstrating the types of cells commonly seen on carbon filaments in this study. Spherical cells are those undergoing cell division. Spindle and sheath cells were seen most often. These cells migrated along the fibers, orienting themselves parallel to the fibers. They appeared to be aggressively attached to the fibers by filopodia-like structures. It is believed that, in vivo, after attaching to the fibers, the cells extrude new collagen parallel to the fibers, producing a new fibrous tissue. This has

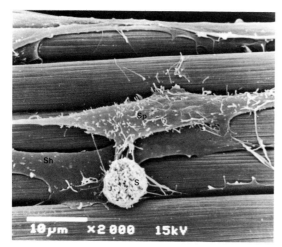

Figure 9–1. Scanning electron micrograph of a neonatal rat-tendon fibroblast cell culture on carbon filaments showing a spherical cell (S), a spindle cell (Sp), and a sheath cell (Sh). (Reprinted, with permission of John Wiley & Sons, Inc., New York, from Ricci et al [35].)

been demonstrated in numerous animal [2, 5] and human [43] specimens.

In Vivo Testing

This device has also been subjected to extensive preclinical animal testing prior to its clinical use. It has been preclinically tested for biocompatibility and in in-use simulation studies in animals. Since the function of ligaments and tendons is to transfer mechanical load, a major evaluation method is to measure the mechanical properties of the replaced structure and compare them with those of the original structure. The implant must also be compatible with the host tissue and not cause excessive adverse tissue response. Therefore histologic evaluation is also of extreme importance. The animal testing performed with this device is listed in Table 9–2. A synopsis of some of the more important animal testing results follows.

TABLE 9–2.
TESTING IN ANIMALS

Systemic injection toxicity
Intracutaneous reactivity
Acute intramuscular tissue toxicity
Long-term rat biocompatibility
C-fiber debris in the synovial joint
Rabbit patellar tendon
Dog patellar tendon
Rabbit Achilles tendon
Dog medial collateral ligament
Dog anterior cruciate ligament
Sheep anterior cruciate ligament

The Effect of Carbon Fiber Debris Within the Synovial Joint

The question of carbon fragmentation and the consequences of the resulting debris residing in the body for long periods remains troublesome. This is particularly true when carbon debris may be released within a synovial joint, as with the repair or replacement of a cruciate ligament. In this environment, there is a concern that carbon-fiber debris may cause direct abrasion of the articular cartilage; or the carbon fragments may be picked up by the synovial lining of the joint. Particulate matter residing in the synovium could potentially produce synovitis. Often, a consequence of synovitis is degradation of the articular cartilage through release of enzymes by the inflamed synovium.

In our study, [31] the consequence of carbon-fiber debris residing within the rabbit knee joint was examined. As a positive control, a well-defined magnesium tetrasilicate (talc) particle–induced synovitis model was used [18].

A dog knee joint with a failed carbon-fiber anterior cruciate ligament was available for histologic study. From examination of the synovium, a carbon fragment size distribution was obtained (range = 10 μm to 80 μm, mean = 50 μm). Carbon fragments having a similar size distribution were produced. Talc particles having a similar distribution were obtained commercially.

In the right knee of 30 white New Zealand rabbits, 0.1 g of sterile carbon particles suspended in 1 cc of saline was injected. In groups of five, these animals were killed at four days, two weeks, four weeks, and eight weeks after injection. Ten animals were killed at 16 weeks after injection. Three additional groups of five rabbits each were treated in a similar fashion. These groups of rabbits, however, received an injection of 0.1 g of talc particles in 1 cc of saline in the right knee. These groups were killed at four days, two weeks, and four weeks.

The medial articular surfaces of the knees of these rabbits were tested mechanically using an indentation technique. The lateral articular surfaces and synovium were examined histologically. No carbon or talc particles were seen to be embedded in the cartilage layer. Instead, most particulate matter appeared to reside in the synovium, particularly in the suprapatellar region and posterior aspects of the knee.

Histologically, all positive controls had talc particles in the synovium. These birefringent particles are easily identified under polarized light. Throughout the study, these particles elicited a strong inflammatory response in the synovial tissue directly adjacent to the particles (Fig. 9–2B) as

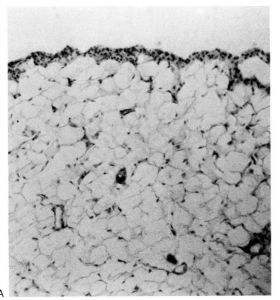

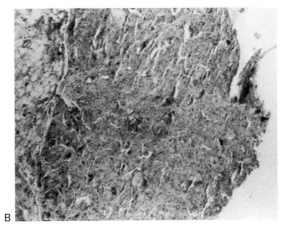

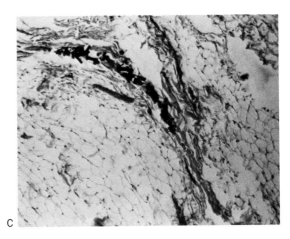

Figure 9–2. Synovial tissues from normal, positive controls (talc) and experimental (carbon) joints were examined histologically. (A) Microscopic examination of normal rabbit synovium revealed a thin layer of synovial cells and underlying fatty tissue (hematoxylin and eosin stain; original magnification, ×100). (B) Talc particles produce an immediate (four days after injection) severe foreign-body reaction, which persists for two to four weeks. By four weeks after injection, the reaction has largely subsided. This micrograph illustrates the severe reaction present two weeks after injection (hematoxylin and eosin stain; original magnification, ×100). (C) Carbon debris produced a foreign-body reaction that was much less severe than that produced by talc. This micrograph illustrates the mild long-term response to carbon debris (16 weeks after injection) (hematoxylin and eosin stain; original magnification, ×100). (Reprinted, with permission, from Parsons et al [31].)

compared with control specimens (Fig. 9–2A). The cartilage from these knees demonstrated some loss of metachromasia at two weeks and four weeks (Fig. 9–3A). This loss of metachromasia (and presumably proteoglycan) was most prevalent near the surface of the cartilage, but varied greatly from animal to animal. Carbon-fiber particles also elicited an inflammatory response from the synovium throughout the study period (Fig. 9–2C). However, the response was relatively mild in comparison to that produced by talc. The cartilage from these joints appeared to be normal (Fig. 9–3B).

At two weeks, the talc-induced synovitis had maximally altered the measured mechanical parameters. At four weeks, the talc synovitis appeared to be resolving and mechanical parameters began to approach normal. Throughout the 16-week study, the cartilage from knees with carbon-fiber debris appeared to be mechanically normal.

Of the parameters measured, none was significantly different ($P < 0.05$) from contralateral controls.

Soft Tissue Attachment—Strength and Ingrowth

The success of this material as a scaffold to replace ligament and tendon deficits depends largely on the development of a rapid, secure soft-tissue filling and anastomosis. Studies were performed that describe the histologic and mechanical characteristics of an anastomosis between an absorbable-polymer–coated carbon-fiber implant and various animal tendon systems. In one study, [5, 29] 54 adult male white New Zealand rabbits were used. The proximal third of the Achilles tendon was removed and replaced by either an absorbable-polymer–coated composite or a control absorbable-polymer–coated Dacron-fiber composite. A 1-cm defect was bridged with one 10,000-fiber implant strand.

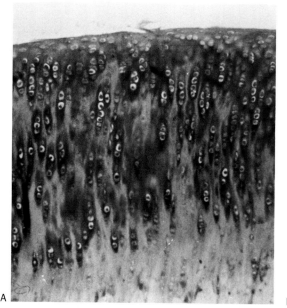
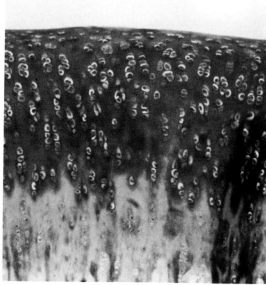

A   B

Figure 9–3. Articular cartilage from knees exposed to talc particulate (positive control) and carbon debris (experimental) were examined histologically. (A) Microscopic examination of articular cartilage from knees exposed to talc revealed a maximal loss of metachromasia, and presumably proteoglycan, two weeks after injection (periodic acid–Schiff–alcian blue; original magnification, ×200). (B) Microscopic examination of articular cartilage from knees receiving injections of carbon particulate revealed normal staining patterns throughout the period of study. This micrograph is from a specimen taken 16 weeks after injection of carbon (periodic acid–Schiff–alcian blue; original magnification, ×200). (Reprinted with permission, from Parsons et al [31].)

At one week, the defect was filled with a space-filling scar. By 12 weeks, it had remodeled into oriented tendonlike tissue. Histologically, at one week, the polymer was still evident and no appreciable ingrowth had occurred. By 12 weeks, significant tissue ingrowth was noted to spread the individual carbon fibers of the implant. The growth was highly cellular. There was minimal foreign-body or inflammatory response present.

Upon mechanical testing, the gastrocnemius mechanisms of the control limbs, which were not operated on, failed in tension by rupture through the belly of the gastrocnemius muscle. The average force of failure was 339 N.

During the early postoperative period (up to two weeks), the gastrocnemius mechanisms with carbon-composite implants failed by pullout of the carbon composite from the proximal soft-tissue anastomosis. At 4 weeks, 8 weeks, and 12 weeks, the carbon composites failed through a mechanism similar to that of the contralateral normal, that is, failure of the gastrocnemius well proximal to the repair site. The Dacron composites at all times were weaker than the repairs receiving carbon-fiber implants. Furthermore, the Dacron composites continued to fail through the area of resection at all times.

The shams always failed by rupture of the paratendinous soft tissue in the region of resected tendon. The mechanical behavior of carbon composites, Dacron composites, and shams are illustrated in Graph 9–1.

In a second study, [2] patellar tendons were removed from adult beagle dogs. They were re-

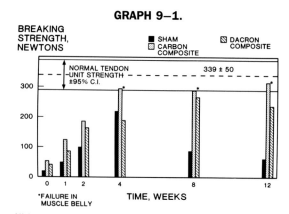

GRAPH 9–1.

Ultimate strength versus time for rabbit Achilles tendon repairs using carbon-fiber–absorbable polymer composites and Dacron-fiber–absorbable polymer composites. The strength of sham procedures (scar) is shown for comparison. C.I. denotes confidence interval. (Reprinted, with permission of Praeger Publishers, New York, from Parsons et al [30].)

placed with absorbable-polymer–coated carbon-fiber implants that were passed through drill holes in the tibia and through the quadriceps tendon above the patella to form a continuous figure-eight repair. Dogs retained for 12 months walked with no discernible limp. Upon mechanical testing, the regrown structures were found to have mechanical properties similar to the contralateral tendons that were not operated on (Graph 9–2).

Scanning electron micrographs of the central tendon region of the patellar tendons regrown about the carbon-PLA scaffold demonstrated extensive ingrowth. A collagen-fiber network similar to that of the corresponding region of a normal patellar tendon was found. The developing collagenous network appeared to grow about the carbon fibers as it would about a naturally occurring collagen-fiber bundle. The normal collagen-fiber bundles of the patellar tendon of the dog were similar in size to the individual fibers.

Ligament Stability

To establish the ability of this device to provide ligament stability, a number of studies were performed. In the first, the medial collateral ligament was chosen for replacement in 32 adult male beagle dogs [6]. After periods of 4 weeks, 8 weeks, 12 weeks, and 26 weeks, the dogs were killed and the regrown medial collateral structures were tested mechanically. Laxity, measured as millimeters of

knee-joint opening in an instrumented valgus stress test, was found to be within the 95 per cent confidence interval of the laxity of the contralateral normal knees by 26 weeks after operation (Graph 9–3).

To evaluate the growth of tissue into the implant within a synovial joint, an anterior cruciate replacement study in dogs was initiated [1]. This study involved eight different experiments in 73 dogs. Various combinations of carbon fiber, polylactic acid polymer, autogenous tissue structures, and fixation methods were investigated. After periods of 4, 8, 12, and 26 weeks, the dogs were killed and the ligament structures were examined grossly and tested mechanically. The mechanical test involved a machine-controlled in vitro anterior drawer test to establish joint laxity, ligament stiffness, and ultimate strength.

In clinical evaluation, almost all of the dogs had minimal anterior drawer signs in their operated legs when compared with their contralateral normal legs. However, upon death, it was found that in many instances this was due to hypertrophy of the medial capsule. This hypertrophy appears to be a natural reaction to anterior cruciate insufficiency in the dog. Gross histologic examination provided extremely variable results. For the early time periods in all experiments (less than eight weeks) and for the later time periods in the fiber-reinforced autogenous-graft experiments, a structurally sound regrown anterior cruciate ligament was noted. However, for later time periods in the non-autogenous-graft experiments, a thin, wispy tissue structure was found.

GRAPH 9–2.

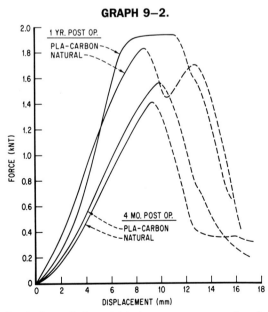

Graph shows the load-extension response comparison for regrown and contralateral natural patellar tendons at 4 and 12 months. (Reprinted, with permission, from Alexander et al [2].)

GRAPH 9–3.

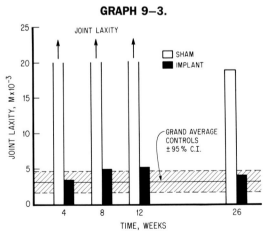

Joint laxity or the "opening" of the joint under low valgus force as a function of postoperative time is illustrated. The "sham" procedure resulted in a lax joint. Use of the carbon-fiber tissue scaffold produced a more stable joint. C.I. denotes confidence interval of the mean. (Reprinted, with permission, from Aragona et al [6].)

Mechanical testing indicated high laxity, low stiffness, and low ultimate strength for the non-autogenous grafts. The reinforced autogenous grafts produced better results. This was particularly true for the primary repairs, for the repairs using the central third of the patellar tendon, and the flexor hallucis longus repairs. However, in the long term these too were only marginally successful with some joint laxity developing and ultimate strengths of 400 to 500 N (compared with 1300 to 1400 N for the contralateral normal legs).

This poor result with the dog model has also been demonstrated by Bejui et al. [8] and Barclay and Barclay [7]. Consequently, another study was performed using a sheep anterior cruciate model. A $\frac{1}{2}$-cm-long section of the anterior cruciate ligament (ACL), near its distal attachment, was removed from 12 skeletally mature, adult female Rambioulette sheep. In an attempt to avoid the need for including autogenous tissue along with the implant in the joint, a bovine collagen sponge-coated absorbable copolymer carbon-fiber ligament prosthesis was used. It was passed through an arthrotomy over the top of the condyle, into the intercondylar notch lateral to the posterior cruciate ligament (PCL), and then through a tibial drill hole. The prosthesis was secured proximally by weaving the implant in and around the biceps musculotendinous junction and overlying fascia. The implant was then secured distally to the tibia with a carbon-PLA fastener. Postoperatively, no form of immobilization was used. Care was taken to ensure that all intra-articular portions of the prostheses remained coated with the bovine collagen. The animals were killed at 3, 6, and 12 months. Specimens were retrieved from the proximal soft-tissue attachment, intra-articular region, tibial bony attachment, popliteal and inguinal lymph nodes bilaterally, and the synovium. For mechanical testing, the femur and tibia were mounted and held at 90 degrees of flexion. Four separate mechanical tests were performed: anterior and posterior drawer signs with all knee structures intact, just the PCL and reconstructed ACL intact, and finally just the reconstructed ACL intact. The fourth test was a test to failure of the reconstructed ACL. Contralateral knees were used as controls.

The sequential maturation of the carbon–host tissue responses in various areas of the knee was followed histologically. At the attachment of the carbon fiber to the biceps muscle and fascia, a clear pattern could be seen upon reviewing the 3-month, 6-month, and 12-month histology. At 3 months, the cross-sections revealed each carbon fiber surrounded by a cylinder of concentrically arranged spindle-shaped cells with flattened nuclei forming separate islands. Between the islands were

TABLE 9–3. MECHANICAL TEST RESULTS

	3 Months	6 Months	12 Months
Drawer at 50 N	5.4 mm	10.6 mm	3.2 mm
Failure force	220 N	135 N	610 N

Normal values: $n = 8$, drawer 2.4 ± 1.0, failure 810 ± 220.

septa of fibroblast-type cells and collagen. The longitudinal cuts at 3 months revealed linearly arranged fibroblasts and occasional giant cells. By 6 months, the linear pattern on the longitudinal cuts was thicker and less cellular. The cross-sections revealed carbon fibers well separated by fibrous ingrowth. By 12 months, the density of the connective component had increased further. The cells now had indistinct nonapparent cell borders and resembled a more mature collagen arrangement.

The intra-articular carbon fiber was coated with a white-gray fibrous tissue reaction. By 3 months, this fibrous reaction had permeated partially into the carbon strand such that the most inner portion of the carbon remained less cellular. At 6 months, the fibroblastic response was more uniformly distributed throughout the carbon forming a carbon–host unit several times thicker than the initial carbon. Some giant cells were present. By 12 months, the areas in between the carbon strands consisted of a more mature collagen arrangement with less nuclei present and indistinct cell bodies, similar to the proximal muscle specimens. Of all of the knees examined, there was only one case of apparent release of carbon within the synovium. There was envelopment of the carbon by the synovial membrane with no giant-cell response. There was no carbon found in any of inguinal or popliteal lymph nodes at 3 months, 6 months, or 12 months (including the case with intrasynovial carbon particles). Table 9–3 compares the mechanical test results for anterior drawer signs and ultimate properties with the contralateral normal controls. Both the amount of drawer and the ultimate strength at 3 and 6 months were inferior to the controls, but by 12 months the values for the reconstructed ACL approached that of the control knees.

CLINICAL TESTING

The implant in clinical use is a double-armed uniaxial tow of 10,000 fibers coated with a copolymer of lactic acid and ϵ-caprolactone. It is 1 m long, 0.5 cm wide, and has a ultimate tensile strength of approximately 425 N. The system had been used initially with soft-tissue attachment

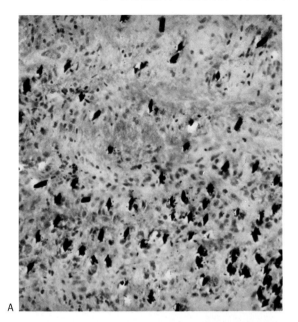

A

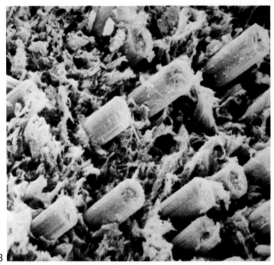

B

Figure 9–4. Light (A) and scanning electron (B) micrographs showing collagenous ingrowth around the carbon fibers in a reconstructed anterior cruciate ligament at 18 months postoperatively. (A, ×100; B, ×1000) (Reprinted, with permission, from Weiss et al [43].)

TABLE 9–5. PERCENT TYPE III COLLAGEN IN VARIOUS TISSUES

Tissue	% Type III Collagen
Skin	24
Joint capsule	51
Healing ACL	44
Joint capsule with carbon	40
Carbon-fiber ACL repair	42
Normal ACL	25
Carbon-fiber MCL repair	52
Normal MCL	11

only, using the locking-weave anastomosis shown in the animal studies. More recently, bone attachment has been accomplished through the use of a newly designed composite material attachment device (expandable fastener).

The most recent compilation of clinical results is presented in Chapter 11. However, in an earlier report, [43] the results from 82 patients treated over a 27-month period for both acute (8 per cent) and chronic (92 per cent) knee-ligament instabilities were presented. Preoperative and postoperative evaluation, consisting of questionnaires, physical examination, and isokinetic testing, revealed significant improvements in categories of stability, pain, function, and strength. Arthroscopic examination and histologic studies of retrieved specimens demonstrated well-vascularized reconstructions of the anterior cruciate ligament with collagenous tissue ingrowth into the carbon–copolymer implants.

The histologic appearance of the regrown tissue was previously presented by Weiss et al [43]. Both light and electron microscopy demonstrated collagenous ingrowth surrounding the carbon fibers used to reconstruct the anterior cruciate ligament (Fig. 9–4). Various samples were enzymatically degraded with pepsin and interrupted gel electrophoresis was performed to characterize the types of collagen present (Table 9–5). The collagenous ingrowth was composed of types I and III collagen in similar proportions to that found in normal healing ligamentous tissue.

Early reports from other clinical centers indicated early results either as good [34, 41, 44] or better than previously used repairs [23]. King and Bulstrode [23] reported that free carbon fibers had been spread in the joint as a result of using a technically incorrect implantation procedure. However, there did not appear to be any clinically deleterious consequences of this fiber spread, corroborating the results of the animal study reported by Parsons et al [31]. Witvoet and Christel, [44] performing a combined reconstruction of the ACL and collateral structures, reported that the use of the implant allowed an earlier return to normal activity than would have been possible with a standard autogenous tissue repair.

DISCUSSION

This series of animal experiments suggests that carbon fiber–absorbable polymer composites are useful in soft-tissue repair. Fibrous tissue ingrowth appears to be consistent with some organization of the tissue evident as early as four weeks. Complete envelopment of the implant by aligned collagen fibers has been noted at eight weeks in animal studies. Bone ingrowth around the carbon fibers in the drill holes in beagle tibias (patellar tendon study) was also evident. However, this process is clearly much slower than soft-tissue ingrowth, requiring upwards of one year. Within the synovial joint, protection of the carbon fiber with autogenous tissue appears to be necessary to counteract the slower growth rates in this environment.

Carbon-fiber composite clinical implants have, to date, demonstrated ingrowth potential similar to that seen in the animal studies. The implant has high strength and reasonable flexibility when woven into soft tissue. It is highly biocompatible and encourages rapid tissue ingrowth. The absorbable polymer coating appears to delay the fragmentation of the fibers, thereby preventing migration. It is anticipated that this new material will soon be a useful addition to the surgeon's armamentarium for the treatment of unstable joints and tendon injuries.

Acknowledgments

This work has spanned an eight-year period and has benefited from the contributions of many individuals. Amos Gona, Ophelia Gona, and Irving Strauchler contributed to much of the early planning of these experiments. Research residents Stephen Corcoran, James Aragona, Richard Fong, Albert Mylod, Richard Rosa, Leigh Ende, Anthony Rosario, Marie Hatam, Teresa Vega, and Andrew Goldstein attended to much of the day-to-day experimental details. Helen Chen and Irene Collins did all of the tissue histology. Robert Ainsworth and Kenneth St. John of Osteonics Biomaterials (formerly Hexcel Medical) prepared the implants.

This project has been funded by the generous support of the William Lightfoot Schultz Foundation through the Foundation of the University of Medicine and Dentistry of New Jersey and the Hexcel Corporation.

REFERENCES

1. Alexander H, Parsons JR, Smith G, Fong R, Mylod A, Weiss AB. Anterior cruciate ligament replacement with filamentous carbon. Trans Orthop Res Soc 1982; 7:45.
2. Alexander H, Parsons JR, Strauchler ID, Corcoran SF, Gona O, Mayott CW. Canine patellar tendon replacement with a polylactic acid polymer-filamentous carbon tissue scaffold. Orthop Rev 1981; 10:41–51.
3. Alexander H, Weiss AB, Parsons JR. Absorbable polymer-filamentous carbon composites—a new class of tissue scaffolding materials. In: Burri C, Claes L, eds. Aktuelle Probleme im Chirurgie und Orthopaedie, Bern: Hans Huber, 1983:83–97.
4. Amis AA, Campbell JR, Kempson SA, Miller JH. Comparison of the structure of neotendons induced by implantation of carbon or polyester fibres. J Bone Joint Surg (Br) 1984; 66:131–139.
5. Aragona J, Parsons JR, Alexander H, Weiss AB. Soft tissue attachment of a filamentous carbon-absorbable polymer tendon and ligament replacement. Clin. Orthop Relat Res 1981; 160:268–278.
6. *Idem*. Medial collateral ligament replacement with a partially absorbable tissue scaffold. Am J Sports Med 1983; 11:228–233.
7. Barclay SM, Barclay WP. Filamentous carbon fiber prosthesis for cranial cruciate ligament replacement in the dog—a pilot study. Cornell Vet 1984; 74:3–7.
8. Bejui J, Vignon E, Hartman D, Bejui-Thivolet F. Intra-articular changes related to carbon fiber reconstruction of the anterior cruciate ligament. Trans World Biomater Congr 1984; 2:270.
9. Bercovy M, Goutallier D, Voisin MC. et al. Carbon-PGLA prosthesis for ligament reconstruction. Clin Orthop Relat Res 1985; 196:159–168.
10. Brady JM, Cutright DE, Miller RA, Battistone GC, Hunsuck EE. Resorption rate route elimination and ultrastructure of the implant site of polylactic acid in the abdominal wall of the rat. J Biomed Mater Res 1973; 7:155–166.
11. Burri C, Henkemeyer H, Neugebauer R. Techniques and results of alloplastic carbon fiber ligament substitution. In: Burri C, Claes L, eds. Aktuelle Problems im Chirurgie und Orthopaedie. Bern: Hans Huber, 1983:146–159.
12. Christel P, Buttazzoni B, Leray JL, Moris C. Tissue tolerance of carbon materials. Trans World Biomater Congr 1980; 1:4, 7, 9.
13. Claes L, Wolter D, Gistinger G, Rose P, Huttner W, Fitzer E. Physical and biological aspects of carbon fibres in the ligament prosthesis. Presented at the Third World Congress on Mechanical Properties of Biomaterials, 1978, Keele University.
14. Cutright DE, Hunsuck EE. Tissue reactions to the biodegradable polylactic acid suture. Oral Surg 1971; 31:134–139.
15. Dandy DJ, Flanagan JP, Steenmeyer V. Arthroscopy and the management of the ruptured anterior cruciate ligament. Clin Orthop Relat Res 1982; 167:43–49.
16. Forster I, Ralis ZA, McKibbin B, Jenkins DHR. Biological reaction to carbon fibre implants. Clin Orthop Relat Res 1978; 131:229–307.
17. Forster IW, Shuttleworth A. Tissue reaction to intra-articular carbon fibre implants in the knee. J Bone Joint Surg (Br) 1984; 66:282.
18. Gershuni DH, Kuei SC, Woo SL-Y, Thibodeaux JI, Akeson WH. Articular cartilage deformation following experimental synovitis in the rabbit hip. Trans Orthop Res Soc 1980; 5:3.
19. Haubold A. Carbon in prosthetics. Ann NY Acad Sci 1977; 283:383–395.
20. Jenkins DHR, The repair of cruciate liagments with flexible carbon fibre. J Bone Joint Surg (Br) 1978; 60:520–522.
21. Jenkins DHR, Forester IW, McKibbins B, Ralis ZA. Induction of tendon and ligament formation by carbon implants. J Bone Joint Surg (Br) 1977; 58:53–57.
22. Jenkins DHR, McKibbin B. The role of flexible carbon fibre implants as tendon and ligament substitutes in clinical practice—a preliminary report. J Bone Joint Surg (Br) 1980; 62:497–499.
23. King JB, Bulstrode C. Polylactate-coated carbon fiber in extra articular reconstruction of the unstable knee. Clin Orthop Relat Res 1985; 196:139–142.

24. Kinzl L, Wolter D, Claes L. Aspects of coated carbon fibres in the ligament prosthesis. Trans Soc Biomater 1979; 3:71.
25. Kulkarni RK, Moore EG, Hegyeli AF, Leonard F. Polylactic acid for surgical implants. Arch Surg 1966; 93:839–843.
26. Neugebauer R, Burri C, Claes L, Helbing G. The trap door: a possibility of fixation of carbon fibre strands into cancellous bone. Trans World Biomater Congr 1980; 1:4, 7, 5.
27. *Idem.* The anchorage of carbon fibre strands into bone: a biomechanical and biological evaluation on knee joints. Trans Eur Soc Biomater 1979; 2:64.
28. Neugebauer R, Burri C, Claes L, Helbing G, Wolter D. The replacement of the abdominal wall by a carbon-cloth in rabbits. Trans Soc Biometer 1979; 3:135.
29. Parsons JR, Alexander H, Ende LS, Weiss AB. Fiber reinforced absorbable polymer tissue scaffolds: a comparison of carbon fiber and dacron fiber systems. Trans Orthop Res Soc 1983; 8:86.
30. Parsons JR, Alexander H, Weiss AB. Soft tissue repair and replacement with carbon fiber-absorbable polymer composites. In: Hunt TK, Heppenstall RB, Pines E, Rovee D, eds. Soft and hard tissue repair: biological and clinical aspects. New York: Praeger, 1984; 417–452.
31. Parsons JR, Bhayani S, Alexander H, Weiss AB. Carbon fiber debris within the synovial joint—a time-dependent mechanical and histologic study. Clin Orthop Relat Res 1985; 196:69–76.
32. Parsons JR, Rosario A, Weiss AB, Alexander H. Achilles tendon repair with an absorbable polymer-carbon fiber composite. Foot Ankle 1984; 5:49–53.
33. Pitt CG, Gratzlk MM, Kimmel GL, Surles J, Schindler A. The degradation of poly (DL-lactide) poly (E-Caprapectone) and their copolymers M-V in vivo. Biomaterials 1981; 2:215.
34. Post M. Rotator cuff repair with carbon filament—a preliminary report of five cases. Clin Orthop Relat Res 1985; 196:154–158.
35. Ricci JL, Gona AG, Alexander H, Parsons JR. Morphological characteristics of tendon cells cultured on synthetic fibers. J Biomed Mater Res 1984; 18:1073–1087.
36. Rice RM, Hegyeli AF, Gourlay SK, et al. Biocompatibility testing of polymers: in vitro studies with in vivo correlation. J Biomed Mater Res 1978; 12:43–54.
37. Rushton N, Dandy DJ, Naylor CPE. The clinical, arthroscopic and histological findings after replacement of the anterior cruciate ligament with carbon fibre. J Bone Joint Surg (Br) 1983; 65:308–309.
38. Schindler A, Jeffcoat R, Kimmel GL, Pitt GG, Wall ME, Zweidinger R. Biodegradable polymers for sustained drug delivery. In: Pearce E, Schaefgen J, eds. Contemporary topics in polymer science. New York: Plenum Press, 1977:II:251–289.
39. Strover AE. Technical advances in the reconstruction of knee ligaments using carbon fiber. In: Burri C, Claes L, eds. Aktuelle Problems im Chirurgie und Orthopaedie. Bern: Hans Huber, 1983:127–134.
40. Strover AE, Firer P. The use of carbon fiber implants in anterior cruciate ligament surgery. Clin Orthop Relat Res 1985; 196:86–98.
41. Strum GM, Larson RL. Clinical experience and early results of carbon fiber augmentation of anterior cruciate reconstruction of the knee. Clin Orthop Relat Res 1985; 196:124–138.
42. Tayton K, Phillips G, Ralis ZA. Long term effects of carbon fiber on soft tissue. J Bone Joint Surg (Br) 1982; 64:112–114.
43. Weiss AB, Blazina ME, Goldstein AR, Alexander H. Ligament replacement with an absorbable copolymer carbon fiber scaffold—early clinical experience. Clin Orthop Relat Res 1985; 196:77–85.
44. Witvoet J, Christel P. Treatment of chronic anterior knee instabilities with combined intra and extra-articular transfer augmented with carbon-PLA fibers. Clin Orthop Relat Res 1985; 196:143–153.
45. Wolter D, Fitzer E, Helbine G, Goldaway J. Ligament replacement in the knee joints with carbon fibers coated with pyrolitic carbon. Trans Soc Biomater 1977; 1:126.

10

INTEGRAFT* ANTERIOR CRUCIATE LIGAMENT RECONSTRUCTION

ROY M. RUSCH, M.D.

BACKGROUND HISTORY

In 1977, Jenkins [17] reported that filamentous carbon showed promise as an orthopedic implant material when used to augment repairs of ligaments and tendons. Jenkins and his coworkers [11, 16–18] demonstrated first in animals and then in clinical applications that filamentous carbon fibers, when woven into soft tissue, provided a scaffold for collagen-forming fibroblasts and formed a neotendon that could physically replace ruptured or lax soft tissue to support the joint. The biocompatibility and effectiveness of the carbon were established [9, 10, 15–25, 27–30]; however, the usefulness of this device was restricted because of fragmentation of the uncoated carbon during surgical implantation. [1–6, 10, 12, 13, 31]

Similarly, Wolter, et al., [31] Claes et al. [10] and Kinzel et al. [19] used thick braided tows of carbon to replace medial collateral ligaments in animals and extra-articular knee and ankle ligaments in human beings. In these studies, the carbon fiber was found to fragment and migrate from the implant site before the new fibrous tissue encapsulated it. Carbon fragments were found in the lymph nodes of the animals in whom uncoated carbon had been implanted. Bercovy et al. [7] and Goutallier et al. [14] showed that uncoated carbon fibers fragmented and migrated to the lymph nodes

in animals but that coating with a polymer prevented this fragmentation.

The research team at the University of Medicine and Dentistry of New Jersey developed a filamentous carbon-fiber implant coated with a biodegradable polymer; this protected the carbon from fragmentation and migration during and after surgical implantation. This biodegradable coating holds the carbon filaments together, preventing fragmentation of the device while weaving through tissue or passing through the joint. Once in the tissue, the polymer degrades and breaks down to lactic acid and ϵ-hydroxycaproic acid, which are metabolized through the body's normal metabolic pathways.

This new device retained the excellent features of biocompatibility and the induction of new tissue structures, which had been reported by previous researchers. [1, 6, 12, 29, 30] It also greatly improved the usefulness of the implant, as a result of minimal fragmentation during handling.

Poly L-lactic acid was originally used to coat the carbon fibers, but proved to be too stiff, and reduced flexibility when passing through tissues such as ligaments and tendons. The researchers at Hexcel Corporation developed a copolymer of lactic acid and ϵ-caprolactone, providing the same protective qualities with vastly improved product-handling characteristics. Animal experiments showed there to be no functional difference between these two polymers, [26] and this copolymer has been used to coat the majority of the products used in the clinical evaluation studies.

---

*Integraft is a trademark of Osteonics Biomaterials, Livermore, California.

52

PRODUCT DESIGN

The Integraft stent is a ribbonlike high-tensile-strength device approximately 1 m long and 5 mm wide, which is fabricated from a tow composed of about 10,000 individual filaments of pure carbon, each about 7 to 8 μm in diameter. A bioabsorbable copolymer of lactic acid and ϵ-caprolactone coats the fibers and the device is supplied with a variety of needle sizes and configurations attached at each end (Fig. 10–1). These different needle designs allow the product to be used for a variety of repairs in multiple sites around the body.

Each tow of the carbon fiber (10,000 filaments) has an ultimate tensile strength of approximately 425 N. It has been documented by Butler et al. [8] that the strength of a young, healthy anterior cruciate ligament (ACL) is approximately 1725 N; therefore four passes of the Integraft carbon fiber stent needs to be woven through the autogenous graft to approximate the natural ACL. One stent can be used to make multiple passes through the tissue. In addition, where there is insufficient tissue length, the stent can compensate.

The Integraft stent is designed to act as a temporary tissue scaffold. The polymer coating protects the somewhat fragile filaments during handling and surgical implantation, and as the polymer is absorbed by the body, new fibrous tissues align along the fibers and form collagen, which gradually assumes the support function.

The Integraft carbon fiber stent is extremely versatile. The surgeon may vary the strength by weaving multiple passes of the carbon fiber into weaker autogenous graft transfers to yield strength equivalent to the tissue it will be replacing.

The Integraft fastener is recommended for use in conjunction with the Integraft stent when fixation to bone is necessary. The fastener is made of car-

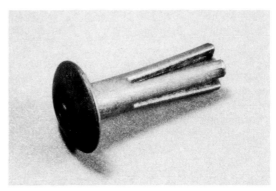

Figure 10–2. Integraft™ fastener

bon fibers that have been chopped, blended with a polymer of lactic acid and formed into a shape similar to an expandable rivet, and is partially absorbable (Fig. 10–2). This combination of materials is designed to provide a compatible attachment device with the Integraft stent.

PRECLINICAL TESTING

In vitro laboratory testing and numerous tests in animals were performed to demonstrate sufficient mechanical strength and biocompatibility of both the Integraft stent and Integraft fastener. Various tests were also performed to establish the noncarcinogenic nature of the material used to produce these devices and included tests to assess the potential of carbon particles, if engulfed by cells, to induce chromosome damage or cellular mutation. These tests, many of which have been described in Chapter 9, also demonstrated the function of the stent as a scaffold, to encourage ingrowth and organized alignment of tissue in the repair of ligament and tendons in a number of anatomic sites. The results obtained from the preclinical testing supported the decision to proceed with controlled clinical testing in human beings.

CLINICAL STUDY

In April 1981, the first human implantation of the Integraft ligament was performed by Dr. Andrew B. Weiss and Dr. Martin Blazina. Phase I of the program was conducted on patients who were severely disabled and whose surgical alternative would be joint fusion, or where conventional treatment would have a small probability of success and the patient may require joint replacement. These repairs took place at the University of Medicine and Dentistry of New Jersey, Newark, N.J.;

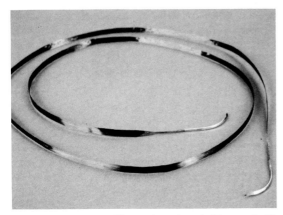

Figure 10–1. Integraft™ stent shown here double-armed with small curved needles

the University of Texas Health Science Center, Dallas; and the Sherman Oaks Community Hospital, Sherman Oaks, Calif.

A second phase of the study was begun in February 1982, in which 240 patients were treated for acute and chronic injuries of the connective tissues of the knee and ankle. For this series the number of clinical centers around the country increased to 12.

For the current phase (Phase III) of the clinical evaluation study, the number of centers increased to 25. These surgeries were performed by 64 surgeons, and included all sites where repairs of ligaments and tendons were indicated.

To date, over 1100 patients have received the Integraft stent system for procedures in and around the knee, ankle, hip, shoulder, elbow, and hand. The results will be reported for only those patients with chronic repairs of the anterior cruciate ligament.

SURGICAL TECHNIQUE

The versatility of the Integraft stent system is such that it can be used to augment any soft-tissue substitutions to repair the ACL-deficient ligament. Four passes of the stent through the autogenous tissue will give the initial strength necessary to compensate for the applied loads during the healing and regeneration stages of the repair process. In the clinical study, a large number of the reconstructions are chronic cases where previous attempts to repair deficient ACLs using the patients own tissue had failed. The ability to provide the necessary tensile strength to any tissue by adding the carbon allowed the surgeon to select an alternative autogenous tissue that alone did not have the mechanical properties necessary for a successful repair.

Reconstructions of the ACL were performed in the majority of cases by augmenting the iliotibial band or central third of the patellar tendon with the Integraft carbon-fiber stent. In all cases, it was recommended that four passes of a carbon stent be made across the joint to provide adequate mechanical properties in the resulting composite graft, and that the carbon be completely buried in tissue. Depending upon the degree of deformity and soft-tissue damage, medial and lateral collateral ligaments were also augmented.

Iliotibial Band

Two techniques that incorporated the iliotibial band were used. In the first technique the anterior two thirds of the iliotibial band is elevated as a fascial strip in a distal-to-proximal direction with the flap remaining attached proximally. A small bone-block 10 mm wide and 15 mm long is removed from Gerdy's tubercle distally and somewhat wider at its proximal attachment. The bone-block is then split longitudinally so that the cancellous surfaces are facing outward. Four passes of the carbon-fiber stent with straight-needle configuration are woven through the fascial strip in a proximal-to-distal direction. The carbon tow is initially drawn through the iliotibial band and underlying the vastus lateralis approximately 2 to 3 cm proximal to the attachment of the flap and brought through the tissue to its midpoint so that half the tow length is exposed on either side. Both ends of the carbon stent are then woven through the fascial strip proximally to distally. The carbon strands should exit the flap on the fascial attachment side of the bone-block, thereby avoiding the cancellous surface of the elevated bone. A second carbon stent is then woven in an identical manner such that there will be four carbon-stent ends exiting distally.

The fascial strip with the interwoven carbon stents is then converted to a tube by folding it longitudinally and suturing the edges together using interrupted nonabsorbable sutures. The bone-block is trimmed to size so that it will pass through a $\frac{3}{8}$-in. (9.5-mm) drill hole. Using a drill guide, a $\frac{3}{8}$-in. (9.5-mm) hole is drilled from a point 1 in. (2.5 cm) distal to the tibial condylar surface into the knee joint to exit just medially and anteriorly to the tibial attachment of the deficient ACL.

The entire implant complex is then passed through the posterior capsule, through the intercondylar notch in a posterior-to-anterior direction using the over-the-top method. The bone-block should be below the level of the tibial plateau within the tibial bone with the four ends of carbon stent exiting through the tibial hole. These are then wrapped around an Integraft carbon-composite fastener placed 1 in. (2.5 cm) distal to the exit hole and with the composite graft pulled tight (the knee in 30 degrees of flexion) the fastener and central pin is at full impact.

In the second technique, commencing at Gerdy's tubercle a 2 cm wide segment of iliotibial band is carefully cut and then extended proximally, widening progressively to achieve a width of 4 cm. A longitudinal or transverse incision is made in the thigh approximately 20 to 22 cm from Gerdy's tubercle and the iliotibial band is cut transversely in that area. The graft is then passed deep to the lateral collateral ligament, maintaining proximity to the femoral attachment as described by MacIntosh. [20] Four passes of the carbon stent are then woven through the posterior third of iliotibial band beginning distally and exiting proximally. The combination is then rolled in such a manner as to enclose fully the carbon fibers and is stitched with absorbable sutures to maintain this form.

Using a drill guide, holes are placed isometrically in the femur and tibia to accept the composite carbon and iliotibial-band graft. After passing the graft through the femoral hole and the joint, exiting from the tibial hole, it is anchored to the tibia using the Integraft fastener, pulling the graft tight with the knee in 30 degrees of flexion. This technique is described more fully in Chapter 12.

Central Third of Patellar Tendon

A 1-cm-wide strip of patellar tendon is harvested, complete with a bone-block at each end. Four passes of carbon stent are woven longitudinally into the graft using the curved-needle configuration, taking care that no carbon is exposed to the outer surfaces. Total encapsulation of the carbon fibers by ligament tissue is ensured by stitching the edges of the tendon graft with absorbable sutures, creating a tubed ligament composite graft. No. 1 nonabsorbable sutures are placed through the bone-blocks to assist in passing the graft through the joint without placing undue tension on the carbon stent as well as retaining the graft under proper tension during final placement.

Using a drill guide, holes are placed isometrically in the femur and tibia, the graft placed through the joint and the excess strands of carbon stent exiting from the femoral and tibial holes. The Integraft composite fastener is used to anchor the graft. The femoral side is attached first and the tibial side secured while the graft is tightened with the knee in 30 degrees of flexion. This technique is described more fully in Chapter 12.

PATIENT DEMOGRAPHICS

The Integraft stent system has been used to repair ACL-deficient knees in 440 patients. Of these, 155 chronic repairs have been followed for two years and are reported on here (Fig. 10–3). Of these ACL chronic patients, 108 (70 per cent) were male, 93 patients (59 per cent) were between 21 and 30 years of age, and 145 (93 per cent) were under the age of 40. As can be expected for this younger group, 94 patients (61 per cent) were operated on as a result of a sports-related injury. Motor-vehicle accidents accounted for 21 patients (14 per cent) with 18 (12 per cent) occurring as a p167result of the patients' occupations. Of these patients, 101 (65 per cent) had at least one previous surgery, with 16 (10 per cent) having had three or more surgeries. The repairs were equally divided between right and left legs.

Cause of Injury	Frequency	Percent
Job related	18	11.8
Sports	94	61.4
Vehicular	21	13.7
Other	20	13.1
Prior Surgeries		
0	54	34.8
1	70	45.2
2	15	9.7
3	5	3.2
4	6	3.9
5+	5	3.2
Age (yr)		
15–20	25	16.1
21–30	92	59.4
31–40	28	18.1
41–50	7	4.5
51 +	3	1.9
Sex		
Male	46	29.9
Female	108	70.1
Side		
Left	76	49.0
Right	79	51.0

Figure 10–3. Patient demographics for multicenter study

RESULTS

Results were assessed for the 155 chronic ACL patients at two years by using two methods: the composite scoring system and objective knee tests.

Composite Scoring System

A composite scoring system was used to assess levels of activity according to pain, function (gait, walking, running), stability, and, because of the initial injury, ability to return to sports (Fig. 10–4). Data forms were completed preoperatively and at intervals of 3, 6, 9, 12, 18, 24, and 36 months postoperatively. Assessment of the baseline improvement from the preoperative score to that at 24 months was recorded for each of the parameters.

For pain (where a maximum score of 5.0 represented no pain) the score increased from a preoperative average of 2.46 to an average score of 4.06 (Graph 10–1) at 24 months.

In the function category (Graph 10–2), gait average scoring (maximum score, 3.0) improved from 1.79 to a 24-month score of 2.72, walking ability from 1.57 to 2.73, and running from 0.8 to 2.17.

The ability to return to sports was very important in view of the percentage of sports-related injuries. In this category, the scoring improved from 0.67 to 3.18 (Graph 10–3). The average stability rating preoperatively was 1.92 and increased to 10.05 at 24 months.

Pain (5 points possible)

No pain during running, stair climbing, or
sports activities 5

Occasional ache; no compromise of activities 4

Mild pain following excessive activities; may
take aspirin 3

Moderate pain with normal activities; may
require pain medicine stronger than aspirin
after excessive or unusual activities that
cause considerable pain 2

Severe pain, but able to walk. Serious
limitation of activities; may need
prolonged medicine stronger than aspirin. 1

Totaly disabled with pain; unable to ambulate 0

Function (9 points possible)

Gait (3 points possible)

No limp 3
Mild to moderate limp 2
Severe limp 1

Walking (3 points possible)

Unlimited range 3
Able to walk one-half mile 2
Indoors only; unable to walk without discomfort 1

Running (3 points possible)

Can run one-fourth mile 3
Can run less than one-fourth mile 2
Unable to run without instability 1

Sport (5 points possible)

Can be active in sports involving "cutting
movements" 5
Can be active in sports not involving "cutting" 3
Unable to participate in sports without
instability 0

Stability (15 points possible) (cruciate ligament laxity)

Negative drawer (no displacement) . . . (0) 15
Mild drawer sign <5 mm (mild
displacement) . . . .(1+). 9
Moderate drawer sign 5 to 10 mm . . . .(2+). 6
Severe drawer sign >10 mm . . . .(3+). 0

Figure 10–4. Rating scale of the composite scoring system

Using this composite scoring system with patient ratings based on percentage improvement
from their preoperative score, the average for all
24-month chronic ACL patients increased from
9.28 to 24.77 at 24 months (Graph 10–4). Eighty-
eight per cent were rated excellent and good 24

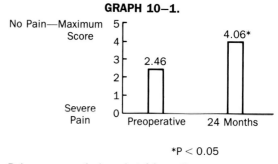

GRAPH 10–1.

*P < 0.05

Pain—preoperatively and at 24 months

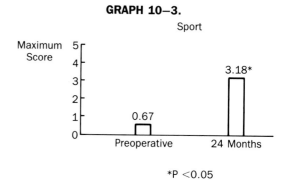

GRAPH 10–3.

*P <0.05

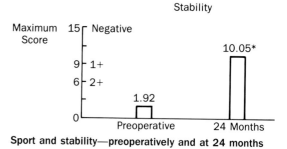

Sport and stability—preoperatively and at 24 months

months postoperatively (Table 10–1). In all of
these composite scoring system categories the increases were statistically significant (P < 0.05).

Objective Knee Tests

Objective knee tests were performed on each
patient at 24 months postoperatively.

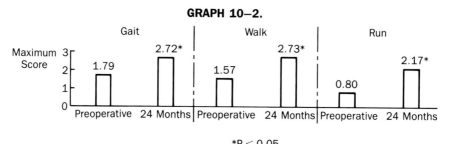

GRAPH 10–2.

*P < 0.05

Function—preoperatively and at 24 months

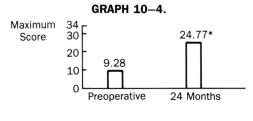

GRAPH 10–4.

*P < 0.05

Average composite score—preoperatively and at 24 months

Lachman Test

For the Lachman test, an anterior drawer test performed with the knee in approximately 25 degrees of flexion, the anterior translation of the tibia with respect to the femur, was graded from 0 to 3. Physiologic laxity was graded as 0, 5 mm or less of measured laxity was graded as 1, 6 mm to 10 mm was graded as 2, and 11 mm or greater of measured laxity was graded as 3.

Preoperatively, 10 per cent of the patients exhibited a Lachman score of 0 to 1+ with 69 per cent at 3+. At 24 months 88 per cent were at 0 to 1+ and only 6 per cent had a 3+ condition.

Pivot-Shift Test

Anterolateral rotary instability was assessed by performing the pivot-shift test (where the knee is brought from flexion into extension) and, if positive, a "jump" is noticed at approximately 30 degrees of flexion. The pivot shift was graded as negative (no "shift"), 1+ (mild), 2+ (moderate), and 3+ (severe).

Preoperatively, 70 per cent had a pivot shift score of 2+ to 3+, whereas at 24 months 95 per cent of the patients had scores of 0 to 1+.

Anterior Drawer Test

The anterior drawer test was performed in 90 degrees of flexion, in neutral rotation. Increased laxity was measured in the same gradations as the Lachman test, where 0 indicates physiologic translation, 1+ indicates 5 mm or less tibial translation, 2 is 6 mm to 10 mm, and a grade of 3+ indicates 11 mm or greater.

TABLE 10–1. CHRONIC RECONSTRUCTION EFFICACY RESULTS IN 104 PATIENTS AT 24 MONTHS (HEXCEL COMPOSITE SCORE)

Excellent } Good	88%
Fair	8%
Poor	4%

TABLE 10–2. ACL CHRONIC RECONSTRUCTION EFFICACY RESULTS IN 104 PATIENTS AT 24 MONTHS (OBJECTIVE MEASUREMENTS)

	Lachman	Anterior Drawer	Pivot Shift
0 } 1+	85%	88%	94%
2+	7%	10%	3%
3+	8%	2%	3%

Over 90 per cent of the patients had a preoperative anterior drawer score of 2+ to 3+; in contrast, at 24 months, 89 per cent of the patients had a 0 to 1+ score.

As for the composite scoring systems, the 24-month improvement in all these objective measurements was highly statistically significant (P < 0.05). These 24-month objective results are shown in Table 10–2.

COMPLICATIONS

When reviewing the individual patient files to obtain the objective test results, all events, no matter how mild, were also reported as potential complications. If a complication of synovitis was reported and with it an associated effusion, this was reported as two complications, synovitis and effusion. Even with this intense reporting of complications, the rates for the reported complications are similar to other reported studies on replacement of the ACL.

Instability was reported in 37 patients. Deep infections were reported in 8 patients and superficial ones in 31. Three patients had synovitis and there were 19 with effusions (Table 10–3).

CONCLUSION

The results of this long-term, multicenter clinical study have demonstrated that functional stabil-

TABLE 10–3. INCIDENCE OF COMPLICATIONS FOR ALL PATIENTS ENTERED INTO STUDY (N = 920)

Complication	Incidence
Instability	37
Infections	
Deep	8
Superficial	31
Synovitis	3
Effusion	19

ity was attained in 88 per cent of all chronic ACL-deficient knees repaired using the Integraft carbon fiber stent as an augmentation device. These results were achieved using several different tissue structures as the autogenous graft and held true despite the inclusion of patients in the early part of the study, who had severe chronically unstable knees with multiple previous surgeries (end-stage knees).

The Integraft stent system is versatile in that it allows the surgeon to use the autogenous technique of his choice. Carbon fiber enhances graft strength, and shares the load with the graft tissues. This coupling of synthetic and graft material enables the physician to achieve this needed earlier mobilization.

REFERENCES

1. Alexander H, Parsons JR, Smith R, Mylod A, Weiss AB. Anterior cruciate ligament replacement with filamentous carbon. Trans Annu Meeting Orthop Res Soc 1982; 5:45.
2. Alexander H, Strauchler IL, Weiss AB, Mayott C, Parsons JR. Carbon-polymer composites for tendon and ligament replacement. Trans Meeting Soc Biomater 1978; 2:123.
3. Alexander H., Weiss AB, Parsons JR, et al. Canine patellar tendon replacement with a polylactic acid polymer-filamentous carbon tissue degrading scaffold. Orthop Rev 1981; 10:41–51.
4. Alexander H, Weiss AB, Parsons JR, Strauchler ID, Gona O. Ligament and tendon replacement with absorbable polymer-filamentous carbon tissue scaffold. Trans Annu Meeting Orthop Res Soc 1979; 4:27.
5. *Idem.* Ligament and tendon replacement scaffolds. Transactions of the Eleventh International Biomaterials Symposium in Conjunction with the Fifth Annual Meeting of the Society of Biomaterials, 1979; 3:72.
6. Aragona J, Parsons JR, Alexander H, Weiss AB. Soft tissue attachment of a filamentous carbon-absorbable polymer tendon and ligament replacement. Clin Orthop Relat Res 1981; 160:268–278.
7. Bercovy M, Goutallier D, Voisin MC, et al. Carbon—PGLA Prostheses for Ligament Reconstruction. Clin Orthop Relat Res 1985; 196:159–168.
8. Butler DL, Grood ES, Noyes FR, Sodd AN. The interpretation of our anterior cruciate ligament data. Clin Orthop Relat Res 1985; 196:26.
9. Christel P, Buttazzoni B, Leray JL, Morin C. Tissue tolerance of carbon materials. Trans World Biomater Congr 1980; 4.7.4.
10. Claes L, Wolter D, Gislinger G, Rose P, Huttner W, Fitzer E. Physical and biological aspects of carbon fibres in the ligament prosthesis. Presented at the Third Conference on the Mechanical Properties of Biomaterials, Keele University, September, 1978.
11. Forster IW, Ralis ZA, McKibbin B, Jenkins DHR. Biological reaction to carbon fiber implants. Clin Orthop Relat Res 1978; 131:299–307.
12. Gona O, Parsons JR, Alexander H, Weiss AB. Tissue in-

growth into polyethylene and polylactic acid coated carbon fibers. Trans Annu Meeting Orthop Soc 1980; 5:358.
13. Goodship AE, Brown PN, Yeats JJ, Jenkins DHR, Silver IA. An assessment of filamentous carbon fiber for the treatment of tendon injury in the horse. Vet Rec 1980; March 106:217.
14. Goutallier D, Bercovy M, Blanquaert D, Voison MC, Gaudichet A, Rouveix B. Clinical applications of biomaterials, John Wiley & Sons, Ltd., 1982.
15. Haubold A. Carbon in prosthetics. Ann N York Acad Sci 1977; 283:383–395.
16. Jenkins DHR. The repair of cruciate ligaments with flexible carbon fibre. J Bone Joint Surg (Br) 1978; 60:520–522.
17. Jenkins DHR, Forster IW, McKibbin B, Ralis ZA. Induction of tendon and ligament formation by carbon implants. J Bone Joint Surg (Br) 1977; 59:53–57.
18. Jenkins DHR, McKibbin B. The role of flexible carbon fibre implants as tendon and ligament substitutes in clinical practice. J Bone Joint Surg (Br) 1980; 62:497–499.
19. Kinzl L, Wolter D, Claes L. Aspects of coated carbon fibres in the ligament prostheses. Trans Annu Meeting Soc Biomater 1979; 71.
20. MacIntosh DL. As described in: Edmonson AS, Crenshaw AH. Campbell's operative orthopaedics. St. Louis: CV Mosby, 1980:967.
21. Minns RJ, Flynn M. Intra-articular implant of filamentous carbon fibre in the experimental animal. J Bioeng 1978; 2:279–286.
22. Neugebauer R, Burri C. Ergebnisse Nach Alloplastischem Bandersatz Mit Kohjenstoffasern. Unfallchirurgie 1981; 7:298–304.
23. Neugebauer R, Burri C, Claes L, Helbing G. The trap door, a possibility of fixation of carbon-fibre strands into cancellous bone. Trans World Biomater Congr 1980; 1:4.7.5.
24. Neugebauer R, Burri C, Claes L, Helbing G, Wolter D. The anchorage of carbon fibre strands into bone, a biomechanical and biological evaluation of knee joints. Trans Meeting Eur Soc Biomater 1979.
25. Neugebauer R, Claes L, Helbing G, Wolter D. The replacement of the abdominal wall by a carbon-cloth on rabbits. Trans Annu Meeting Soc Biomater 1979; 4:135.
26. Parsons JR, Alexander H, Ende LS, Weiss AB. A comparison of carbon fiber and Dacron fiber tissue scaffolds. Trans Int Biomater Symp 1983; 6:53.
27. Tayton K, Phillips G, Ralis Z. Long term effects of carbon fiber on soft tissue. J Bone Joint Surg (Br) 1982; 64:112–114.
28. Valdez H, Clark RG, Hanselka DV. Repair of digital flexor tendon lacerations in the horse, using carbon fiber implants. J Am Vet Med Assoc 1980; 177(5):427–435.
29. Weiss AB, Alexander H, Blazina M, Parsons JR. Ligament replacement with absorbable polymer-carbon fiber scaffolds—early clinical experience. Trans Annu Meeting East Orthop Assoc 1982.
30. Weiss AB, Alexander H, Parsons JR. Ligament replacement with absorbable polymer carbon fiber scaffolds—early clinical experience. Trans Annu Meeting Soc Biomater 1983; 6:54.
31. Wolter D, Fitzer E, Helbing G, Goldaway J. Ligament replacement in the knee joint with carbon fibers coated with pyrolytic carbon. Trans Annu Meeting Soc Biomater 1977; 1:126.

11

INTEGRAFT* ANTERIOR CRUCIATE LIGAMENT RECONSTRUCTION: ARTHROSCOPIC TECHNIQUE

ROY M. RUSCH, M.D.
ELVERT F. NELSON, M.D.
DONALD NOEL, O.P.A.

INTRODUCTION

It is not the intent of this chapter to teach the technique of arthroscopy, but to show, by careful planning, appropriate instrumentation, and good surgical technique, how anterior cruciate ligament (ACL)-deficient knees can be reconstructed arthroscopically with a composite of autogenous tissue and the carbon-fiber Integraft system.

I will describe the harvesting of two autogenous tissues, either of which could be used for the repair. Harvesting of a section of iliotibial band or of the central third of patellar tendon, its reinforcement with carbon fiber, and finally, the arthroscopic insertion of the composite device with attachment to bone will be described.

It has been documented by Butler et al. [1] that the strength of a young, healthy ACL is approximately 1725 N. Each strand of carbon fiber has a tensile strength of 425 N. Therefore to match closely the strength of the natural structure, four strands of carbon should be woven within each of the autogenous tissue grafts before passing through the joint.

---

*Integraft is a Trademark of Osteonics Biomaterials, Livermore, California.

HARVESTING OF AUTOGENOUS GRAFT

Iliotibial Band

With the patient in a supine position and the table adjusted to allow the knee to be flexed more than 90 degrees, an incision is made starting proximally to Gerdy's tubercle and extending proximally for a distance of 5 to 6 cm. Care must be taken so as not to penetrate the iliotibial band. A 2-cm-wide segment of iliotibial band is carefully cut distally and then extended proximally, progressively widening to achieve a width of 4 cm. A longitudinal or transverse skin incision is then made in the thigh approximately 20 to 22 cm from Gerdy's tubercle and the iliotibial band is cut transversely at that location. The deep soft-tissue attachments are mobilized from the deep aspect of the band and the graft is pulled distally, exiting through the distal wound. If the band's attachment to the intermuscular septum distally must be divided, care must be taken to establish hemostasis of the vessels in this area.

The anterior and posterior margins of the lateral collateral ligament are identified and dissected and the graft is then passed deep to the lateral collateral ligament (Fig. 11–1), maintaining proximity to the femoral attachment as described by MacIntosh [2].

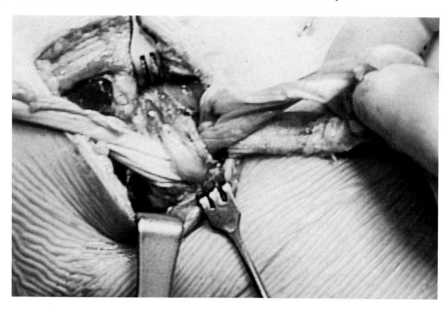

Figure 11–1. Passing of the iliotibial graft beneath the lateral collateral ligament.

Four passes of the carbon stent are then woven through the posterior third of the iliotibial band, beginning distally and exiting proximally (Fig. 11–2). To assist the passage of the carbon through the tissue, it is helpful to keep the area moist. Care must be taken in handling the carbon fiber so that the carbon portion of the stent is never grasped with metal instruments, but only held gently with the gloved hand or with rubber-coated instruments.

The iliotibial band with the carbon stents in place is then rolled in such a manner that the carbon fibers are totally enclosed within the composite graft with none being exposed externally. An absorbable suture is then used to maintain the graft in this tubular form (Fig. 11–3). A No. 1 nonabsorbable traction suture is placed through the free end of the completed graft and will be used to assist in passing the graft through the joint without placing undue tension on the carbon stent. Final diameter of the graft is then checked using a graft-sizing guide to determine the drill size for the femoral and tibial alignment holes. It is usually between 6 and 8 mm.

The composite graft is now ready for arthroscopic placement into the joint. But before progressing to this part of the procedure, the preparation technique for harvesting a bone–tendon–bone

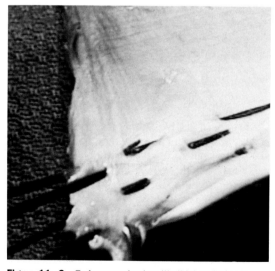

Figure 11–2. Carbon weaving into iliotibial graft (fourth pass shows moist tissue).

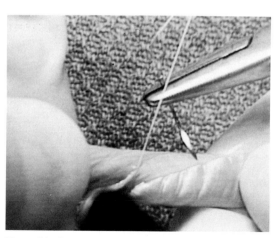

Figure 11–3. Tubing of iliotibial graft with absorbable suture to completely encapsulate the carbon fiber stent.

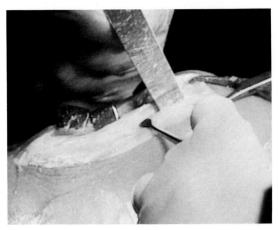

Figure 11—4. Harvesting of central third of patellar tendon with bone wedge.

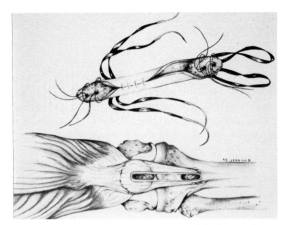

Figure 11—6. Schematic representation of the harvested central third of the patellar, partially tubed with absorbable suture.

graft of the central third of the patellar tendon, reinforced with the carbon fiber stent, will be described.

Central Third of Patellar Tendon

With the patient in the supine position, an incision is made along the medial aspect of the patellar tendon and extended distally to the proximal medial tibia. The distal aspect of the patella, the patellar tendon, and the tibial tubercle are exposed. The central third of the patellar tendon, along with a triangle-shaped portion of the bone, is obtained proximally and distally (Fig. 11–4). Considerable care must be taken to ensure that the tendinous attachment of the bone wedges is not compromised. Four passes of the carbon stent are placed within the patellar tendon, using a stent that is double-armed with curved needles, commencing at the bone–tendon attachment site. The carbon fiber is placed longitudinally within the graft, using a

weaving technique such that no carbon is exposed to the outside surfaces (Fig. 11–5). This is technically possible if care is taken to begin the suture at the site of bone attachment and if the needle is maintained within the substance of the tendon during passage. Total encapsulation of the carbon fibers by ligament tissue is ensured by suturing the edges of the tendon graft with continuous or interrupted absorbable suture, creating a round ligament composite graft (Fig. 11–6).

The completed bone–tendon graft with the carbon fiber stents in place is then lifted from its bed. Small 1-mm-diameter holes are drilled through each bone end and one or two No. 1 nonabsorbable sutures are placed through the holes to assist in passing the graft through the joint without placing undue tension on the carbon stent, as well as retaining the graft under proper tension during final placement. The correct diameter of the entire composite graft is ensured by placing it through a graft-sizing guide (Fig. 11–7).

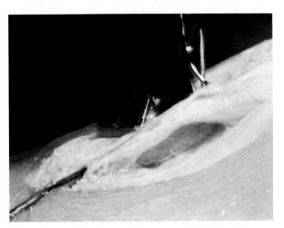

Figure 11—5. Weaving technique of carbon fiber into the central third of the patellar graft, showing no carbon exposed.

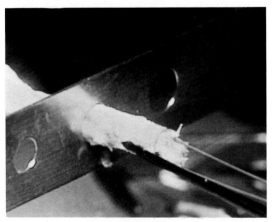

Figure 11—7. Completed graft being passed through a sizing guide to determine the femoral and tibial drill-hole size.

ARTHROSCOPIC GRAFT-INSERTION PROCEDURE

The arthroscopic portal holes should be made close to the patellar tendon both medially and laterally (Fig. 11–8) in order to properly visualize the intercondylar-notch region. Arthroscopically, the status of the meniscii are assessed and corrected appropriately, along with any other apparent mechanical derangements. Under arthroscopic visualization, the intercondylar notch is enlarged and debrided to the extent that the posterior capsule can be easily identified. This allows the precise location of the drill hole for the femoral attachment of the cruciate ligament to be established. A 2.5-mm-diameter Steinmann pin is used initially through the drill guide to ensure that the precise location within the posterior intercondylar notch is achieved (Fig. 11–9). The position of the Steinmann pin should be approximately 5 mm anterior to the posterior margin of the femur.

Attention is then directed to the proximal tibia. Within the joint, the drill guide is positioned on the tibial plateau to ensure isometric placement of the graft; again, a Steinmann pin is used through the drill guide to confirm this precise intra-articular location. At this point the isometricity of the femoral and tibial holes is checked using an appropriate tensioning instrument. If corrections are necessary, these are made by repositioning the Steinmann-pin exit points within the knee joint until the isometric location is attained. When correct isometric placement has been established, both holes are enlarged by overdrilling the Steinmann pins with a cannulated drill (Fig. 11–10), to match the diameter of the composite graft (normally, 6 to 8 mm). To reduce stress on the resulting repair, it is important that all margins of the drill holes are radiused using a chamfering-tool curette or rasp to remove sharp bony edges.

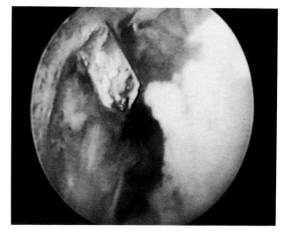

Figure 11–9. Femoral Steinmann pin exiting into the joint.

Of particular benefit in the passage of the graft through the bone holes of the femur and tibia is a thin-walled presized plastic tube (Osteonics Biomaterials, Livermore, Calif.), which has within it a loop of umbilical tape used to draw the graft into the tube. This provides for passage through the joint without impingement against bone, thus eliminating damage to the delicate tissue. The tube is passed through the joint, entering at the tibial hole, progressing through the joint, and partially exiting from the femoral hole (Fig. 11–11). The ends of the carbon fiber stents and the composite graft are partially drawn into the body of the tube (Fig. 11–12), and together they are drawn through the joint with minimal resistance from the bone tunnel, bone edges, or change in angles.

Techniques of proximal and distal fixation of the graft vary according to the surgeon's choice. The

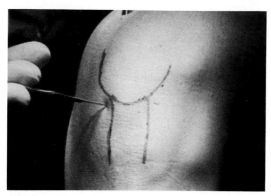

Figure 11–8. Positioning of portal holes.

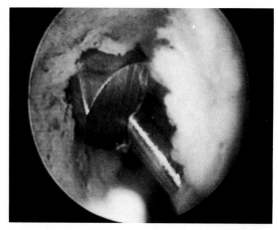

Figure 11–10. Cannulated drill overdrilling the femoral Steinmann pin into the joint.

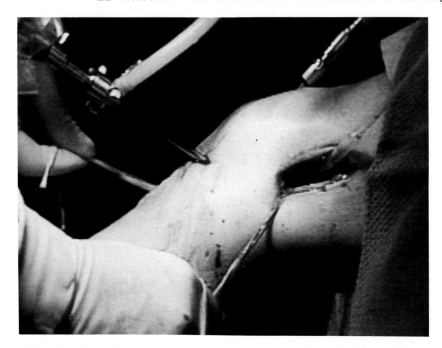

Figure 11–11. Graft passing tube shown traversing the joint, exiting both femur and tibia.

Integraft stent system uses a carbon-fiber and bio-degradable-polymer composite fastener in the shape of an expandable rivet (Fig. 11–13). A hole is drilled 1 cm proximally (femur) and distally (tibia) from the graft drill holes using the combination drill and radius tool (Fig. 11–14). The fastener is partially inserted into the hole in the femur, with its central peg inserted until some resistance is met. The carbon stent and traction sutures are wrapped around the fastener body at least 1 to $1\frac{1}{2}$ turns, with each limb of the stent wrapped in opposite directions (Fig. 11–15), before driving the fastener and then the central pin home using the special insertion instrument (Fig. 11–16). This procedure is repeated on the tibial side and the graft tightened with the knee in 30 degrees of flexion. No attempt is made to close the defect in the

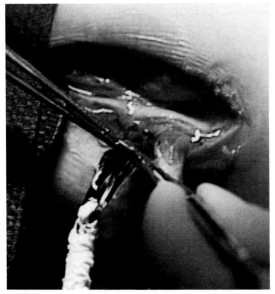

Figure 11–12. Graft being drawn into the passing tube.

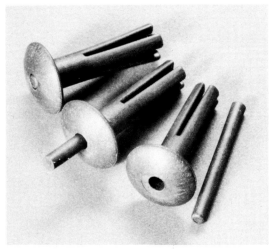

Figure 11–13. Integraft carbon fiber/PLA fastener.

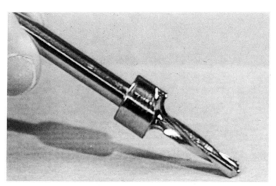

Figure 11—14. Drill bit for precise drilling and radiusing of the bone to accept the Integraft fastener.

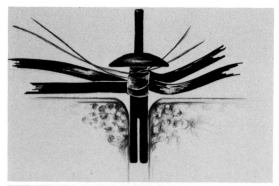

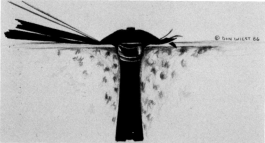

Figure 11—16. Schematic representation showing the wrapping of the carbon stent and stay suture around the fastener in the partially inserted condition, and the assembly completely inserted in its final position.

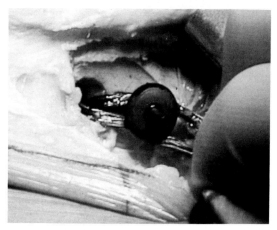

Figure 11—15. Integraft carbon fiber stent being wrapped around the fastener partially inserted into bone.

patellar tendon or iliotibial band. The wounds are closed after appropriate hemostasis has been obtained following release of the tourniquet.

REHABILITATION

Immobilization of the knee in a compression dressing or half splints for a period of 24 to 48 hours is followed by CPM for the duration of the hospital stay, which is generally three to four days. The patient is discharged wearing a knee brace with motion restricted to between 20 and 60 degrees of flexion.

RESULTS

The number of patients and duration of follow-up using this procedure is too small to report meaningful results at this time. Our initial impression is that there has been less morbidity and a shorter hospital stay using this arthroscopic procedure. The complications appear to be no different from those seen in the study, as a whole, using the Integraft carbon-fiber system to augment autogenous tissue in the repairs of anterior cruciate ligaments.

REFERENCES

1. Butler DL, Grood ES, Noyes FR, Sodd AN. The interpretation of our anterior cruciate ligament data. Clin Orthop Relat Res 1985; 196:26.
2. MacIntosh DL. As described in: Edmonson AS, Crenshaw AH. Campbells operative orthopedics. St. Louis: CV Mosby, 1980:967.

12

SYNTHETIC AUGMENTATION OF BIOLOGIC ANTERIOR CRUCIATE LIGAMENT SUBSTITUTION

DALE M. DANIEL, M.D.

C.L. VAN KAMPEN, Ph.D.

The standard of ligament reconstruction surgery is to replace the disrupted structure with a collagenous one of similar size and strength to the original one, protect the joint during the period of soft tissue healing to bone, and gradually increase joint motion and load over a period of 6 to 12 months while the biologic tissue is going through the stages of necrosis, revascularization, and reorganization [2]. The advantage of using a biologic replacement is that the structure can remodel and repair. The disadvantages of using a biologic structure are donor-site morbidity (autograft), transmittal of disease process or host rejection (allograft), and graft disruption or elongation during the process of surgical implantation, healing, or remodeling.

Synthetic augmentation of the biologic graft has been proposed as a method of improving the results of biologic reconstruction [7]. The goals of augmentation are to

1. Improve the initial strength of the biologic graft in order to decrease the risk of graft disruption when tensioning the graft and evaluating joint laxity after graft fixation, and decrease the risk of graft elongation or disruption during the initial healing stage while initiating a program of early joint motion.

2. Protect the biologic graft from elongation or disruption during the period of graft remodeling and increasing limb activity.

3. Share ligament load with the biologic graft to enhance the ligament-remodeling process.

BIOMECHANICS OF AUGMENTATION

A critical aspect of synthetic augmentation of a biologic graft is the recognition that long-term remodeling of the biologic graft is dependent on the tissue carrying a portion of the load. Biologic tissues remodel according to the loads they carry; therefore the biologic graft must be subjected to appropriate loading in order to develop a strong biologic reconstruction [1]. Thus it is essential to the remodeling process that load sharing occurs between the augmentation device and the biologic graft. The following techniques are methods that might be used to ensure load sharing.

1. Mechanically couple the augmentation device and biologic tissue, but secure the augmentation device to the bone at only one end.

2. At the initial surgery, secure both the augmentation device and the biologic tissue skeletally at both ends; at a second surgery release the augmentation device at one or

65

both ends or remove it, thereby placing full load on the biologic graft.

3. Design an augmentation device that biologically degrades and becomes more compliant, thereby increasing the load to the biologic graft.

The technique of ligament augmentation proposed by Kennedy et al. [7], and used in the U.S. and Canadian clinical studies reported in Chapters 13 and 14, is to couple the augmentation device to the biologic graft with sutures and secure the composite graft to the bone at only one end. Load transmission with this arrangement may be analyzed by a simple mechanical model in which the components of an augmented ligament reconstruction are represented by spring elements. As shown in Figure 12–1, the biologic graft, the synthetic augmentation device, and the suture connection between them can each be assigned a spring constant K, which approximates the relative stiffness of these components. The load transmitted from the femur to the tibia is distributed between the augmentation device and the biologic graft by the sutures along the length of the reconstruction. The augmentation device is not anchored to the bone at one end, in this case the tibia; therefore a short length of unaugmented tissue is present.

The application of basic spring theory to the model in Figure 12–1 gives the following mathematical expression for the ratio of forces in the biologic graft and the synthetic augmentation device:

$$\frac{F_{\text{graft}}}{F_{\text{device}}} = \frac{K_g}{K_a K_s / (K_a + K_s)}.$$

This simple analysis indicates that the ratio of force is dependent only upon the relative stiffness of the components. Assumptions may now be made regarding the relative stiffnesses in order to analyze load sharing in the composite reconstruction. First, let us assume that the tissue is relatively compliant and assign the following values to the spring constants.

$$K_g = K$$
$$K_a = 10K$$
$$K_s = 10K$$

Using the above spring constants, the ratio forces in the composite reconstruction is calculated:

$$\frac{F_{\text{graft}}}{F_{\text{device}}} = \frac{1}{5}.$$

Thus the augmentation device is carrying about five times more load than the biologic graft. If the graft were a stiffer structure or became a stiffer structure, it would carry an increasing proportion of the load.

This model may be used to demonstrate the effect of anchoring the augmentation device directly to the bones at both ends of the device. Such a configuration would result in two separate, parallel pathways for carrying the load. The following expression would describe the ratio of the forces in this situation:

$$\frac{F_{\text{graft}}}{F_{\text{device}}} = \frac{K_g}{K_a}.$$

In the case where $K_g = K$ and $K_a = 10K$, the ratio of forces in the biologic graft and the synthetic augmentation device would be calculated:

$$\frac{F_{\text{graft}}}{F_{\text{device}}} = \frac{1}{10}.$$

Thus if the augmentation device is fixed to bone at both ends of the device, the augmentation device would be carrying 10 times more load than the

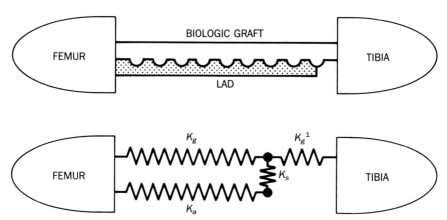

Figure 12–1 Spring model of the components in an augmented ligament reconstruction. Relative stiffnesses of the biologic graft, the ligament augmentation device (LAD), and the suture connection between them are given by K_g, K_a, and K_s, respectively.

biologic graft. As the biologic tissue softened during the revascularization stage an increasing load would be transmitted by the augmentation device, perhaps stress-shielding the tissue too much to allow for proper tissue reorganization. In addition, the higher load on the augmentation device may overload the synthetic material.

As diagrammed in Figure 12–1, there is a segment of graft that is not augmented. The entire graft load must be transmitted through this segment, so graft strength can be no greater than the strength of this graft segment and its attachment.

Further analysis of the expression for the ratio of forces between the graft and the device indicates the importance of the suture between the biologic tissue and the device. The load transmitted to the augmentation device may be no greater than the load that the suture bond will transmit. If the mechanical coupling by the suture is very compliant, such that $K_s = K$ instead of $10K$, then the loads would be approximately evenly distributed between the biologic graft and the synthetic augmentation device, potentially overloading the biologic graft.

MATERIAL REQUIREMENTS FOR SYNTHETIC AUGMENTATION

The material used for a synthetic augmentation device must be strong and flexible in order to withstand the loading and bending of an anterior cruciate ligament (ACL) reconstruction. In addition, the material must be resistant to creep, fatigue, and abrasion under cyclical loading. However, the material requirements for a synthetic augmentation device are not as stringent as for a total ACL prosthesis. The augmentation device is planned to be a short-term stent, functioning only for a period of months (maximum of 12 to 18 months), during the initial period of ligament healing and remodeling. The number of cycles to which the knee joint is exposed during a year of normal activity is estimated at 3.5 to 4 million [3]. So the synthetic device should withstand approximately 5 million cycles. It is estimated that the typical working load on the ACL during normal activity is 500 N [5,9]. The load is shared between the augmentation device and the biologic tissue. During the initial healing period the load carried by the composite graft would be reduced, because to some extent the patient would be protecting the knee that had been operated on. Thus a synthetic augmentation device must withstand loads of less than 500 n for about 5 million cycles. This is in contrast to a total prosthesis, with may need to withstand loads of 500 N for well over 100 million cycles.

While the issues of material creep and fatigue are less critical for a synthetic augmentation device than for a total prosthesis, these properties cannot be ignored. The material must not stretch out or break before the biologic tissue has substantially healed. An important material consideration is abrasion resistance. Rubbing of the device against bone or abrasion of fibers against one another may lead to failure of the device and shedding of debris into the joint, which may provoke an inflammatory response.

The Kennedy ligament augmentation device (LAD) used in the Canadian and U.S. clinical trials (Chapters 13 and 14) is a flat braid of high-tenacity polypropylene yarn. Details of the mechanical properties of the device (tensile strength, fatigue properties, and cyclical-creep behavior) have been published previously [8]. The ultimate tensile strength of the polypropylene braid is approximately 1700 N, which is similar to the strength of the natural ACL [6,10]. Dynamic loading to 500 N results in 9 per cent strength loss and 3 per cent creep after 1 million cycles.

ANIMAL STUDIES OF THE KENNEDY LAD

The ACL was excised in one knee of young adult goats [8]. The ligament was reconstructed with the central third of the patellar tendon–prepatellar fascia–rectus femoris tendon. In half of the goats the graft was augmented with a 6-mm polypropylene braid. In each case the graft was passed through a bone tunnel in the tibia, through the joint, and over the top of the lateral femoral condyle to the lateral aspect of the femur, where it was fixed with a screw and metal bushing. Knees were immobilized with an external fixer for six weeks. Six animals from each group were killed at 0, 3, 6, 12, and 24 months—three for mechanical testing and three for histologic evaluation. Mean values for load-to-failure testing for stiffness and strength of the bone–ligament–bone preparations are presented in Graphs 12–1 and 12–2. Note that between zero and six months there is a marked increase in graft strength and stiffness in both the augmented and nonaugmented grafts. The levels at one year are about 50 per cent of normal values for the goat [8]. The augmented graft is significantly stronger and stiffer than the nonaugmented graft only at time zero.

Histologic studies revealed that the augmentation device was well tolerated and the biologic graft went through the normal tissue-remodeling process without significant signs of foreign-body reaction or inflammation [8].

GRAPH 12–1.

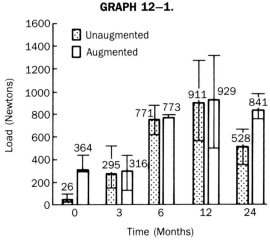

Failure loads of goat knees receiving augmented and nonaugmented transplants. Mean values are given, three animals per group. The bars indicate the range of values. Loaded under tension at an elongation rate of 2.5 mm/sec.

CADAVERIC STUDIES OF GRAFT SUTURING

In the Canadian and U.S. clinical trials (Chapters 13 and 14), the LAD was sutured to the biologic graft and fixed to the bone at only one end. The load that may be transmitted from the biologic graft to the LAD is limited by the strength of the

GRAPH 12–2.

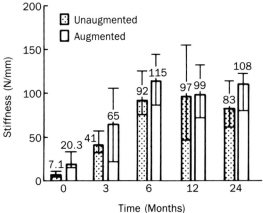

Stiffness of goat knees receiving augmented and nonaugmented transplants. Stiffness was defined as the slope of the load–elongation curve in its linear region. Mean values are given, three animals per group. The bars indicate the range of values. Loaded under tension at an elongation rate of 2.5 mm/sec.

suture bond coupling the two structures. Also, as discussed above, a factor in the compliance of the composite graft is the compliance of the suture bond. We performed a study in our laboratory to evaluate the strength and compliance of the composite graft attached so that all of the load was transferred from the LAD to the biologic tissue through the suture bond.

Materials and Methods

Cadaveric knee specimens from elderly subjects were frozen at −20°C until the time of testing. The patellar tendon was left attached to the tibia and a graft was harvested consisting of one third of the patellar tendon with prepatella fascia and quadriceps tendon. The LAD was sutured to the biologic graft by an orthopedic surgeon with 00 ethibond in the distal 5 cm of the graft and 00 Dexon more proximally. During the suturing process the LAD and the biologic graft were tensioned equally with a load of about 10 N. Sutures were placed at 1-cm intervals as interrupted sutures, continuous running sutures, or a combination of these, as shown in Figure 12–2. Sutures were tied with three square knots. The composite graft was passed through a tunnel in the tibia and secured with a hook attached to a load cell. The tibia was clamped securely in an orientation that allowed loading the graft in a direction that simulates in vivo conditions. Cylical loading at eight cycles per minute were carried out for 5 to 15 minutes at each of several increasing load levels until graft failure. Force data was collected on a strip-chart recorder. The specimen was measured under a 10-N load. A total of 20 composite grafts were tested.

Results

1. There was a mean 4 per cent graft elongation during the first 10 cycles at 90 N. After 15 minutes of cycling at 90 N, there was an additional elongation of 2 per cent (range, 0.5 to 3). With progressive loading there was a progressive increase in elongation.
2. There was no significant difference in elongation or load to failure that could be attributed to the suture method. All sutures remained securely tied at load levels up to 180 N. At 270 N, 13 per cent of sutures untied or pulled out of the tendon. The sutures did not break. The failed sutures were all at the distal LAD attachment.
3. The mean graft failure load was 275 N (range, 100 to 404; S.D., 82). The usual mechanism was failure of the distal sutures with progression proximally until there was failure through a weak portion of the biologic graft or complete detachment of the LAD.

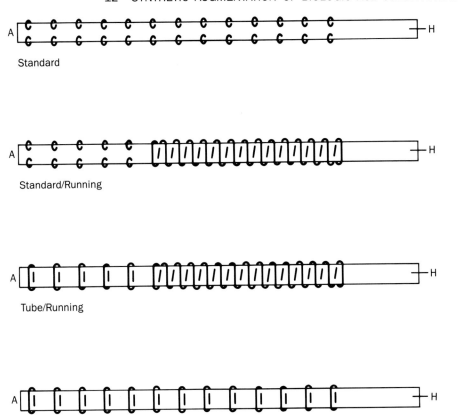

Figure 12–2. Suturing methods used to attach the LAD to the biologic tissue. Sutures were placed at 1-cm intervals. A indicates the end at which the patellar tendon was attached anatomically to the tibia. H indicates the end at which the LAD was attached via a hook to the load cell. The five sutures (or pairs of sutures) closest to A were 00 ethibond. The other sutures were 00 Dexon.

This study measured the load that may be transmitted through the suture bond. Fixation of biologic tissue with the LAD proximally, as is done clinically, will allow direct load bearing through the biologic tissue as well as load transfer to the LAD through the suture bond; therefore the total graft strength will be higher. This study was performed in cadaveric tissue from elderly subjects. Undoubtedly, the tissue in young patients undergoing ligament reconstruction surgery will be stronger.

Composite-ligament failure may occur at the biologic-tissue anatomic attachment site, through the unaugmented biologic tissue, at the LAD–biologic tissue suture bond, and at the proximal attachment site. Limited studies in our laboratory using cadaveric bone from elderly subjects revealed failure of the LAD biologic graft fixed with a double-barbed staple, as was used in the U.S. and Canadian clinical trial, to be at 300 N. Soft tissue fixed with a barbed staple alone fails at 81 N [11].

The composite graft is only as strong as its weakest link. The augmented patellar tendon–prepatellar fascia–quadriceps tendon graft is not strong enough to withstand normal cruciate loading. But this graft is strong enough to allow graft tensioning without fear of graft failure on passive motion of the isometrically placed graft (Chapter 4).

CONCLUSIONS

Augmentation may strengthen a biologic graft with a weak segment and improve fixation strength of the graft. The added strength and stiffness of the composite graft contributed by the augmentation device will depend largely on the suture bond between the two structures. To minimize the compliance of this link it is recommended that both structures be equally tensioned at the time of suturing and that the composite graft be cyclically loaded 10 times at a 90-N (20 lb) load prior to graft fixation.

The benefit of augmentation of a biologic structure beyond the operative period has not been demonstrated. The important suture bond between the biologic tissue and augmentation device will undoubtedly weaken with tissue necrosis and revascularization in the postoperative and remodeling period [12]. However, it is likely during a number of days to weeks after surgery that the augmented graft will be stronger than the nonaugmented graft. Remodeling of the augmented graft proceeds in a similiar fashion to that of a nonaugmented graft. Load-to-failure testing in a goat model months after surgery did not demonstrate a difference in strength and stiffness between the augmented and nonaugmented grafts.

REFERENCES

1. Akeson WH, Frank CB, Amiel D, Woo S. Ligament biology and biomechanics In: Fineman G, ed. AAOS Symposium on Sports Medicine: the knee Editor 6. Fineman St. Louis: CV Mosby, 1985.
2. Arnoczky SP, Tarvin GB, Marshall JL. Anterior cruciate ligament replacement using patellar tendon. J Bone Joint Surg (Am) 1982; 64a:217.
3. Chen EH, Black J. Materials design analysis of the prosthetic anterior cruciate ligament. J Biomed Mater Res 1980; 14:567.
4. Chiroff RT. Experimental replacement of the anterior cruciate ligament. J Bone Joint Surg (Am) 1975; 57a:1124–1127.
5. Grood ES, Noyes FR. Cruciate ligament prosthesis: strength, creep, and fatigue properties. J Bone Joint Surg (Am) 1976; 58a:1083.
6. Kennedy JC, Hawkins RJ, Willis RB. Strain gauge analysis of knee ligaments. Clin Orthop Relat Res 1977; 129:225.
7. Kennedy JC, Roth JH, Mendenhall HV, Sanford JB. Intra-articular replacement in the anterior cruciate ligament-deficient knee. Am J Sports Med 1980; 8:1.
8. McPherson GK, Mendenhall HV, Gibbons DF, et al. Experimental mechanical and histologic evaluation of the Kennedy ligament augmentation device. Clin Orthop Relat Res 1985;196:186.
9. Morrison JB. Bioengineering analysis of force actions transmitted by the knee joint. Biomed Eng 1969; 4:573.
10. Noyes FR, Grood ES. The strength of the anterior cruciate ligament in humans and rhesus monkeys. J Bone Joint Surg (Am) 1976; 58a:1074.
11. Robertson DB, Daniel DM Biden E. Fixation of soft tissue to bone. Am J Sports Med.
12. Urbaniak JR, Cahill JD, Mortenson RA. Tendon suturing methods: analysis of tensil strengths. In: AAOS Tendon surgery in the hand. St Louis: CV Mosby, 1975.

13

THE MARSHALL/MACINTOSH ANTERIOR CRUCIATE LIGAMENT RECONSTRUCTION WITH THE KENNEDY LIGAMENT AUGMENTATION DEVICE: REPORT OF THE UNITED STATES CLINICAL TRIALS

DALE M. DANIEL, M.D.
E. PAUL WOODWARD, M.D.
GARY M. LOSSE, M.D.
MARY LOU STONE, R.P.T.

INTRODUCTION

Numerous surgical procedures have been performed to decrease the pathologic anterior laxity and improve the function of the patient with a chronic anterior cruciate ligament (ACL) disruption. Marshall [6] and MacIntosh [4] described an intra-articular ACL reconstruction that used as the graft source the middle third of the patellar tendon, prepatellar retinaculum, and the middle third of the quadriceps tendon. The graft was left attached to the tibia, passed through a tibial drill hole, and then passed over the top of the lateral femoral condyle. Because of the weak prepatellar retinaculum, the graft was at risk of disruption while it was being passed through the joint and tensioned

[3,7,8]. Postoperatively, biologic grafts go through stages of tissue necrosis, revascularization, and remodeling [1]. During the early period of remodeling the graft becomes weaker and even minimal stresses to the knee could result in rupture or elongation of the autograft, rendering it functionally deficient [3].

Kennedy et al. [3,7] proposed that coupling the autogenous graft tissue with a synthetic material would provide greater graft strength. Load sharing between the synthetic device and the biologic graft would allow biologic-graft healing and remodeling (Chapter 12). The greater composite graft strength would permit adequate graft tensioning to eliminate pathologic anterior laxity and allow more secure graft fixation as well as potentially diminish the tendency of the graft to elongate in the early postoperative period.

PATIENT POPULATION

A total of 157 patients from 17 centers were entered in the prospective ligament augmentation device (LAD) study. A total of 148 patients are included in this review. Prior to participating in the LAD study, between November 1980 and October 1983, author E. Paul Woodward performed nonaugmented Marshall/MacIntosh ACL reconstructions. A total of 29 patients with nonaugmented grafts were reviewed. Demographic data and history of knee surgery are presented in Tables 13–1 and 13–2. Operative findings are noted in

Table 13–3. Entry requirements for the Marshall/MacIntosh LAD prospective study patients and the retrospective nonaugmented controls are listed below.

1. Closed or nearly closed growth plates.
2. Period of six months or more between injury and ligament surgery.
3. Contralateral normal knee.
4. Preoperative pathologic anterior laxity of 3 mm or greater. (Anterior knee laxity was measured with the KT-1000 Arthrometer. The laxity test was performed with the knee in 20 to 40 degrees of flexion with a 20-lb anterior displacement force [2,5]. Pathologic laxity is defined as the laxity in the involved knee minus the laxity in the contralateral normal knee.)

TABLE 13–1. PATIENT POPULATION

	LAD Patients			Nonaugmented Controls		
	Males	**Females**	**All Patients**	**Males**	**Females**	**All Patients**
Total number of patients (%)	106 (72)	42 (28)	148 (100)	21 (72)	8 (28)	29 (100)
Mean age	27	25	26	28	27	28
Mean weight (kg)	80	62	75	79	62	74
Mean height (cm)	179	166	176	177	162	173
Mean age of injury (mo)	39	41	39	50	58	52
Mean no. of months after operation				33	29	32

TABLE 13–2. PREVIOUS SURGERY

	LAD Patients ($n = 148$)		Nonaugmented Controls ($n = 29$)	
	No. of Patients	**Percent**	**No. of Patients**	**Percent**
Number of patients with prior surgery (all types)	121	82	15	52
Number of patients with prior ligament surgeries				
None	119	80	21	72
One	25	17	8	28
Two	4	3	0	0

TABLE 13–3. OPERATIVE FINDINGS

	LAD Patients ($n = 148$)		Nonaugmented Controls ($n = 29$)	
	No. of Patients	**Percent**	**No. of Patients**	**Percent**
Meniscal condition normal				
Medial	52	35	12	41
Lateral	82	56	20	69
Cartilage surface normal				
Medial	82	55	21	72
Lateral	116	79	23	79
Patellofemoral	106	72	25	86

SURGICAL PROCEDURE

The surgical procedure performed in the LAD augmented and nonaugmented control patients were nearly identical. All reconstructions were performed using an arthrotomy. Meniscus repairs or resections and joint-debridement procedures were performed as needed at the time of the arthrotomy or at a previous arthroscopy. Surgery performed in addition to the Marshall/MacIntosh LAD procedure is listed in Table 13–4.

The autogenous graft was prepared by harvesting the middle third of the patellar tendon, central two third of the prepatellar retinaculum, and the middle third of the quadriceps tendon. The graft was left attached to the tibial tubercle. In the patients with augmented grafts an 8-mm-wide LAD of appropriate length was sutured to the autogenous graft using interrupted 00 nonabsorbable sutures in the proximal and distal thirds of the graft and interrupted 00 absorbable sutures placed in the middle third. The sutures were placed at 1-cm intervals. Tubing of the graft to cover the intra-articular portion of the LAD was performed as width of graft tissue allowed.

The graft was routed through a 9-mm tibial drill hole and then through the posterior capsule and over the top of the lateral femoral condyle to reach the lateral aspect of the distal femur [3]. With the knee in about 30 degrees of flexion, the graft was tensioned and fixed to the lateral aspect of the femur with two barbed staples. In the augmented cases the composite graft was tensioned to a measured 10 to 20 lb. The joint was placed through a range of motion of 0 to 90 degrees to check for possible areas of graft impingement at the anterior portal of the intercondylar notch. Bone excision was performed as indicated, to prevent graft impingement. Edges of the drill hole were contoured to prevent abrasion of the graft. Sixteen of the 29 patients with nonaugmented grafts were immobilized in a cast for seven to eight weeks. The remaining nonaugmented cases and all augmented cases were immobilized in a cast or a brace for three weeks. A limited and protected motion program in a postoperative brace was then used for three to five weeks, followed by a progressive activity program as directed by the patient's physician. Walking with the aid of crutches after surgery was recommended for 6 to 10 weeks.

EVALUATION SYSTEM

With respect to the prospective multicenter LAD study a standard questionnaire, clinical examination, and anterior/posterior (A/P) laxity measurements (KT-1000 Arthrometer) were performed preoperatively and at 6, 12, 18, and 24 months postoperatively. A laxity examination was also performed under anesthesia prior to the ligament reconstruction and after wound closure. The evaluation was performed by staff at each of the study sites using an evaluation protocol provided by the 3M Company. At least one examiner at each study site received instruction in A/P laxity measurement with the KT-1000 Arthrometer by a member of the team from San Diego who developed the device [2,5]. The retrospective analysis of the controls with nonaugmented grafts utilized the same evaluation protocol as used in the prospective Marshall/MacIntosh LAD study.

INTRAOPERATIVE GRAFT TENSIONING AND FIXATION

During the LAD surgical procedure the surgeon tensioned the composite graft with the use of a tensiometer. The surgical goal was to establish an-

TABLE 13–4. ADDITIONAL OPERATIVE PROCEDURES

| Procedure | LAD Patients (n = 148) | | Nonaugmented Controls (n = 29) | |
	No. of Patients	Percent	No. of Patients	Percent
Meniscus repair				
Medial	12	8	0	0
Lateral	1	1	0	0
Meniscectomy	30	20	8	28
Medial	30	20	8	28
Lateral	30	20	6	21
Extra-articular ligament procedures (patients)	50	34		
Posterior/medial procedures	31	21		
Lateral procedures	46	31		
Medial procedures	2	7		

terior laxity (with a 20-lb displacement) in the knee that was operated on within 3 mm of the patient's normal knee, as well as to eliminate the pivot shift. The mean graft load was 16.2 lb (range, 10 to 22). In no case did the composite graft disrupt while being passed or tensioned. In one case, the tibial attachment site of the graft was attenuated during the harvesting process and it was reinforced with a 6.5-mm screw with a soft-tissue washer. Laxity measurements after wound closure revealed that the pivot-shift sign was negative in all patients. Ninety-nine percent of the grafts were tightened to +3 mm or less than the noninvolved knee.

IN-HOSPITAL COMPLICATIONS

In-hospital complications were reported in five patients with augmented grafts. Three patients developed a notable hematoma and one underwent a wound exploration. None were infected. One patient had elevated blood pressure and one patient had superficial cellulitis treated with antibiotics administered intravenously.

POSTOPERATIVE EVENTS AND COMPLICATIONS

A list of reported postoperative events and complications for all patients with augmented grafts are presented in Table 13–5. Arthroscopy or surgery has been performed subsequent to the ligament-reconstruction procedure in 28 patients (19 per cent) for the treatment of a subsequent injury or the evaluation of restriction of knee motion, pain, effusion, or pathologic laxity (Table 13–6). In four patients, LAD breakage was confirmed arthroscopically (at 12, 14, 18, and 27 months postoperatively) in all cases through the intra-articular segment. Synovial biopsies were performed in 10 pa-

TABLE 13–5. POSTOPERATIVE EVENTS AND COMPLICATIONS IN LAD PATIENTS (N = 148)

Event	No. of Events	No. of Patients	Percent
Manipulations	7	6	4
LAD breakage	4	4	3
Graft retensioning	4	4	3
Superficial infection	5	5	3
Deep infection	1	1	1
Patellar-tendon rupture	4	4	3
Other operative procedures	29	24	16

TABLE 13–6. SUBSEQUENT SURGERY OF THE KNEE IN LAD PATIENTS

Surgery	No. of Events	No. of Patients	Percent of All Patients
Partial meniscectomy	6	6	4
Meniscal repair	2	2	1
Diagnostic arthroscopy	23	21	14
Debridement	10	9	6
Staple or screw removal or replacement	8	7	5
Extra-articular procedure	2	2	1
Tightening of ACL graft	2	2	1
Release of adhesions	1	1	1
Scar revision	1	1	1

tients at the time of subsequent surgery and foreign particles were observed in two patients.

A deep infection was diagnosed in one patient with an augmented graft (0.7 per cent). The patient presented with a swollen joint after being involved in a fight three months after surgery. Arthroscopy, retensioning of the LAD, and an Arnold–Kocker ITB procedure were performed five months after the LAD reconstruction. Cultures taken at the time of the LAD retensioning grew *Staphylococcus epidermidis*. The patient was taken back to surgery, the joint debrided and the LAD removed. The infection cleared with intravenous antibiotics.

Four patients with augmented grafts (2.7 per cent) sustained a postoperative rupture of the patellar tendon. All ruptures resulted from hyperflexion of the knee during minor injury events at two, three, five, and six months after surgery. The patellar tendon avulsed off of the inferior pole of the patella. The ruptures were surgically repaired and have healed satisfactorily. None of these patients developed problems with range of motion after their subsequent surgery. All patients exhibited a range of motion of 140 degrees or greater at the time of their last follow-up visit.

In four patients with augmented grafts (2.7 per cent) who developed postoperative pathologic laxity the graft was surgically retensioned by exposing the femoral fixation site, removing the staples, freeing the graft from the surrounding tissues, tensioning the graft, and stapling it in the new position. This was performed at two, four, five, and eight months after surgery. The status of these patients at their last visit is shown in Table 13–7.

At the time of the single evaluation visit for the control or nonaugmented group, the patients were questioned if they had experienced any major reinjuries to either knee or if they had any surgeries after their nonaugmented ACL reconstruction.

TABLE 13–7. STATUS OF LAD PATIENTS WITH ACL COMPOSITE GRAFT RETENSIONING

Patient	Month Retensioned	Month Examined	Pivot Shift (I–N)	Lachman Test (I–N)	KT-1000 20-LB Anterior Displacement (I–N)
C001	3	10	0	0	1.5
E027	5	LAD removed at 6 months			
M035	2	14	0	0	1.5
P006	8	17	2	0	8.5

Two patients (7 per cent) had had a subsequent surgery.

RESULTS

A comparative evaluation between the 24-month U.S. study results (17 investigative sites) and the control patients from the single center (E.P.W.) is presented in Table 13–8.

Comparing pivot-shift scores between the patients with augmented and nonaugmented grafts, 82 per cent of the LAD patients were rated grade 0 versus 59 per cent of the control patients (nonaugmented). Comparing patients with grade 0 or 1 pivot shift, 93 per cent of the LAD patients were rated grade 0 or 1, while 89 per cent of the control patients were graded 0 or 1. The overall mean values for the LAD patients and the control patients were 0.2 and 0.5, respectively.

A Lachman test was not performed on the control patients, thus a comparison to the augmented group is not possible. However, the patients with augmented grafts had a preoperative mean Lachman value of 1.95, while the mean score at two years of follow-up was 0.40 (grade 0 to +3).

TABLE 13–8. SUMMARY OF OBJECTIVE MEASUREMENTS

		24-Month LAD Patients	Nonaugmented Controls
Number of patients		75	29
Flexion contracture	$\bar{x}$	1.64°	4.04°
	>5°	8%	33%
Pivot shift (I–N)	$\bar{x}$	0.24	0.52
	0	82%	59%
	1	11%	30%
	2	7%	11%
	3	0%	0%
Anterior laxity	$\bar{x}$	1.47	1.90
20-lb I–N	≤3 mm	84%	76%
Range of motion	$\bar{x}$	137.0°	136.4°
	>120°	99%	96%

KT-1000 Arthrometer 30°/20 lb anterior tibial displacement measurement showed a side to side difference (I–N) of 3 mm or less in 84 per cent of LAD patients and 76 per cent of control patients. The mean side-to-side difference was 1.5 mm for the LAD and 1.9 mm for the control patients.

Serial 20-lb anterior displacement measurements and pivot-shift tests for the augmented two-year follow-up examination are given in Graphs 13–1 and 13–2. Note that anterior laxity increased postoperatively between 0 and 12 months but did not increase significantly between 12 and 24 months.

Flexion contracture of more than 5 degrees was identified in 8 per cent of the LAD patients, while 33 per cent of the control patients exhibited greater than 5 degrees of flexion contracture. The mean overall flexion contracture values were 1.6 degrees for the LAD group and 4.0 for the control group. The mean range of motion for the LAD group was 137.0 versus 136.4 for the control patients. Ninety-nine per cent of LAD patients and 96 per cent of control patients exhibited more than 120 degrees range of motion.

Ten of 75 patients with augmented grafts (13 per cent) had evidence of an effusion at 24 months (eight graded mild and two graded moderate). Two of 29 control patients (with nonaugmented grafts) (7 per cent) had evidence of an effusion (both graded mild) at a mean follow-up time of 31.6 months.

With respect to patellofemoral signs of dysfunction, 60 per cent of augmented patients had crepitus, while 57 per cent of the control patients experienced crepitus at the follow-up evaluation. Preoperative pain with patellar compression was experienced by 12 per cent of LAD patients and by 17 per cent of the control patients at 24 months.

Table 13–9 presents the assessment of function in patients with augmented and nonaugmented grafts. Subjective evaluation by the patient of present knee function compared to preoperative function revealed that 90 per cent of the patients with augmented grafts and 96 per cent of those with nonaugmented grafts felt that their knee was better. In respect to specific activities (running, jump-

GRAPH 13—1.

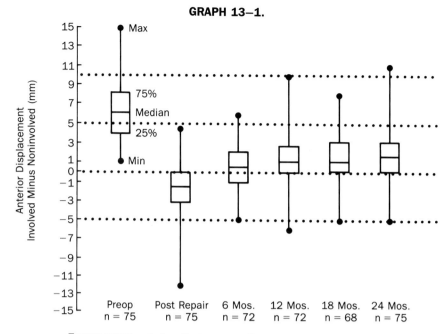

Twenty-pound anterior displacement (I–N) versus time since surgery

ing, and cutting) the two patient groups' evaluations were similar. The patients' assessments of swelling were also similar—68 per cent in the nonaugmented group versus 63 per cent in the augmented group. Awareness of pathology was also similar in the two groups.

DISCUSSION

It is difficult to compare reports of ligament-reconstruction procedures. Treatment outcome de-

pends not only on the surgical procedure performed, but also on the surgeon, patient population, knee pathology, and rehabilitation program. The reported results also depend on the evaluation protocol, evaluators, and interpretation and presentation of the data. In this report, a retrospective review of patients with nonaugmented grafts, treated in nearly the same manner and evaluated using the same protocol as the patients with augmented grafts, has been carried out to present a comparison group. It should be remembered, however, that the controls were from one center (four

GRAPH 13—2.

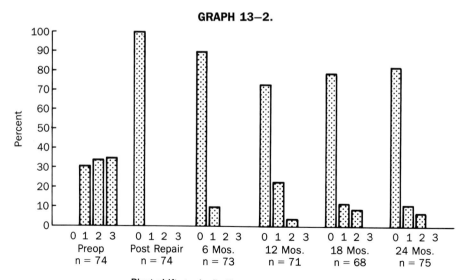

Pivot-shift grade (I–N) versus time since surgery

TABLE 13–9. KNEE FUNCTION BASED ON PATIENT QUESTIONNAIRE

	24-Month LAD Patients	Nonaugmented Controls
Number of patients	75	29
Knee function is better	90%	96%
Knee does not swell	63%	68%
Unaware or occasionally aware of pathology	57%	58%
Stable running on uneven surface	85%	73%
Stable jumping	73%	65%
Stable cutting	80%	77%

TABLE 13–10. PARTICLES VERSUS PERSISTENT EFFUSION ($N = 10$)

		Particles	
		Yes	No
Persistent Effusion	Yes	0	4
	No	2	4

TABLE 13–11. PARTICLES VERSUS SYNOVITIS ($N = 10$)

		Particles	
		Yes	No
Synovitis	Yes	2	6
	No	0	2

evaluators) and the LAD patients were from 17 centers and tested by numerous evaluators. It is recognized that these patients do not form an ideal control group. Nevertheless, the patients with non-augmented grafts reported in this study and evaluated with the same protocol provide a better comparison than using data published from other centers using different evolution protocols.

In both the augmented and nonaugmented groups there was general patient satisfaction and the majority of the patients felt that postoperatively they could run, jump, and cut better than before surgery. The 75 patients with augmented grafts were noted to have a significant reduction of their 20-lb anterior laxity, the mean injured minus normal knee anterior tibial displacement was 6.2 mm preoperatively and 1.5 at two years of follow-up. By comparison, the 29 patients with non-augmented grafts had a mean laxity value of 1.9 at a mean follow-up time of 32 months. Sixteen per cent of the LAD patients and 24 per cent of the patients with nonaugmented grafts had a persistent pathologic laxity (I–N)* of greater than 3 mm. A comparative analysis between LAD patients and control patients with respect to pivot shift reveals that the LAD patients were significantly better statistically. An additional difference between the two groups, which may have an effect on the pivot shift, is that none of the control patients had an extra-articular procedure, while 31 per cent of the LAD patients had an extra-articular procedure.

The LAD is used to augment and strengthen a weak biologic graft [8]. At the time of surgery, this strengthening allows adequate tension (mean, 16.2 lb) to be placed on the graft to allow elimination of pathologic laxity. The knee laxity may be tested at the time of surgery without fear of rupturing or stretching the graft. The additional graft

strength provided by augmentation may allow an early knee-motion program with less risk of graft disruption. The ultimate graft strength is dependent upon graft revascularization and remodeling, as with other autogenous grafts.

The risks of using the polypropylene braid appear to be low. A low incidence of joint effusion is present but decreases with time (25 per cent at 6 months, 14 per cent at 24 months). Comparing this incidence of effusion with that in the control patients, we noted a 7 per cent mild effusion rate at the single mean follow-up time of 32 months. There was no significant difference in effusion rates between LAD and control groups. Particulate debris was noted in two patients on biopsy. These particles may result from the graft rubbing against bone. This would emphasize the importance of good surgical technique to reduce the chances of bone impingement. With the limited data available, the presence of particles does not correlate to either persistent effusion or a diagnosis of synovitis (Tables 13–10 and 13–11).

The Marshall/MacIntosh operation is perceived critically by some surgeons today because of graft-source morbidity and the fact that the Marshall/MacIntosh operation uses the prepatellar retinaculum intra-articularly. In this report, both the patients with augmented and those with non-augmented grafts show good clinical results.

REFERENCES

1. Chiroff RT. Experimental replacement of the anterior cruciate ligament. J Bone Joint Surg (Am) 1975; 57:1124–1127.

*(injured laxity minus normal laxity)

2. Daniel DM, Malcom LL, Losse G, Stone ML, Sachs R, Burks R. Instrumented measurement of anterior laxity of the knee. J Bone Joint Surg (Am) 1985; 67:720–726.
3. Kennedy JC, Roth JH, Mendenhall HV, Sanford JB. Intra-articular replacement in the anterior cruciate ligament-deficient knee. Am J Sports Med 1980; 8:1.
4. MacIntosh D. Acute tears of the anterior cruciate ligament: over the top repair. Presented at the Annual Meeting of the American Academy of Orthopaedic Surgeons, Dallas, Texas, 1974.
5. Malcom LL, Daniel DM, Stone ML, Sachs R. The measurement of anterior knee laxity after ACL reconstructive Surgery. Clin Orthop 1984; 186:35–41.
6. Marshall JL, Gurgis FG, Al Monajem ARS. The anterior cruciate ligament. Clin Orthop 1975; 106:216–231.
7. McPherson GK, Mendenhall HV, Gibbons DF, et al. Experimental mechanical and histologic evaluation of the Kennedy ligament augmentation device. Clin Orthop Relat Res 1985; 196:186.
8. Noyes FR, Butler DL, Grood ES, Zernicke RF, Hefzy MS. Biomechanical analysis of human ligament grafts used in knee-ligament repairs and reconstructions. J Bone Joint Surg (Am) 1984; 66:344–352.

Acknowledgments

The authors wish to acknowledge the following investigators, who allowed their clinical data to be used in this report: John Callahan, John Callander, Jay Cox, Dale Daniel, Harold Halvorson, Larry Hull, Walter Krengel, Robert Larson, Robert Lehmer, J. Lee Leonard, Paul K. Lim, Gary Losse, Robert Meisterling, Wm. Mohlenbrock, Frank Pettrone, Ray Sachs, Dennis Walker, and Paul Woodward.

This review was funded by the 3M Company.

14

POLYPROPYLENE-BRAID–AUGMENTED ANTERIOR CRUCIATE LIGAMENT RECONSTRUCTION

JAMES H. ROTH, M.D., F.R.C.S.(C.)
JOHN C. KENNEDY, M.D., F.R.C.S.(C.)

INTRODUCTION

Chronic anterior cruciate ligament insufficiency of the knee remains an enigma for the present-day orthopedic surgeon. Diagnostic tests such as the Lachman [1] and pivot shift [2] signs, as well as arthroscopic examination have improved our ability to diagnose this common condition. However, a multitude of operative procedures have been described to manage the symptomatic ''giving way'' that these patients experience. None of these has stood the test of time. The late Dr. J.C. Kennedy devoted the majority of his research activities to solving the problem of the anterior cruciate ligament (ACL)-deficient knee. The purpose of this chapter is to review the work initiated and stimulated by Dr. Kennedy at our center and to outline our present surgical technique.

INTRA-ARTICULAR AUTOGRAFTS

A one-year study evaluating intra-articular autogenous semitendinosus reconstruction of the excised anterior cruciate ligament in 64 New Zealand white rabbits demonstrated that the autograft underwent degeneration that was still present at the one-year autopsy [3] (Figs. 14–1, 14–2, 14–3).

Mechanical testing revealed that on the average the normal anterior cruciate ligament failed at 4.5 and 5.9 kg. Thus at 52 weeks the transfer retains 50 per cent of its original tensile strength, which is only 15 per cent of the tensile strength of the anterior cruciate ligament that it is replacing.

It was found microscopically that the autogenous intra-articular transfer underwent degeneration that was still present at one year after operation (Figs. 14–4 and 14–5). It is postulated that an autograft must initially degenerate, revascularize, and, finally, recollagenize before it has enough tensile strength to withstand the stress of everyday life. If unprotected stress is applied to the autograft when it is in a degenerative and weakened state, it will probably elongate or rupture, thereby making it unusable.

Based on this study, it was felt that the long-term success of autogenous intra-articular grafts for reconstruction of the anterior cruciate ligament is uncertain at best. Another solution to the problem should be sought.

PROSTHETIC ANTERIOR CRUCIATE LIGAMENT REPLACEMENT

A study was undertaken in large dogs to replace the excised anterior cruciate ligament with a total

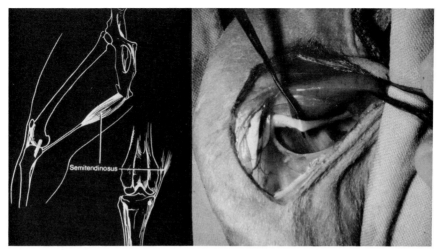

Figure 14–1. The semitendinosus musculotendinous unit is a definite anatomic structure in the rabbit and seems a very suitable autograft for ACL reconstruction.

prosthesis [Mendenhall HV, et al.: unpublished data]. A 3.6-mm diamond-braided cylindrical prosthesis of polypropylene was used (Fig. 14–6). Necropsies were performed at 3, 6, and 10 months. Varying degrees of destruction of the device occurred in all but one animal (Figs. 14–7 and 14–8). The prosthesis was grossly loose in 30 per cent of the animals, resulting in considerable edema of the soft tissues. A persistent acute inflammatory reaction characterized by eosinophils, lymphocytes, and plasma cells was present around individual filaments of the device in these animals (Fig. 14–9). Considerable ''drift'' of the prosthesis on its compressive side was present.

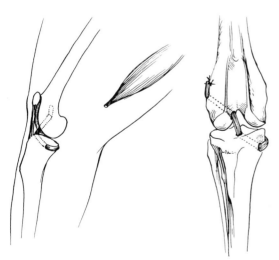

Figure 14–2. The anterior cruciate ligament was excised. Bone tunnels were created in the proximal tibia and distal femur. The autograft was left attached to the proximal tibia and sutured to the periosteum of the distal femur.

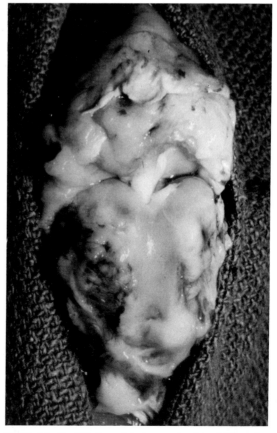

Figure 14–3. This is an intact reconstruction at 26 weeks. Note that the fat pad seems attached to the graft and that it has a visible covering of synovium.

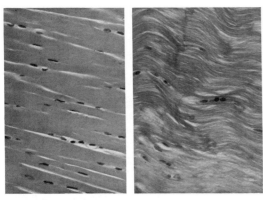

Figure 14—4. The microscopic picture of a normal semitendinosus tendon on the left shows parallel arrangement of fibers and normal cellularity. In contrast, in the figure on the right, there is fragmentation of fibers and less-than-normal cellularity in a 26-week reconstruction.

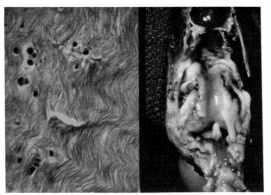

Figure 14—5. On gross appearance, this reconstruction at 52 weeks was graded excellent; however, the microscopic picture was that of severe degeneration. Mechanical testing demonstrated that reconstructions at one year retained only 50 per cent of their original tensile strength.

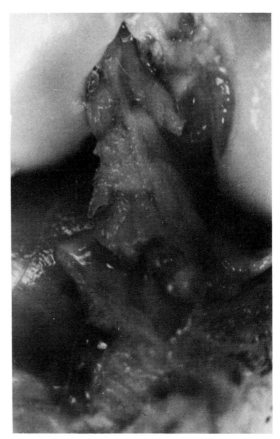

Figure 14—7. This total prosthesis had been implanted three months previously. Note the near-complete destruction of the intra-articular portion.

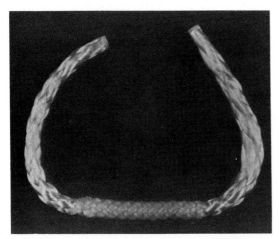

Figure 14—6. A cylindrical, braided polypropylene prosthesis was chosen. Note the tightly braided center and loosely braided ends. The prosthesis was passed through a tunnel in the proximal tibia and routed over the top of the lateral femoral condyle. The prosthesis was internally fixed to bone at both ends.

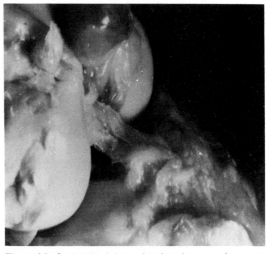

Figure 14—8. Prosthesis in another dog, demonstrating severe fraying of the artificial ligament at 10 months postimplantation.

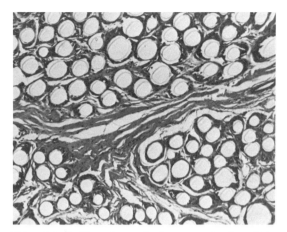

Figure 14—9. Photomicrograph of a cross-section through the prosthesis just after it entered the joint through the posterior capsule, 192 days after implantation. There is little ingrowth between filaments and each filament is surrounded by edema and dead macrophages.

Based on this study, it was felt that total prosthetic ligament replacement would inevitably result in drift, eventually resulting in device laxity even with a material that has low viscoelasticity. If drift did not occur, the prosthesis would likely fail intra-articularly from fatigue. Another solution was sought.

SYNTHETIC AUGMENTATION OF AN INTRA-ARTICULAR AUTOGRAFT

The concept of synthetic augmentation of an autograft was born from the failures of the intra-articular autogenous and total prosthetic replacement of the anterior cruciate ligament in animals. A composite graft is fabricated consisting of an autograft and a synthetic augmentation device. In theory, the synthetic device reinforces the autogenous tissue until recollagenization and strengthening occur. Once this occurs, the autogenous tissue reinforces the synthetic device, limiting adverse cyclic-load problems and preventing drift or fatigue failure. The 3M Company has developed a polypropylene braid to function as a ligament augmentation device (LAD) [4] (Figs. 14–10 and 14–11).

The surgical principles involved in using the polypropylene braid include composite graft formation, direct bone fixation of the braid at one end only, and intra-articular placement. A composite graft of the autogenous tissue and the polypropylene braid is formed using multiple sutures. The initial strength of the composite graft is dependent on the securely tied sutures. It is imperative that the composite graft be directly fixed to bone at one end only. The other end of the composite graft is

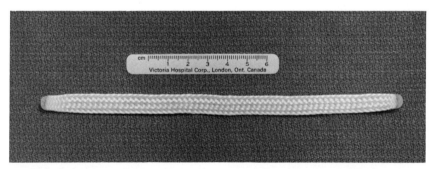

Figure 14—10. Polypropylene braid consisting of high-tenacity polypropylene yarn. It is a flat, straplike device with heat-sealed ends, available in various lengths.

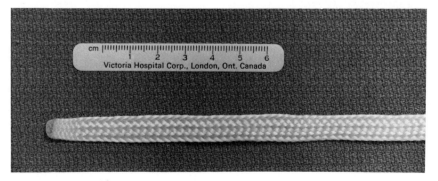

Figure 14—11. Closer view of the polypropylene braid. It comes in 6- and 8-mm widths.

attached to bone only by soft-tissue attachment of the autograft. If the polypropylene braid is internally fixed to bone at both ends, it becomes a frank prosthesis rather than an augmentation device. Such incorrect usage results in total stress-shielding of the autogenous tissue, preventing its proper reorganization. The entire strength of the composite graft then becomes dependent on the polypropylene braid. We feel that the braid is a poor model for an ACL prosthesis, and will fail because of fatigue or drift. The polypropylene braid has been designed and tested for intra-articular use only. Provided that the above principles are adhered to, any existing intra-articular autogenous procedure used to reconstruct the anterior cruciate ligament can be modified to utilize the polypropylene braid.

A two-year study in goats was undertaken to investigate the polypropylene braid for safety and efficacy [5] (Figs. 14–12 and 14–13). The polypropylene braid was found to be safe, without adverse reactions. The augmented reconstructions had better mechanical properties at the time of surgery and again at two years than the nonaugmented reconstructions (Fig. 14–14 and Graph 14–1). Clinically, the knees with the polypropylene-braid–augmented reconstructions had better

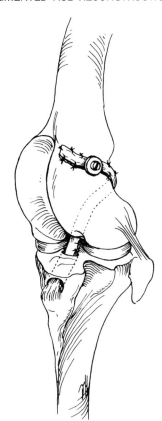

Figure 14–13. The composite graft was passed through a tunnel in the proximal tibia and over the top of the lateral femoral condyle. It was internally fixed to the lateral and distal aspect of the femur with a screw and bushing.

stability and less degenerative change than the knees with the nonaugmented reconstruction. The augmented reconstructions demonstrated insertion fibers between the autogenous tissue and bone (Fig. 14–15).

The conclusion of this study was that the polypropylene braid combined with the autograft described was safe. Efficacy over the nonaugmented procedure was suggested when it was used to reconstruct the excised anterior cruciate ligament in a goat.

POLYPROPYLENE-BRAID—AUGMENTED AND NONAUGMENTED INTRA-ARTICULAR RECONSTRUCTION OF THE ANTERIOR CRUCIATE LIGAMENT IN HUMAN BEINGS

Prior to June 1979, the late Dr. J.C. Kennedy was reconstructing chronic ACL-deficient knees using an intra-articular autograft composed of the central one third of the full-thickness quadriceps tendon, central two thirds of the prepatellar perios-

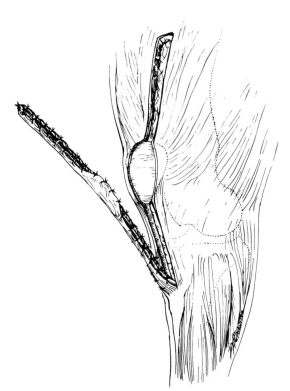

Figure 14–12. The polypropylene braid was sutured to an autograft consisting of the quadriceps aponeurosis, prepatellar periosteum, and central portion of the patellar tendon.

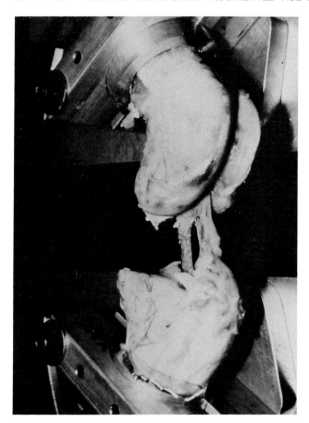

Figure 14–14. Failure loads were evaluated on bone–ligament–bone preparations. The nonaugmented reconstructions failed in the intra-articular portion of the autograft in midsubstance. The polypropylene-braid–augmented reconstruction failed by tibial pullout.

GRAPH 14–1.

TENSILE FAILURE LOAD
in Goat Knees (N = 3 Per Group)

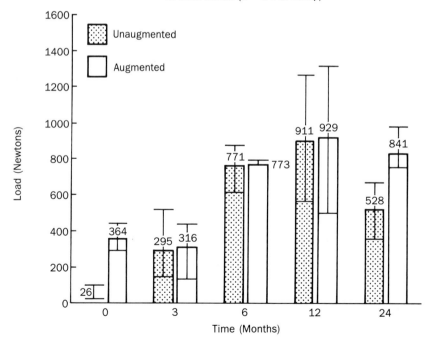

Failure loads were increased in the polypropylene-braid–augmented reconstructions at the time of surgery and at two years. Clinically, the augmented knees were more stable and had less degenerative change on gross inspection than did the nonaugmented knees.

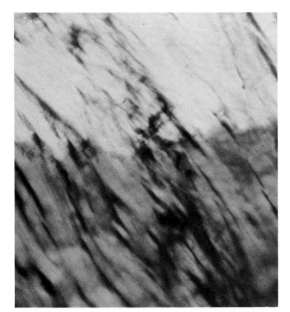

Figure 14—15. Insertion fibers between the autogenous portion of the composite graft and the tibial bone tunnel and distal femur were seen in the 24-month polypropylene-braid–augmented reconstructions only.

same autograft, but with synthetic augmentation (Fig. 14–16). Between January 1, and June 30, 1984, Dr. Kennedy's augmented and non-augmented reconstructions were reviewed simultaneously [6]. As well as the subjective evaluation and physician's examination objective testing, including testing with the KT1000 arthrometer [6], Cybex isokinetic strength analysis [7], and one-leg horizontal hop for distance, was performed. Radiographs of each knee operated on were obtained. This simultaneous clinical review demonstrated that the polypropylene-braid–augmented reconstructions were significantly better subjectively and on physical examination and improved with respect to objective testing. No adverse effects of the polypropylene braid were seen on follow-up for up to 57 months. This review in human beings confirmed the safety and suggested improved efficacy of the augmented procedure, as had the long-term study in goats.

MODIFIED KENNEDY TECHNIQUE TO DIMINISH PATELLOFEMORAL MORBIDITY

teum, and central one third of the full-thickness patellar tendon. This autograft was left attached distally to the tibial tubercle. This particular autograft has an obvious area of weakness centrally in the region of the prepatellar periosteum. The autograft was routed through a tunnel in the proximal tibia and then over the top of the lateral femoral condyle. Once the polypropylene braid became available for investigation in human beings in June 1979, all reconstructions were performed using the

Although we were pleased with stability results in the patients who had undergone polypropylene-braid–augmented ACL reconstruction, we were concerned with the high incidence of patellofemoral morbidity and arthrofibrosis. The incidence was similar in the patients with nonaugmented grafts suggesting that the addition of the polypropylene braid was not the source of the problem. We felt that this morbidity was secondary to the operative technique and postoperative regimen. Dr. Kennedy's original technique involved dislo-

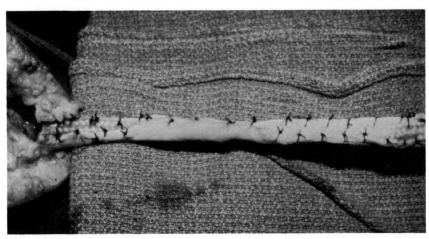

Figure 14—16. An autograft consisting of the central one third of the quadriceps tendon, central two thirds of the patellar periosteum, and central one third of the patellar tendon was augmented synthetically with a polypropylene braid. There is a biologic fixation only at the distal end of the composite graft.

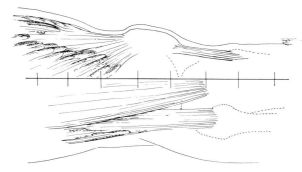

Figure 14–17. The modified technique utilizes a single lateral incision.

cating the patella laterally, possibly damaging the retropatellar articular cartilage. Full-thickness quadriceps tendon defects were created, violating the suprapatellar pouch. Also, the quadriceps and patellar tendon defects were closed with sutures, possibly increasing the patellofemoral compression forces. Perhaps most significant was the six-week immobilization of the knee in a long leg cast prior to starting a rehabilitation program.

We have modified Dr. Kennedy's original technique, hoping to diminish the patellofemoral morbidity. The procedure is performed through a single longitudinal lateral incision centered between the fibular head and the lateral border of the patella (Fig. 14–17). The anterior skin and subcutaneous flap are elevated to expose the quadriceps tendon, prepatellar periosteum, and patellar tendon. The central 1 cm of the quadriceps tendon is elevated, taking only partial thickness. The deepest third of the quadriceps tendon is left intact. The suprapatellar pouch is not entered. The central 2 cm of the prepatellar periosteum is carefully dissected from the patella. The central 1 cm of the patellar tendon is elevated and its biologic attachment to the tibial

tubercle is left intact (Fig. 14–18). A lateral arthrotomy is performed, in which the appropriate length of polypropylene braid is chosen and sutured to the autograft. The autograft is "tubed" around the synthetic device (Figs. 14–19 to 14–21).

An 8-mm hole is drilled from the tibial tubercle into the intercondylar region exiting just anterior and medial to the previous insertion of the anterior cruciate ligament. This hole is radiused proximally and distally with a curette or burr to avoid composite-graft abrasion. The vastus lateralis is elevated from the intermuscular septum and the intramuscular septum is incised distally. This allows entrance of the surgeon's index finger to sweep all soft tissues off the lateral gastrocnemius tendon and muscle over the lateral femoral condyle and to palpate the posterior capsule, knowing that a posterior tibial neurovascular bundle is out of harm's way (Fig. 14–22). A special wire passer is used to create a passageway over the top of the lateral femoral condyle. The patella is not dislocated or subluxed. The composite graft is routed through the tibial tunnel into the intercondylar region. The composite graft is then passed through the defect in the posterior capsule and over the top of the lateral femoral condyle. With the knee at 20 to 30 degrees of flexion the composite graft is tensioned with enough force to eliminate the pivot shift and to return the Lachman sign to normal. The composite graft is internally fixed to the lateral and distal aspect of the femur (Fig. 14–23). After fixation,

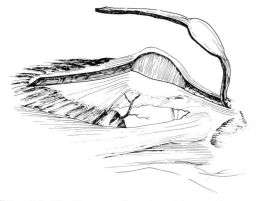

Figure 14–18. The autograft consists of the central 1 cm of the partial-thickness quadriceps tendon, the central 2 cm of the full-thickness prepatellar periosteum, and the central 1 cm of the full-thickness patellar tendon. The autograft is left attached distally to the tibial tubercle.

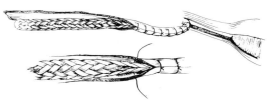

Figure 14–19. The autograft is "tubed" around the polypropylene braid to ensure that autogenous tissue is in contact with bone in the tibial tunnel and the femur.

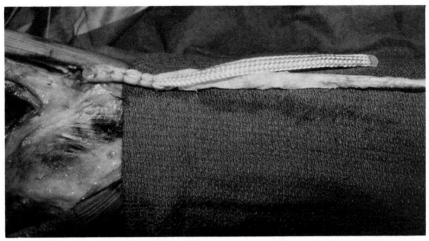

Figure 14—20. The polypropylene braid is partially sutured to the autograft. The suturing technique is important. The initial strength of the composite graft is dependent on a strong bond between the autograft and the synthetic device.

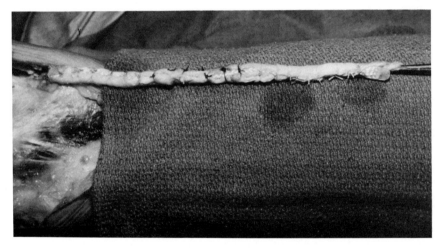

Figure 14—21. The completed composite graft.

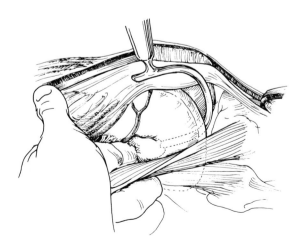

examination should reveal that the knee can be fully extended. The retinaculum is left open to function as a lateral retinacular release. The subcutaneous tissue and skin are closed and a long bulky leg dressing is applied to keep the knee at 30 degrees of flexion.

Four days after the procedure, the bulky dressing is removed and replaced with the patient's

Figure 14—22. The vastus lateralis is elevated from the intermuscular septum and the septum is detached from the distal femur. This allows entrance of the surgeon's index finger to sweep all soft tissues off the lateral gastrocnemius and posterior capsule, thus protecting all neurovascular structures from damage.

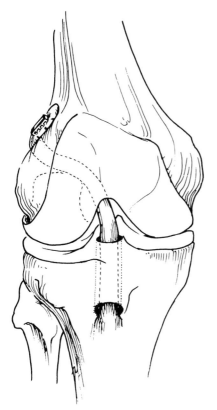

Figure 14–23. The composite graft is passed through a tunnel in the proximal tibia and over the top of the lateral femoral condyle. It is tensioned to return the Lachman sign to normal and to eliminate the pivot shift sign. The composite graft is internally fixed to the distal femur but there is biologic attachment only of the patellar tendon portion of the autograft to the tibial tubercle.

ACL-stabilization brace, which has built-in blocks to motion in a range of 30 to 90 degrees (Fig. 14–24). The patient then starts on gentle active range-of-motion exercises. The knee is brought passively into full extension daily by the therapist. The patient remains on crutches for three months, and active terminal extension exercises are prohibited for six months.

It is our impression that we are seeing less frequent and less severe patellofemoral problems and arthrofibrosis using this modified technique and postoperative regimen. However, we have not formally reviewed this patient group.

REFERENCES

1. Torg JS, Conrad W, Kalen V. Clinical diagnosis of anterior cruciate ligament instability in the athlete. Am J Sports Med 1976; 4:84–93.
2. Galway RD, Beaupre A, MacIntosh DL. Pivot shift: a clinical sign of symptomatic anterior cruciate insufficiency. J Bone Joint Surg (Br) 1972; 54:763.
3. Kennedy JC, Roth JH, Mendenhall HV, et al. Intra-articular replacement of the anterior cruciate ligament deficient knee. Am J Sports Med 1980; 8:1–8.
4. McPherson GK, Kennedy JC, Roth JH, et al. Experimental, mechanical and histologic evaluation of the Kennedy ligament augmentation device. Clin Orthop 1985; 196:186–195.
5. Roth JH, Kennedy JC, Lockstadt H, et al. Polypropylene braid augmented and non-augmented intra-articular anterior cruciate ligament reconstruction. Am J Sports Med 1985; 13:321–336.
6. Daniel DM, Malcolm LL, Lossee G, et al. Instrumented measurement of anterior laxity of the knee. J Bone Joint Surg (Am) 1985; 67:720–726.
7. Watkins MP, Harris BA. Evaluation of isokinetic muscle performance. Clin Sports Med 1983; 2:37–53.

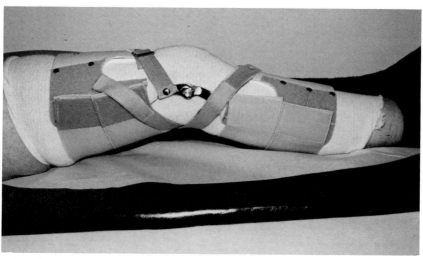

Figure 14–24. An ACL-stabilization brace with metal welds to limit range of motion to 30 to 90 degrees is applied on the fourth postoperative day and physiotherapy is commenced. The welds are removed with a file six weeks after surgery.

15

BIOMECHANICS PROFILE OF THE PROCOL CRUCIATE BIOPROSTHESIS

WILLIAM C. MCMASTER, M.D.

Determining the biomechanical parameters of a prosthetic ligament is mandatory because of the load-bearing role the device will undertake. Concerns about the fatigue potential, stress elongation, load–deformation pattern, and ultimate failure load of such devices are important.

One particular difficulty has been uniformity of testing parameters, which would allow for a logical comparison to be made among various materials, devices, and testing laboratories. In the past, each testing laboratory performed biomechanical characterizations under different conditions and reporting of data was nonuniform, leaving critical gaps that made comparisons among materials and laboratories impossible. Great strides have been made in the field of biomechanics to unify testing parameters and thus eliminate these variances.

In the specific area of ligament testing, problems have been encountered in many areas. Reports on ligament strength have come from tensile tests of bone–ligament–bone preparations, and from various materials removed from the in vivo environment and tested in vitro [1, 2]. This has led to variances in data that are difficult to reconcile and has led to much confusion for the observer of these values. For instance, the age of the ligament will affect the results no matter what the preparation is [3]. In addition, even within the substance of the ligament itself there appears to be a regionalization of mechanical properties such as strain [4].

When one departs from the testing of natural ligaments and looks at various prosthetic devices,

additional constraints are introduced, which must be reconciled. These technical problems are particularly tedious when working with a biologic device. One major technical problem yet to be resolved is the mechanical grips used to secure the material being tested. All currently available prototypes of such grips allow some slippage or crushing of the material, creating a stress riser within it. This will contribute to premature failure of the material, which will bias the results when attempting to profile the mechanical properties of such devices.

These problems have not been unique to the testing of the ProCol CLR bioprosthesis. A number of mechanical grips have been used by various laboratories and include standard crushing types, roller types, and a wedge type. In spite of the improved mechanical advantage of each refinement of these grips, the ultimate problem has not been solved. In large measure the problem arises from the compression exerted by the grips in an attempt to grasp and maintain the material securely during the tensile testing procedure. The forces applied to the material are great. This crushes the material and leads to a concentration of stress at the edge of the grip, where the maximum compression force is being applied. This crushing force weakens the material and provides a point of premature failure. This results in a failure load that is much lower than would be anticipated for the material based on its known potential. These problems were manifest in the fact that during testing, failures occurred at the grip junction rather than in the midsubstance of the ligament test material. As a consequence, the biomechanical properties that can be identified under these testing circumstances are felt to represent minimum values because of these artificially induced failure points. The true biomechanical properties of the materials being tested are thus likely to be considerably higher in value.

Any material or device that is to function as a ligament prosthesis must approximate certain mechanical characteristics described for the natural ligament if the device is to have the potential for long-term use under loaded circumstances. Previous failed clinical devices have been analyzed and demonstrated poor mechanical properties, which were probably responsible for the failure [5].

Any potential device must demonstrate sufficient maximum strength to withstand the high load forces that may be applied during sudden movement or to withstand the application of stress, as would occur in sports or injury-producing events. In addition, the material must exhibit adequate fatigue resistance. Under circumstances of high cyclic loads, the material must maintain its biomechanical properties.

When one reviews the profile of a ligament under tensile load, it is seen that a characteristic load–deformation relation can be identified. In particular, there is a toe region of the curve that is nonlinear, and usually in the 0 to 3 per cent strain area. Here, the curve of a natural ligament demonstrates disproportionate elongation with respect to applied load. Once the material has strained about 4 per cent, the curve assumes a new relation and the linear portion of the curve is entered. This toe region is highly typical of natural ligamentous tissue and extremely important in preventing failures of the ligament material during physiologic function.

The toe region occurs as a consequence of a physical configuration of the collagenous tissue that makes up the ligament. When viewed under high magnification, the collagen bundles can be noted to form a pleated or crimped pattern. Unfolding of the crimp in the initial application of load to the ligament provides a mechanism for ligament elongation without an increase in stress within the ligament tissue. This property protects the ligament against internal damage in the functional load range. Materials that do not have a crimped pattern, or some other attribute to produce a toe region, will be subject to high internal stresses immediately upon application of tensile load. Because the toe region is such an integral identifier of a natural ligament and seems so important to the maintenance of form and function of

the ligament, it is logical that any prosthetic device should, in some way, reproduce this type of load relation. As a consequence, our initial attention turned toward the biologic material as a ligament substitute, affording us the opportunity to take advantage of the natural configuration of a collagenous tensile structure. The material is processed in a nontensed state, thus preserving the inherent crimped pattern.

The Xenotech ProCol CLR Bioprosthesis has undergone several independent assessments. Technical grip problems have been encountered with each of these assessment techniques. However, refinements in equipment, particularly the grip configurations, have continued to improve the quality of results.

The initial assessment of these materials, was performed using the 1122 Instron manufactured by Instron Corp., N.Y., N.Y. (McMaster WC: unpublished data). The materials were production-quality ProCol CLR Bioprostheses. The material was held in the mechanical crushing type of grips with the Instron machine. The extent of exposed material between the grips was 5 cm. The amount of exposed collagen material was kept at a uniform length, avoiding a variable that might be imposed by differences in length of the test specimens. The specimens were kept moist during the procedure to prevent desiccation. Tension was applied by a cross-head travel of 1000 m per minute. This rate will produce a 1.667-cm-per-second distance change between the cross heads and in the exposed 5-cm segment of test material will produce a 33 per cent strain potential per second. Under these testing parameters the CLR ProCol ligament demonstrated an ultimate failure load of about 1000 N. This test was unsatisfactory from many aspects and in particular from the grip point of view. Significant crushing of the materials occurred and visible slipping of the specimens within the grips was identifiable. Failures occurred routinely at the grip edge, indicating that they had induced a significant stress riser. The ultimate loads recorded in these tests were unexpectedly low and indicated the inadequacy of the preparation.

Further tests were performed by the Cleveland Research Institute, which has previously described their results [6, 7]. In order to overcome the mechanical testing problems encountered with the grips, they developed a roller type of grip, which was adapted to the MTS (Material Test Systems, Minneapolis) testing equipment. The roller grip was akin to the Chinese-finger-trap concept in that the applied tensile force resulted in an increased clamping effect in the grip. In addition, the material exited the grip over a rounded edge, thereby attempting to eliminate the edging effect caused by the crushing clamp.

A series of production-grade ProCol CLR specimens were tested. Three loading rates were evaluated—0.5, 5.1, and 50.8 cm per minute. The cross-sectional area of the test specimen was determined using a vernier caliper and a thickness-measuring device whose concept was previously described by Woo et al [8]. The specimens were tested in a thermally equilibrated saline bath at $37°C$. Specimen strain was measured using an exstensometer applied directly to the test material.

The results showed no significant difference in material properties based on load-application rate within the parameters described. Test results of the CLR model ProCol ligament demonstrated a maximum load at failure of 1027 ± 152 N. A maximum tensile strength of 27 ± 8 mPa, and an Elastic modulus of 2500 ± 600 mPa were recorded.

These results reflected the improved test parameters, which allowed the material to exhibit higher strength characteristics under tensile load-to-failure testing. The mechanical grips, in spite of their improved design, were still the weak link in the system and produced a pinching action, resulting again in uniform failure at the grip edges. There was a feeling among the authors that, as a result of these experimental constraints, the reported maximum loads and tensile-strength data were conservative [6, 7].

The most recent reassessment of the ProCol CLR Bioprosthesis has been performed by the biomechanical group at Mayo Clinic Foundation under the direction of K. An, Ph.D. An attempt was made to improve the previous techniques, again concentrating on the grip failure problem [9]. Taking these technical difficulties into consideration, a wedge-type clamp was designed with a self-tightening mechanism. The mechanical efficiency of this grasping device seemed to improve fixation, reduce the tendency for slippage within the clamps, and reduce clamp-induced failures secondary to the crushing mechanism. As a result, preliminary results of tensile tests with this clamp showed tensile failure loads that were higher than had been previously reported. It was felt that this design would be better suited to the ProCol Bioprosthesis in view of its specific constraints, and would result in a more realistic assessment of its biomechanical properties. These clamps were modified to interface with the MTS hydraulic material-testing machine (Material Test Systems, Minneapolis). A series of tests were designed to assess complete tensile failure, creep, and tensile cycles of a fatigue nature. A standard MTS strain-gauge extensometer with a modification of attachment was used to monitor the strain or deformation of the specimens during testing. A Lebow load cell was used to monitor the force application during testing. The analog signals of force from the load cell, strain from the extensometer, and displacement on the test machine were recorded on a Hewlett–Packard recorder and, when appropriate, by a digital computer through AD (Analog to Digital) conversion, and recorded in appropriate units of proper scale factors.

To obtain the material property of the specimens, the test data were normalized by geometric measurements such as cross-sectional area of the midsubstance of the material under test within the extensometer gauge length. The pretest cross-sectional area measurement was computed by approximating the specimen cross-sectional area. The major diameter A and the minor diameter B were measured with a micrometer and the area was computed by $\pi AB/4$ with the cross-sectional configuration of the specimen being roughly an ellipse. Using a micrometer to measure these distances seemed quite adequate in the glutaraldehyde-treated bioprosthesis, as these specimens had sufficient surface rigidity so that the amount of force applied during measurements produced only small variations or error in repeated measurements.

The procedure for testing was as follows: The specimens were selected from production materials, the middle 10-cm portion of the specimen to be tested was wrapped with a saline-saturated tissue paper and then wrapped with waxed paper. The specimens were then left for two to three hours in room air so that the exposed ends would desiccate. Testing caps were attached to these desiccated ends and then the capped ends were placed in the wedge-action grips on the MTS machine. The protective waxed paper and tissue was then removed from the midportion of the specimen and the major and minor diameter of the middle substance of the test specimen was measured as noted above. The exstensometer was then placed and checked. The tensile testing procedure was carried out with the cross heads of the MTS machine separating at the rate of 0.3 in. per second or 46 cm per minute. The load applied and strain were continuously monitored and recorded until the sample failed. All specimens were kept moist with saline during testing. Two testing temperatures were evaluated, 24 and $37°C$. The maximum failure load, the slope of the linear region and the strain at the transition toe region were measured and documented from the load-strain curve.

Creep testing was also deemed to be important in regard to any polymeric material, including collagen materials. As opposed to synthetic polymeric materials and elastomers, the collagen polymer is highly resistant to the creep phenomenon, an intrinsic property that makes it ideal as a tensile-load–transferring device.

Creep tests were performed in two modes—static and dynamic. The static conditions were simply carried out by attaching the specimen to a hanging dead weight of 100 lb. A fixed-length extensometer was attached to the specimen prior to application of load force and the elongation or deformation of the specimen under the applied weight load were recorded. The load was observed over a period of up to 360 minutes. During this time the specimens were constantly irrigated with a saline solution maintained at 37°C.

Creep potential during the dynamic load situation was monitored during the cyclic tensile-load–testing evaluations. This was assessed by monitoring both maximum and minimum peak strains, which were recorded during load tests carried out on the MTS machine, with loads up to 200 lb being applied and the specimen cycled up to 20,000 times.

The results of these tests were also affected by the mechanical problems encountered in the previously described tests assessing mechanical properties of the ProCol CLR Bioprosthesis. Although the mechanical grips designed in the Mayo Clinic assessment performed superiorly to previous designs, failures of the materials at the grip site were still seen, and this problem could not be completely resolved. Thus in any of the evaluations carried out so far, improvements in the design of the mechanical testing grips has consistently resulted in increases in the ultimate load exhibited by the device. It is therefore important to understand that the failure loads observed during each of these test circumstances is not a duplication of the ultimate load of the material. The results are a conservative estimate of the ultimate load.

There was no statistical difference between the failure load of the CLR device when comparison was made between room-temperature and body-temperature tensile failure testing. Neither was a statistical difference noted when properties such as stiffness, strength, and modulus of elasticity were compared. In these tests, the ProCol CLR Bioprosthesis demonstrated a mean failure load of 2160 ± 400 N, a modulus of elasticity of 2172 ± 112 mPa, and a failure strength of 90 ± 17 mPa. Under these failure tests, the strain observed in the toe region was 2.2 ± 1 per cent and the strain at 100 lb. of force application 3 ± 1.2 per cent. It is of interest that the mechanical properties of unfixed bovine tendon with a cross-sectional area equal to the test specimens showed a failure load of 1800 ± 430 N,

a modulus of elasticity of 2327 ± 285 mPa, and a failure strength of 74 ± 20 mPa. It would appear from this that the glutaraldehyde cross linking of the collagen material has produced a 17 per cent increase in the failure-load strength while the modulus of elasticity was essentially unchanged.

DISCUSSION

Mechanical testing of the ProCol CLR Bioprosthesis has been done under a variety of circumstances, using sophisticated test devices and equipment. As previously noted, evaluation of biologic specimens is difficult because of the mechanical effects of the gripping devices used to hold the test samples. The grips crush the material, producing a stress riser within it, and negatively affect the results.

In spite of these constraints, all methods of testing the ProCol CLR Bioprosthesis have indicated a material with a high load capability and sufficient margin to carry the loads that have been described for the human anterior cruciate ligament. The demonstrated load to failure of the ProCol CLR Bioprosthesis is 2158 N, which is greater than has been described for human anterior cruciate ligaments [1]. An estimation of the potential strength of the ProCol CLR Bioprosthesis can be made by assuming that the ultimate tensile strains of the collagenous fibers range from 10 to 18 per cent [10]. This would result in an ultimate load for this device between 3000 and 4000 N.

It has been estimated by many authors that the loads applied to the human anterior cruciate ligament in a variety of activities, including ADL (Activities of Daily Living) activities as well as sports activities do not exceed 1000 N. At a load of 1000 N and above, failures of the human anterior cruciate ligament occur. Thus this device has a demonstrated safety factory of 2:1 against that failure load. Using the theoretical ultimate load potential for the device, a safety factor as high as 4:1 could be expected.

The ProCol CLR Bioprosthesis is stiffer than the natural cruciate ligament. When the stiffness is assessed as a unit of force per strain rather than as force over a unit of length, the necessity for normalizing the initial length of the specimen is eliminated. The average stiffness by this method for the CLR Bioprosthesis is 52 kN per strain, which is about three times as high as that reported for the human anterior cruciate ligament by Noyes and Grood [3]. One must allow that this stiffness occurs in the more linear portion of the load–deformation curve well above the toe region. As this progresses, early fiber rupture within the tissue begins and failures will occur [10, 11]. The implanted device, however, would not be expected to function, under normal load circumstances, in this linear range where failure would occur. This is supported by Armes and Claes and their colleagues, who showed that during normal knee motion, the anterior cruciate ligament has been estimated to exhibit a maximum strain of 3.5 per cent [12, 13]. This strain area corresponds to the toe region of the force-elongation curve in both the natural cruciate ligament and the ProCol CLR Bioprosthesis. Thus in the physiologic working region of the cruciate ligament, both the natural ligament and the ProCol Bioprosthesis exhibit similar patterns (Graph 15–1).

Excessive creep of a ligament material under tensile load would lead to stress elongation of the material, development of plastic strain within it, and resultant clinical laxity. This is not a desirable characteristic for a load-bearing device. In materials, creep is load- as well as temperature-dependent [14]. The creep load in this circumstance was at the upper border of that in the anterior cruciate ligament during activities of daily living. Under static load circumstances, with the load applied up to 360 minutes, an average creep of 0.24 per cent was noted, which would imply that the device has excellent protection against creep under physiologic load circumstances. The creep factors were also not dependent upon the ambient temperature during testing. Under dynamic loading circumstances, the ProCol CLR Bioprosthesis was highly resistance to work-induced creep. After 20,000 cycles, creep was less than 0.2 per cent. In long-term studies of up to 10 million cycles with load between 445 to 890 N, no additional creep could be measured. This data is superior to that reported in the literature for other ligament devices" [15, 16].

The ability of a ligament device to retain tensile load characteristics after it has been worked is extremely important. Fatigue or work hardening of the device may result in failure. When ProCol CLR Bioprosthetic devices were cyclically loaded up to 10 million cycles at 0 to 890 N, then subjected to tensile failure tests, they demonstrated an averaged load of 2513 N. This was not significantly different from the value reported for the virgin, noncycled, devices. On the basis of the testing, accepting approximately 1 million cycles per year of implant life, such a device could have a potential for lasting 10 years.

SUMMARY

Based on the biomechanical studies completed by a variety of laboratories, the ProCol CLR Bioprosthetic ligament device has exhibited excellent strength, resistance to creep, and fatigue life. With strength reserves potentially three to four times that of the natural anterior cruciate ligament, it has excellent potential to substitute for the cruciate ligament. These assumptions are based on in vitro testing methods and one must maintain perspective as to device alterations, either enhancement or degradation, which could occur in an in vivo environment. The clinical and laboratory data, however, acquired from longer-term animal and human clinical studies, will prove the adequacy of the device based on its long-term maintenance of knee stability and function.

GRAPH 15–1.

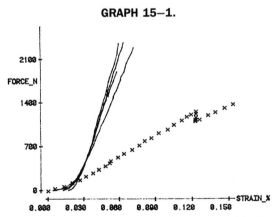

The human ACL tensile test curve is represented by the xxxxx line. The ProCol CLR Bioprosthesis is represented by the —— lines. The toe region is represented in the 0 to 3 per cent strain area, and the overlap of the two curves in this area can be appreciated.

REFERENCES

1. Noyes FR, Butler DL, Grood ES, Zernick RF, Hefzy MS. Biomechanical analysis of human ligament grafts used in knee ligament repairs and reconstructions. J Bone Joint Surg (Am) 1984; 66a:344–352.
2. Kennedy JC, Hawkins RJ, Willis RB, Danylchuk KD. Tension studies of human knee ligaments. J Bone Joint Surg (Am) 1976; 58a:350–355.
3. Noyes FR, Grood ES. The strength of the anterior cruciate ligament in humans and rhesus monkeys. J Bone Joint Surg (Am) 1976; 58a:1074–1082.
4. Woo SL. Mechanical properties of tendons and ligaments I. Quasistatic and nonlinear viscoelastic properties Biorheology 1982; 19:385–396.
5. Grood ES, Noyes FR. Cruciate ligament prosthesis: strength, creep, and fatigue properties. J Bone Joint Surg (Am) 1976; 58a:1083–1088.
6. Berg WS, Starhurski TM, Moran JM, et al. High loading rate and osillatory evaluation of bovine xenografts. Trans Ann Meeting Orthop Res Soc 1984; 9:381.

7. Berg WS, Starhurski TM, Moran JM, et al. Mechanical properties of bovine xenografts. Orthop Trans 1983; 7(2):279–280.

8. Woo SL, Akeson WH, Jermmont GF. Measurement of nonhomogeneous, directional mechanical properties of articular cartilage. J Biomechanics 1976; 9:758–791.

9. An K. Xenotech ligament: biomechanics. Presented at the Second Annual Conference on Prosthetic Ligament Reconstruction of the Knee, Palm Springs, Calif., March 21 to 24, 1985.

10. Viidik A. A rheological model for uncalcified parallel-fibered collagenous tissue. J Biomechanics 1968; 1:3–11.

11. Butler DL, Grood ES, Noyes FR, Ziernicke RF. Biomechanics of ligaments and tendons. In: Exercise and Sports Science Review, vol. 6, Hutton R, ed. Philadelphia: Franklin Institute Press, 1978:125–182.

12. Armes SW, Renstrom P, Stanwyk TS, Hogan M, Johnson RJ, Pope MH. Strain within the anterior cruciate ligament during hamstring and quadriceps activity. Proc Annu Meeting Orthop Res Soc 1985; 10:139.

13. Cleas LE, Durselen L, Kiefer H. Influence of load, flexion, and muscle forces on the stress and strain of knee ligaments. Proc Annu Meeting Orthop Res Soc 1986; 11:238.

14. Cohen RE, Hooley CJ, McCrum G. Viscoelastic creep of collagenous tissue. J Biomechanics 1976; 9:175–184.

15. Bolton WC, Bruckman WC. The Gore-Tex™ expanded polytetrafluoroethylene prosthetic ligament: an in vitro and in vivo evaluation. Clin Orthop 1985; 196:202–214.

16. McPherson GK, Mendenhall HV, Gibbons DF, et al. Experimental, mechanical, and histologic evaluation of the Kennedy ligament augmentation device. Clin Orthop 1985; 196:186–195.

16

OPEN ANTERIOR CRUCIATE LIGAMENT RECONSTRUCTION WITH PROCOL BIOPROSTHESIS: RESULTS AT 24 MONTHS—U.S. SERIES

WILLIAM C. MCMASTER, M.D.

INTRODUCTION

Disabling symptomatic instability associated with the anterior cruciate ligament (ACL)-deficient knee poses a significant management challenge to the orthopedic surgeon. Procedures for stabilizing ACL deficiency continue to be advocated, coming full circle from the teachings of the pioneers, such as Hey Groves, who conceived early techniques for ACL reconstruction [15, 16, 23]. The proposed procedures for treatment have swung from substitution to repair to neglect and back again [6]. Recent approaches include attempts at acute repair with augmentation, if necessary [17]. There is a better identification of the patient population that would benefit from ACL reconstruction [14]. While not all such knees are significantly symptomatic, the group with disabling instability may benefit from reconstruction. [8, 30].

Currently there is no technique that can reliably reestablish stability of ACL-deficient knees. The usual reconstruction employs autologous material harvested in and about the knee. The results of these techniques at three to five years after operation may be disappointing [11]. As a consequence, a variety of cruciate ligament prostheses have been developed are under clinical investigation according to the Investigational Device Exemption (IDE) regulations of the Food and Drug Administration (FDA). No ligament prosthesis material has received full FDA premarketing approval and thus none are available for use by surgeons. The proposed prosthetic devices vary widely and include carbon fibers [18, 26, 28], Dacron-based products [10, 24], Gore-Tex [3], and collagen materials from various sources. Freeze-dried allograft materials have been used in several centers and are not regulated by FDA. Early results are mixed [5].

One collagen-based material is a bioprosthesis of bovine origin known as a bovine xenograft (Procol Bioprothesis, Xenotech Laboratories, Inc., Irvine, Calif.) A native tendon harvested from a bovine source is specially prepared by a proprietary glutaraldehyde cross-linking process, which renders the material sterile and chemically stable. Animal evaluation of this material has demonstrated the biologic response and efficacy in those animal models [13, 19–22]. Biomechanical data confirm that this bioprosthesis is capable of functioning in the anterior cruciate position [1, 2]. Under FDA IDE regulations, a clinical trial was begun in human beings with the Procol xenograft prosthesis in February 1982. I report here on patients in the United States with anterior cruciate implants placed through an open technique.

BIOMATERIAL CHARACTERIZATION

The xenograft collagen bioprosthesis is a Y-shaped bovine tendon with an average 8-mm diameter. The collagen molecule consists of three amino acid chains bound in a helical pattern organized by intermolecular cross-links [27]. These are vital to the maintenance of the collagenous form, its function, and chemical stability against enzyme attack. Increasing the number of these cross-links should increase the molecular stability, particularly if the cross-links are of a covalent nature. Glutaraldehyde, a dialdehyde, is one of the most effective known cross-linking agents for collagen [7]. The bonds created have high chemical stability. Glutaraldehyde-stabilized collagen is resistant to mechanical, chemical, and biologic degradation [4, 9, 25, 29].

The weak immunogenicity of tendinous (Type I) collagen is further reduced by cross-linking, which probably alters antigenic sites. If the density of cross-linking is not controlled, the treated material will be rendered unacceptably stiff and brittle. The proprietary Procol xenograft bioprosthesis process avoids this and preserves most of the material's natural resilience. The Procol bioprosthesis is durable and exhibits host acceptance with the biomechanical characteristics of a suitable material for ligament substitution.

STUDY GROUP PROFILE AND PROTOCOL

This presentation is an extraction of the Pre-Market Approval Request submitted to the FDA in July 1986. The total number of patients worldwide receiving xenograft implants for any indication during that investigational period was 811, with a total of 915 xenografts implanted. Some patients had more than one device implanted. Sex distribution of the patient population was about 1:2 females:males.

This report will review the subgroup of patients in the United States who received xenograft bioprosthesis implants in the anterior cruciate position by open techniques; these were implanted between February 1982 and September 1984. This device has been implanted predominantly in chronic ACL-deficient knees although a few acute ACL repairs and augmentation have been done. Many patients had undergone previous unsuccessful procedures. This group of patients was reviewed as

of September 1986; thus all devices had been in place for at least 24 months. Ninety-three patients in the United States received an open anterior cruciate xenograft ligament prosthesis in that period.

The operative, postoperative, and reporting protocols were established with the FDA prior to the initiation of the study and reflected prevailing practices. Since then, some new concepts have appeared. The original postoperative protocol called for eight weeks of plaster immobilization at 45 degrees of flexion, followed by brace-protected range of motion allowing 10 degrees of additional extension per month. Weight bearing was allowed once 20 degrees of extension had been reached. There have been variations to this protocol dictated by recent developments and the introduction of arthroscopic techniques of implantation. Mostly, the trend has been toward earlier (restricted) knee motion, avoiding active terminal quadriceps contractions.

As agreed upon in the original protocol with the FDA, the clinical outcome of anterior cruciate implants was to be documented by comparing preoperative and 6-, 12-, and 24-month postoperative data using a knee-assessment score. This score is the combined total of six objective clinical tests using a 0 to 4 rating spread for each test. In this test, a score of 24 represented the worst possible result. It has been determined that a score of approximately 2 points was most consistent with that seen in an uninjured knee. The score was determined by the observer's grading of six clinical signs: Lachman, 90-degree neutral anterior drawer, Slocum's test at 90 degrees for both anterior lateral and anterior medial rotational instabilities, the pivot shift, and effusion. The resultant score is heavily weighted toward stability factors (Table 16–1). Student's t-test was used to analyze results with $P < 0.05$ considered significant. For comparison of the individual components of the

TABLE 16–1. COMPONENTS OF THE COMBINED FUNCTIONAL SCORE FOR ASSESSMENT OF OUTCOME IN PROCOL BIOPROSTHESIS ACL RECONSTRUCTION

Criteria	Best To Worse
Lachman	0–4
Anterior drawer	0–4
Anterior lateral rotational instability	0–4
Anterior medial rotational instability	0–4
Pivot shift	0–4
Effusion	0–4
Total	0–24

composite score, the Fisher exact test was used. The null hypothesis tested is that there is no difference between the populations. The null hypothesis was rejected by a P value <0.05.

RESULTS

As of September 1986, 93 patients were beyond 24 months from the time of implantation. Seventeen patients (18 per cent) of that group had had explantation of the device while 2 (2 per cent) had had an explantation and underwent immediate re-implantation of a xenograft, which has been retained. Twenty-three patients (25 per cent) had been lost to follow up.

Of the original 93 patients, 52 (56 per cent) had complete documentation beyond the 24-month period for reporting purposes. Thus stability results are based on these 52 patients with surviving implants. In order to gain a perspective on the data, and in particular reference to any temporal deterioration of stability results, the patient's stability data is presented for each required testing marker they had passed—i.e., 6, 12, or 24 months—and broken down into the components of the stability test group. The six-test composite score for the 52 patients can be broken down according to postoperative time preoperative = 11.4, 6-month = 1.1, 12-month = 2.3, and 24-month = 2.6. The knee assessment score data in Graph 16–1 show a statistically significant increase between 6 and 12 months (P > 0.04). The additional change between 12 and 24 months is not significant (P = 0.26). The composite score was also assessed according to its various components using the Fisher exact test.

Looking at the Lachman test, the results indicated an average preoperative score of 2.8 with scores of 0.6 at 6 months, 0.9 at 12 months, and 0.9 at 24 months. The greatest change occurred between the preoperative and postoperative scores as would be expected (P = 0.0000). Between 6 to 12 months and 12 to 24 months no further significant changes occurred (P = 0.073 and P = 0.602, respectively). The 90-degree anterior drawer test showed similar results with an average preoperative score of 2.6 and 6-, 12-, and 24-month scores of 0.5, 0.9, and 0.9, respectively. The P values for these comparisons were preoperative to 6 months, P = 0.0000; 6 to 12 months, P = 0.131; and 12 to 24 months, P = 0.429. Similarly, for the pivot-shift test, the preoperative average score was 2.2 and the 6-, 12-, and 24-month scores were 0.1, 0.2, and 0.1, respectively. The respective P values for these comparisons were preoperative to 6 months, P = 0.0000; 6 to 12 months, P = 0.658; and 12 to 24 months, P = 0.381. All other components of the composite test score showed similar statistically improved test results postoperatively with the results maintained until the 24-month time frame (Graph 16–2). While the statistical results are not compiled beyond the 24-month observation cycle, patients who have been reviewed at 36 months and beyond have demonstrated maintenance of stability.

Complications have been divided into three categories. The first includes graft-related incidents; the second, clinical infection; and the third, non-grafted-related clinical complications. Of 10 total graft-related complications, 7 consist of postoperative effusion and/or graft rupture. Three other graft-related complications include synovial fistula at the opening of a bone tunnel and extra-articular synovial-fluid accumulation.

Five infections were documented. There is no evidence that any of the clinical infections were related to product sterility problems. All infections manifested within three months. An overall infection rate of 5.0 per cent (5 of 93) was seen for the open anterior cruciate group.

Complications considered to be non-graft-

GRAPH 16–1.
Data from the clinical series of open ACL reconstructions done in the United States (follow-up at least two years).

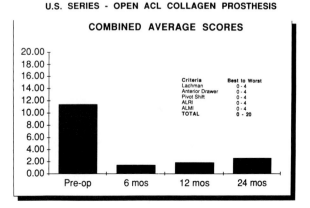

U.S. SERIES - OPEN ACL COLLAGEN PROSTHESIS

COMBINED AVERAGE SCORES

Criteria	Best to Worst
Lachman	0 - 4
Anterior Drawer	0 - 4
Pivot Shift	0 - 4
ALRI	0 - 4
ALMI	0 - 4
TOTAL	0 - 20

U.S SERIES - OPEN ACL COLLAGEN PROSTHESIS

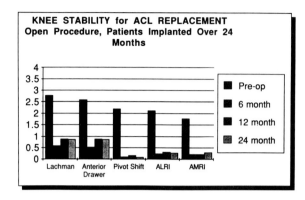

GRAPH 16–2.
Graphic representation of the individual components of the combined score with preoperative averages compared to postoperative assessments at the time intervals indicated.

related were due to reinjury, inadequate surgical technique, or inappropriate patient selection. Thirteen such occurrences have been documented. Six cases involved reinjury, usually a fall, resulting in graft rupture. Seven cases included restricted motion due to incorrect (usually excessive) tensioning of the graft, nonisometric tunnel placement, or poor patient cooperation, resulting in problems during rehabilitation.

Graft-related complications and infections have been tracked by six-month intervals from study onset. Each six-month study interval was considered a distinct population and all complications were assigned to the six-month interval in which the implantation occurred. Over the course of the study, there has been a steady reduction in the number of graft-related complications and infections. During the most recent six-month implant interval the incidence of graft-related complications and infections have been reduced to the 2.5 per cent level.

DISCUSSION

While this interim report is not definitive in regards to long-term (three- to five-year) assessment of open ACL reconstruction results with bovine xenografts, the two-year trends are encouraging. This biomaterial provides excellent initial stability. Although the data show a statistically significant change in stability between the 6- and 12-month assessment, this is felt to be the result of joint capsule and scar resilience changes occurring as a part of normal postoperative recovery, which should stabilize by the 12th month. This concept is supported by the 24-month retest, which showed no significant additional change.

As with any prosthetic implant, complications that compromise results are always of concern. In this review, complication rates show a decreasing temporal trend, which suggests that a learning-curve phenomenon is operating. Improved procedural guidelines based on early experience have lessened the potential for complications for investigators during the latter part of the study. As would be expected, all infections manifested within the first three months after implantation. The decreasing rate of infection was presumably due to improved intraoperative techniques and surgeon awareness of the potential for infection, which prompted the use of prophylactic intravenous antibiotics and care in handing the prosthesis prior to implantation.

For the most part technique-related complications have occurred early and have decreased during the course of the investigation. This may be consequent to the appreciation that technical aspects of the prosthetic cruciate ligament procedure are crucial to success. The bovine xenograft is a true prosthesis and, by virtue of the stable chemical cross-linking employed and unlike autologous tissue, its collagen matrix is resistant to a rapid remodeling phase. The tendency to apply high tension during graft implantation, as one might with autologous tissue, presumably to compensate for graft elongation during the remodeling process, is not appropriate for the xenograft. A full range of motion of the joint must be possible at the time of final fixation of the xenograft. Like autologous tissues and other repair materials, xenografts are susceptible to abrasion caused by impingement on bone surfaces as a result of suboptimal tunnel position, intercondylar-notch encroachment, or poor radiusing of bone tunnel mouths. A more vertical femoral tunnel orientation is better. The optimal position for the tunnels is the isometric position. This needs to be accurately assessed at the time of surgery to ensure that no pistoning or moving of the graft material occurs during a full range of knee motion. Radiusing of the tunnel edges is important to avoid abrasion of the graft material or the creation of a stress riser. Abrasion of the graft will result in minute particulate matter being released into the environs of the knee, which may result in a nonspecific irritating synovitis.

Bony attachment and fixation within the tunnels is extremely important; therefore every effort is made to match carefully the caliber of the tunnel with the cross-sectional area of the graft material. It is naive to expect that adequate host-tissue fixation will occur if large gaps are present between graft and the bony tunnel. Such a gap may, in fact, promote synovial-fluid tracking along the graft material, accumulating subcutaneously at the openings of the bony tunnels, particularly at the tibia. This may lead to "blister formation" as a consequence of the artificially induced synovial fistula.

Clearing the intercondylar notch is necessary to ensure adequate visualization for optimal positioning of the femoral port. In the chronic ACL-deficient knee, osteophytic encroachment on the intercondylar notch may occur. This may cause graft impingement, particularly as the knee comes to full extension, resulting in either premature rupture of the graft or abrasion-wear debris within the knee joint. Therefore a notchplasty or condyle osteotomy is important [12]

This in-progress review supports the efficacy of the xenograft bioprosthesis to stabilize the ACL-deficient knee initially. For the subgroup of patients with at least a 24-month follow-up, it is demonstrated that joint stability is maintained.

SUMMARY

Management of the symptomatic ACL-deficient knee employing autologous reconstruction techniques is often clinically disappointing. Scientific focus has been placed on other materials as substitutes. A bovine tendon material treated by a glutaraldehyde-based process is currently under FDA IDE clinical evaluation. This report on the open ACL xenograft implants was extracted from data on implants placed from February 1982 to September 1984. There were 93 isolated ACL implants placed by open technique.

Follow-up testing has been done at 6, 12, and 24 months, utilizing a knee-assessment score derived from six objective clinical tests. The averaged preoperative score was 11.4. The postoperative scores were 1.1 at 6 months, 2.3 and 12 months, and 2.6 at 24 months. Individual components of the combined stability-test score also demonstrated a similar maintenance of improvement through the review period. Complications were divided into three categories: graft related [11], infections [5], and non-graft-related [13]. More complications were encountered early and have decreased with further experience. There are technical considerations that must be followed carefully to avoid problems. These preliminary results demonstrate that excellent joint stability can be achieved with the xenograft prosthesis, and this has been maintained in the group of patients followed beyond two years.

REFERENCES

1. Berg WS, Starhurski TM, Morgan JM, et al. Mechanical properties of bovine xenografts. Orthop Trans 1983; 7(2):279–280.
2. Idem. High loading rate and osillatory evaluation of bovine xenografts. Trans Annu Meeting Orthop Res Soc 1984; 9:381.
3. Bolton WC, Bruckman WC. The Gore-Tex™ expanded polytetrafluoroethylene prosthetic ligament: an in vitro and in vivo evaluation. CORR 1985; 196:202–214.
4. Bowes J, Cater C. The interaction of aldehydes with collagen. Biochim Biophys Acta 1968; 168:341–352.
5. Bright RW, Green WT. Freeze-dried fascia lata allografts: a review of 47 cases. J Pediatr Orthop 1981; 1:13–22.
6. Burnett QM, Fowler PJ. Reconstruction of the anterior cruciate ligament: historical overview. Orthop Clin North Am 1985; 16(1):143–158.
7. Chvapil M, Owen JA, Clark DS. Effect of collagen crosslinking on the rate of resorption of implanted collagen tubing in rabbits. J Biomed Mater Res 1977; 11:197–314.
8. Clancy WG. Intra-articular reconstruction of the anterior cruciate ligament. Orthop Clin North Am 1985; 16(2):181–190.
9. Deshmukh K, Nimni M. A defect in the intra molecular and inter molecular cross linking of collagen caused by penicillimine. II. Functional groups involved in the interaction process. J Biol Chem 1969; 244:1787–1795.
10. Fijikawa K. Leeds–Keio ligament. Presented at the Second Annual UCLA Conference on Prosthetic Ligament Reconstruction of the Knee, Palm Springs, Calif. March 22 to 24, 1985.
11. Friedman MJ, Sherman OH, Fox JM, et al. Autogenic anterior cruciate ligament (ACL) anterior reconstruction of the knee: a review. Clin Orthop 1985; 196:9–14.
12. Fullerton LR, Andrews JR. Mechanical block to extension following augmentation of the anterior cruciate ligament: a case report. Am J Sports Med 1984; 12:166–168.
13. Gabbardella R, Jurgutis J, Nimni M, et al. The replacement of anterior cruciate ligaments with xenograft implants. Orthop Trans 1984; 8(2):248.
14. Godehon DL, Warren RF, Wickiewicz TL. Acute repairs of the anterior cruciate ligament—past and present. Orthop Clin North Am 1985; 16(1):111–126.
15. Grood ES, Noyes FR. Cruciate ligament prosthesis: strength, creep, and fatigue properties. J Bone Joint Surg (Am) 1976; 58:1083–1088.
16. Hey Groves EW. Operation for the repair of cruciate ligaments. Lancet 1917; 2:674–674.

17. Holden DL, Jackson DW. Treatment selection in acute anterior cruciate ligament tears. Orthop Clin North Am 1985; 16(1):99–110.

18. Jenkins DH. Ligament induction by filamentous carbon fiber. Clin Orthop 1985; 196:86–87.

19. McMaster WC. A histologic assessment of canine anterior cruciate substitution with bovine xenograft. Clin Orthop 1985; 196:196–201.

20. McMaster WC, Kouzelos J. Liddle S, et al. Tendon grafting with glutaraldehyde and fixed material. J Biomed Mater Res 1976; 10:259–271.

21. McMaster WC, Liddle S, Anzel S, et al. Medial collateral ligament replacement in the rabbit: a preliminary report. Am J Sports Med 1975; 3:271–276.

22. Idem. Bovine xenograft collateral ligament replacement in the dog. J Orthop Res 1985; 3:492–498.

23. Noyes FR, Grood ES. The strength of the anterior cruciate ligament in humans and rhesus monkeys. J Bone Joint Surg (Am) 1976; 58:1074–1082.

24. Park JP, Grana WA, Clintwood JS. A high strength Dacron augmentation for cruciate ligament reconstruction: a two year canine study. Clin Orthop 1985; 196:175–185.

25. Richards F, Knowles J. Glutaraldehyde as a protein cross-linking reagent. J Mol Biol 1968; 37:231–233.

26. Strover AE, Firer P. The use of carbon fiber implants in anterior cruciate ligament surgery. Clin Orthop 1985; 196:88–98.

27. Viidik A. Functional properties of collagenous tissues. Int Rev Connect Tissue Res 1973; 6:127–215.

28. Weiss AB, Blazina ME, Goldstein AR, et al. Ligament replacement with an absorbable co-polymer carbon fiber scaffold—early clinical experience. Clin Orthop 1985; 196:77–85.

29. Wold F. Bifunctional reagents. Methods Enzymol 1972; 25:623–651.

30. Zarins B. Combined intra-articular and extra-articular reconstructions for anterior tibial subluxation. Orthop Clin North Am 1985; 16(2):223–226.

17

CLINICAL EXPERIENCE IN CORRECTION OF CHRONIC ANTERIOR CRUCIATE LIGAMENT DEFICIENCY WITH BOVINE XENOGRAFTS: A 5-YEAR STUDY

E. PETER ABBINK, M.D.

INTRODUCTION

Chronic instability of the knee poses surgical dilemmas, particularly when prior attempts at reconstruction using different autologous materials have failed. Bovine xenografts (Model CLR, Xenotech Laboratories, Inc., Irvine, Calif.) seemed to offer the potential for overcoming some of these problems in that they are a strong (at least 2500 N load to failure), natural material that could be expected to have desirable biocompatibility properties. Studies in the dog had shown this material to be well incorporated in osseous tunnels and to be slowly invaded intra-articularly by host tissue after eight months [1]. These xenografts are treated with glutaraldehyde to improve in vivo longevity, as evidenced by a complete lack of susceptibility to collagenese, and to eliminate the weak immunogenicity of the bovine type I collagen.

No evidence of immunogenicity could be found in this clinical study. It must be emphasized that sophisticated chemical procedures are required to obtain complete and uniform cross-linking of bovine tendinous collagen, while retaining most of the original suppleness and the natural complex

stress–strain curve with the associated toe region. Any prosthetic device must be judged from many viewpoints to determine its true usefulness. Implantation must not result in allergic or rejection reactions, must not require inordinate immobilization of the joint, and must be biomechanically effective. While these criteria were shown to be met in this study, the primary objective was to determine the longer-term (over two years) functional and stability characteristics of this prosthesis and to refine the appropriate surgical techniques beyond the level that can be learned from animal models.

INDICATIONS

Giving way, with clinical evidence of a marked positive pivot shift, during competitive and recreational athletics and even during activities of daily living indicates the necessity of a reconstruction procedure, extra-articular, intra-articular, or both, depending on the kind of instability.

An extra-articular procedure on the lateral side will be insufficient to obtain long-term stability in cases of complex rotatory instability, especially when prior meniscectomies at both sides have been performed. It will also be insufficient in cases of long-standing chronic anterior cruciate ligament (ACL) insufficiency, with subsequent stretching of the remaining capsular ligaments, showing a marked anteroposterior drawer sign exceeding 10 mm with a positive pivot shift in internal and external rotation.

An intra-articular procedure on its own in these cases is deemed to become insufficient in time because of the above-mentioned overstretching of the remaining structures and the complexity of the femoral anchorage site, which allows some kind of compromise between the normal anatomy and surgical fixation sites, suffering their own biomechanical insufficiencies.

An anatomical tibial attachment for a graft is almost reproducible by the use of a bone tunnel through the tibial head.

In our first series of patients, all implantations except two over-the-top procedures used the bovine xenograft model CLR in a double-bone-tunnel procedure, with the femoral tunnel positioned posteriorly and as vertically as possible. It originated distally from the original femoral attachment site. The tibial tunnel started from the anteromedial aspect of the tibia about 1 cm proximal to the superior border of the pes anserinus and approximately 2 cm medial from the tibial tubercle. The center of

the intra-articular tunnel port was located at the anterior border of the original ACL attachment site.

Extra-articular procedures were not routinely included. Tunnel diameters closely approximating the variable graft diameter (6 mm minimum to 9 mm maximum) were used and the xenografts were stapled at the distal and proximal points of emergence, leaving minimal graft material outside the staple.

SURGICAL TECHNIQUE SERIES II (SEPTEMBER 1982 TO JANUARY 1986)

Use of only the above methods in the first series of patients yielded poor results, primarily attributable to graft rupture. Serious consideration had been given to terminating the series earlier but the problems seem to revolve primarily around surgical technique, which was believed to be improvable. Careful attention was paid to isometric tunnel positioning, since it was becoming known that as little as a 2 to 3 mm malpositioning of the femoral tunnel could create inordinate stresses in full extension and deep flexion, together with pistoning in the tunnels, which could impede the biologic fixation process of the bovine xenograft.

In the second series the center of the tibial tunnel was located in the center (or slightly posterior to it)

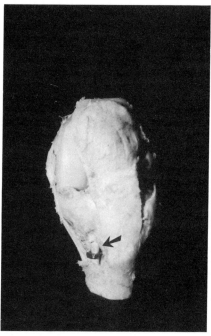

Figure 17–1. Extra-articular tunnel exit at the anteromedial site of the proximal tibia.

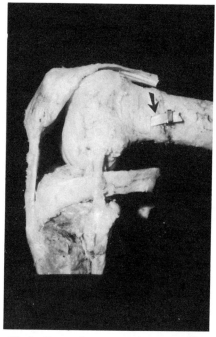

Figure 17–2. Extra-articular tunnel exit at the lateral side of the distal femur.

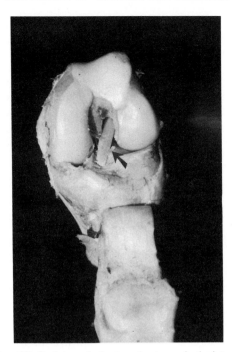

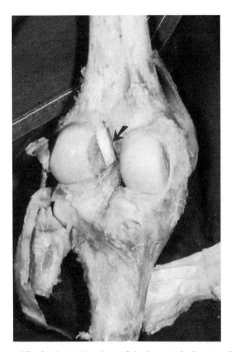

Figure 17–3. Intra-articular tunnel entrance in the intercondylar notch and at the tibial plateau.

Figure 17–4. Posterior view of the intra-articular tunnel entrance at the lateral femoral condyle.

of the native ACL. The femoral tunnel started slightly posterior to the midline of the femoral shaft from an area where small periosteal vessels cross the distal femur. The center of the tunnel was aimed at a point superior and posterior in the notch located on the original insertion site of the native ACL (approximately 4 mm anterior to the posterior margin).

An extensive notchplasty was done, with special attention to the anterior and superior part of the notch. The notch had a somewhat conical shape

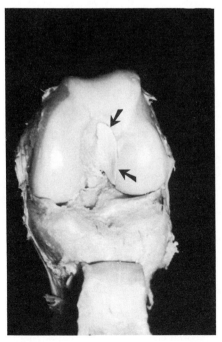

Figure 17–5. Anterior view of the intercondylar notch plasty.

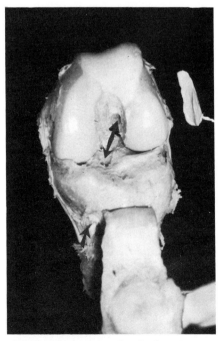

Figure 17–6. A bone cement plug simulates the preoperative lining of the notch and the extension of the notch plasty into the lateral condyle.

with its apex toward the entrance of the femoral tunnel and well into the adjacent lateral condyle (up to 6 mm). This notchplasty, together with a careful chamfering of the condylar tunnel entrances, seems necessary to avoid shearing forces along the femoral condyle, abrasive forces at the tunnel ports, and guillotinelike impingement of the graft by the anterior radius of the notch.

The extent of the notchplasty is related to the local anatomy and placement of the intra-articular tibial tunnel port. Accordingly, tunnel placements were made isometrically to within 2 mm over the full range of motion.

The results of a computer analysis of ligament-length relationships in the moving knee are reported by John Sidles, University of Washington, Seattle. This report presents an investigation of potential ligament attachment sites for surgical reconstruction of the ACL-deficient knee. The motions of more than 5 million potential graft attachment sites for the anterior and posterior cruciate ligaments, as well as for the lateral extra-articular iliotibial band tenodesis were analyzed. All of the ligament insertion sites, which were nearly isometric for motion of the intact knee, were quantitatively and graphically described. (Attachment sites are called isometric whenever they remain equidistant from each other throughout the knee range of motion.) For any specific pair of femoral and tibial insertion sites the distance between these sites could be computed as a function of the knee flexion angle, referred to as length pattern.

Clinically relevant features of a length pattern can be quantified in terms of a measure called the maximum absolute value of strain (MAS). For a given length pattern, MAS values are computed as follows: First, for a full range of knee motion, the maximum length between the femoral and tibial insertion sites is computed. Then for a specified partial range of motion, the minimum length between femoral and tibial insertion sites is computed.

In terms of these minimum and maximum lengths the MAS value is defined to be (maximum length − minimum length)/(maximum length + minimum length) and are thus determined by the length pattern of a pair of insertion sites and any specific partial range of motion.

The MAS value resulting from the above formula indicates the length changes in percentage relative to the mean of the two lengths. Small MAS values indicate near isometry over the specified partial range of motion. Laxity, but not additional tightening, may occur in the remaining range of motion.

Figures 17–8 and 17–9 illustrate a graphic technique for showing MAS values. The most nearly isometric femoral insertion sites for 0 to 110 degrees of flexion were posterosuperior in the notch for central tibial insertion (approximately 6 mm anterior to the posterior margin) [Fig. 17.10], less superior for anterior tibial insertions [Fig. 17.11], and less posterior for posterior tibial insertions [Fig. 17.12].

Not shown in the figures, but worth mentioning here: ACL MAS contours were computed for 0 to 30 degrees of flexion and central or posterior. Tibial insertions had additional, nearly isometric insertions, which included the over-the-top area. For anterior tibial insertions the over-the-top area was not isometric even for this restricted range of mo-

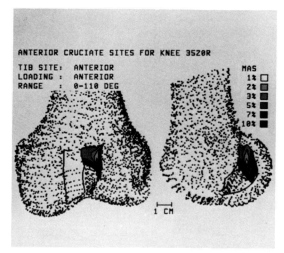

Figure 17–8. Bone anatomy and anterior cruciate MAS contours. Left: The posterior aspect of the distal femur and the lateral half of the distal femur. Right: Enlarged views of the notch from the same perspectives without other anatomic details (superior to inferior: anterior to posterior) *See also Fig 17.9.*

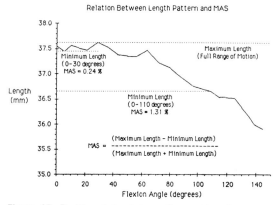

Figure 17–7. The relation between ligament length patterns and MAS values. MAS values are indicated for two ranges of flexion angle: 0–30 degrees and 0–110 degrees. (MAS = maximum absolute value of strain.)

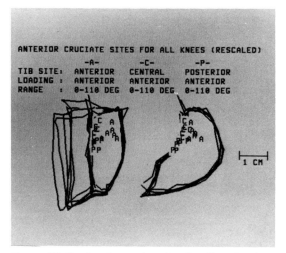

Figure 17—9. Anterior cruciate sites for all used cadaver knees rescaled (*n* = 6).

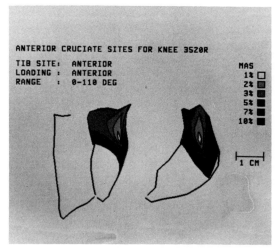

Figure 17—11. Anterior cruciate MAS contours in a representative knee for anterior tibial placement, anterior loading, and 0–110 degrees of flexion.

tion. Tibial insertion sites at the anterior margin of the anatomic attachment suffered notch impingement near full extension.

In my opinion this study covers retrospectively the technical refinement used in the second series, which started in September 1982.

As an additional rotational reinforcement, an iliotibial band tenodesis was performed in all cases in the second series. A strip of iliotibial band 2-cm-wide was passed underneath the collateral lateral ligament; the dorsolateral capsule and lateral margin of the lateral gastrocnemius muscle, and pulled through a superficial bone tunnel in the metaphysis of the lateral condyle. A staple was used to prevent the bony bridge from pulling out.

CLINICAL TRIAL

The clinical trial began in January 1981. Of 226 patients entering the program, all but one have been followed up (because of accidental death) and 252 grafts were implanted. Sixty-eight patients received xenografts for the posterior cruciate ligament or mediodorsal complex or combination of ligament insufficiencies with generally excellent results, but will not be reported on here, since ACL insufficiency is regarded as the most severe test of a candidate reconstruction material.

One hundred fifty-eight patients presented with a positive pivot shift, along with other clinical evi-

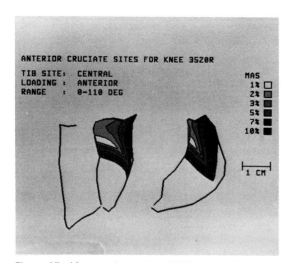

Figure 17—10. Anterior cruciate MAS contours in a representative knee for central tibial placement, anterior loading, and 0–110 degrees of flexion.

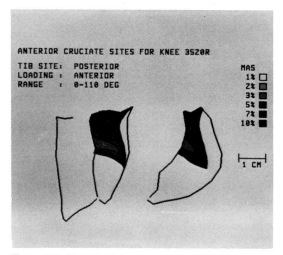

Figure 17—12. Anterior cruciate MAS contours in a representative knee for posterior tibial placement, anterior loading, and 0–110 degrees of flexion.

dence of chronical ACL insufficiency. No acute cases were included, as the use of prosthetic devices in such cases is not deemed appropriate.

Excluded from the series were patients with arthrosis and postfracture incongruence of the articular cartilage. Series I is made up of 57 patients operated on from January 1981 to September 1982 (mean age, 28 yr, average time lapse between injury and reconstruction, 3.1 yr). Series II comprises 101 patients operated on from September 1982 to January 1986 (mean age 27 yr, average time lapse between injury and reconstruction, 1.8 yr).

REHABILITATION

A well-controlled postoperative regimen is necessary, particularly when additional procedures are used to correct multirotational instabilities. The average immobilization time is two weeks, with passive 20 to 70 degrees of flexion allowed immediately after operation. Functional bracing, using a hinged orthosis is applied at two weeks, with passive and guided active exercises allowed (hamstring stretches, leg lifting within 20 to 70 degrees) and partial weight bearing. After 12 weeks, full extension is achieved; thereafter full weight bearing is allowed when quadriceps strength is sufficient. Running is allowed after four to six months and return to recreational sports after one year. All patients were advised preoperatively not to expect to return to competitive athletics.

RESULTS

The primary objective of this study was to evaluate stability of the joint over a minimum two-year interval. The evaluation criteria employed are shown in Table 17–1. Graph 17–1 depicts average combined functional scores (both series) versus postimplantation time period. All patients were recently evaluated quantitatively, using the MedMetric KT-1000 knee arthrometer (MedMetric Corp., San Diego, Calif).

Table 17–2 illustrates the results using the KT-1000 knee arthrometer in both series. Less than 2 mm anteroposterior drawer at 20 degrees of flexion is observed between knees operated on and those not operated on.

In patients where graft was explanted and the knee stabilized by an extra-articular procedure alone, the anteroposterior drawer difference be-

TABLE 17–1. EVALUATION OF JOINT STABILITY

Criteria	Best	Worst
Lachman test	0	4
Anterior drawer	0	4
Anterolateral rotational instability	0	4
Anteromedial rotational instability	0	4
Pivot shift	0	4
Effusion	0	4
Total points possible	0	24

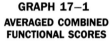

GRAPH 17–1
AVERAGED COMBINED
FUNCTIONAL SCORES

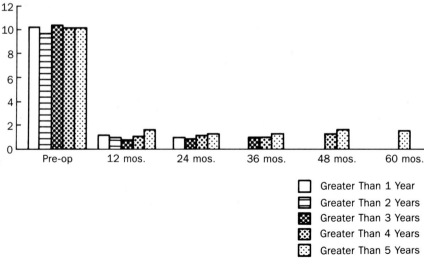

□ Greater Than 1 Year
▤ Greater Than 2 Years
▨ Greater Than 3 Years
▨ Greater Than 4 Years
▨ Greater Than 5 Years

**TABLE 17–2. KNEE ARTHROMETER (KT-1000) TEST RESULTS
(TIBIAL DISPLACEMENT IN MILLIMETERS)**

| | First Series 44 Patients (Average Scores) | | Second Series 90 Patients (Average Scores) | |
	15-lb Passive Drawer	20-lb Passive Drawer	15-lb Passive Drawer	20-lb Passive Drawer
Nonoperated	4.1	5.3	3.4	4.4
Operated	4.5	5.9	4.2	6.2

**TABLE 17–3. WT 1000 ARTHROMETER RESULT IN PATIENTS AFTER
REMOVAL OF THE ACL GRAFT
(TIBIAL DISPLACEMENT IN MILLIMETERS)***

	15-lb Positive Drawer	20-lb Positive Drawer
First series (13 patients)		
Nonoperated	3.2	3.9
Operated	6.0	7.5
Second series (9 patients)		
Nonoperated	3.9	4.5
Operated	6.4	2.0

*Third series, 22 patients (average scores). Lemaire lateral reconstruction; no ACL graft.

tween knees operated on and those not is averaged 3.5 mm [Table 17–3]. This illustrates the need to complement extra-articular procedures with an intra-articular reconstruction because of insufficiency in eliminating the pivot shift or stress to menisci.

Table 17–4 illustrates the result of the Lysholm score. This subjective scoring system shows a marked difference in both series between knees stabilized by ACL and ACL plus extra-articular reconstruction and knees stabilized only by an extra-articular reconstruction.

Satisfactory improvement in stability resulted from the procedure refinements and good stability appears to be maintained over the maximum five-year postoperative interval (Graph 17–2).

Graph 17–3 shows the evaluation of joint function. Again, note that the functional results improved markedly as a result of the technique refinements of Series II (Graph 17–3).

From Series I about 45 percent of the patients with a function score of good to excellent have returned to their preoperative level of recreational and/or competitive athletics (55 percent in Series II).

Complications

Twenty patients (35 percent) in Series I and four (4 percent) in Series II presented with a synovial

**TABLE 17–4. LYSHOLM SCORES
(AVERAGE (SUBJECTIVE) SCORES)***

	Series I		Series II
44 Patients (revisions included)	87.9	92 Patients (revisions included)	92.1
13 Patients (failed; graft removed; Lemaire)	75.4	9 Patients (failed; graft removed; Lemaire)	76.1

*80 to 100 points is excellent to good, 60 to 80 is fair, and <60 is poor.

reaction. Only a slight to moderate effusion and hyperemic synovial membrane was found in the majority of these patients and all showed a loss of stability consistent with graft rupture, which was ultimately verified by diagnostic arthroscopy. In four of these cases (all in Series I), a severe synovial reaction occurred. Cloudy synovial fluid, fibrin, and pannus tissue covering the articular cartilage was observed at reoperation. Histologic examination of the synovial membrane revealed proliferation of lymphocytes, plasma cells, and some giant cells with particles of xenograft material embedded within their cystoplasm.

Synovial-fluid cultures for aerobic and anaerobic microorganisms were negative. Immunologic screening revealed only focal deposition of non-

GRAPH 17–2
STABILITY

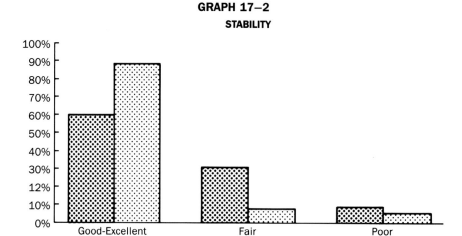

Series I: Original Procedure
Series II: Improved Technique

Rating	Series I (57 patients)	Series II (101 patients)
Good to excellent	34 (60%)	88 (88%)
Fair*	18 (31%)	7 (7%)
Poor†	5 (9%)	5 (5%)

*Residual laxity (all patients in this category had previous total meniscectomies).
†Failed. Graft explanted.

specific IgA in the synovial biopsy specimens. No glutaraldehyde was detected in either the synovial fluid or the ruptured xenograft fragments by means of high-pressure liquid chromatography.

A synovial cyst formation was observed in one patient at the tibial tunnel end, suggesting an oversized tibial tunnel that had allowed the passage of synovial fluid.

One superficial wound infection of *Staphylococcus aureus* was cultured, which responded readily to systemic antibiotics.

Several ruptures (15 grafts) were ascribed to incorrect (nonisometric) tunnel placement and there were 10 and 5 reinjuries in Series I and II, respectively. A total of 32 patients required reoperation, during which 15 new xenografts were implanted.

In support of the validity of the techniques used in the second series, two complications have occurred (reinjuries) in the last 12 months and the majority of patients in Series II have exceeded the time after implantation at which complications occurred in Series I.

DISCUSSION

At the time this study was initiated, the prevailing opinion was that xenografts should be used surgically in the same manner as autologous tissue transplants. In addition to the results of this study, there is now substantial evidence that this opinion is incorrect.

Experience with synthetic material as well as with xenografts has confirmed the link of successful performance to precise positioning of the prosthesis.

The crucial difference between xenografts and autologous tissue is that the former do not stretch during the biologic remodeling process. This desirable attribute of autologous tissue in mitigating short-term problems is, I believe, more than offset by the biologic stability of xenografts, which are thus less likely to become lax during the many months required for remodeling. The high consistency of the two-through-five-year stability results of this study support this hypothesis.

This study shows that any impingement of xenografts on bone must be rigorously avoided. The majority of the complications trace to the violation of this dictum. Tendinous collagen is highly fibrous and any shearing forces will cause fibers to separate from the graft. This can ultimately lead to rupture, but even mild abrasion of the graft can cause an inflammatory reaction, such as a synovitis. This observation is supported by the fact that

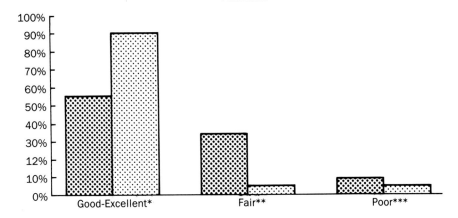

GRAPH 17–3
FUNCTION

■ Series I: Original Procedure
▣ Series II: Improved Technique

*No functional problems
**Some patellofemoral pain
***Giving way and pain

Rating	Series I (57 patients)	Series II (101 patients)
Good to excellent*	31 (55%)	91 (90%)
Fair†	21 (36%)	5 (5%)
Poor‡	5 (9%)	5 (5%)

*No functional problems, although some slight flexion deficits.
†Pain in patellofemoral region and mild effusion after strenuous exercises, with recovery in hours.
‡Giving way and pain, marked loss of function due to progressive degenerative change in the joint.

two patients with mild effusion, 12 and 15 months after operation, were found arthroscopically to be lacking a small anterior portion of the typical synovial covering of the xenograft. Mini-arthroplasties were performed to deburr the offending bone at the point of impingement. Six weeks after this simple procedure, all symptoms of effusion had subsided.

The inflammatory tendency of ruptured or frayed xenografts has been the subject of speculation as to the exact origin. Studies performed by independent researchers indicate that no immunologic or chemical origins could be substantiated and the histology showed the acute-phase inflammatory reaction known to be typical in the presence of particulate matter within the highly sensitive synovial environment.

Specific immunologic rejection requires participation of macrophages, T cells, B cells, and memory cells to stimulate antibody production, especially after a second implantation. These cellular elements were not seen to participate in the inflammatory reaction observed after graft rupture or abrasion. Also, no patients have exhibited sensitivity

to the graft after reimplantation, nor has selective staining for IgG antibodies revealed a significant positive response (Lanzer W: unpublished data). Therefore in neither series has there been an allergic or specific immunologically mediated response to this material.

The unfortunate necessity for reoperation in this study offered the opportunity to examine microscopically the host reaction to the xenograft. Figure 17–13 shows the microanatomy of a bovine xenograft before implantation. Figure 17–14 shows the typical synovial covering visible three to six months (here, three months) after implantation.

Figures 17–15 and 17–16 illustrate the dense collagenous tissue surrounding the graft within the bone tunnel. This type of fixation is believed to distribute the fixation stress throughout the tunnel area, as opposed to concentrating the stress at a single point or small area. Figure 17–17 shows a cross-section of an extra-articular portion of a xenograft after six months in vivo. Host vessels and fibroblasts can be observed invading the interfibrillar septa of the graft. Figure 17–18 shows host

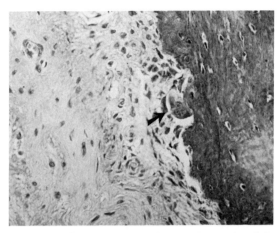

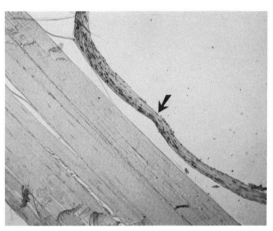

Figure 17–13. Microanatomy of a bovine xenograft before implantation.

Figure 17–16. Osteoblastic activity at the tunnel wall in higher magnification. (See arrow.)

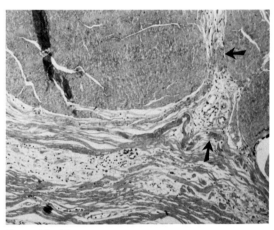

Figure 17–14. Thin synovial lining of a bovine xenograft (CLR) after a 3-month implantation period in the intra-articular environment of the knee joint.

Figure 17–17. Cross section of an extra-articular part of the xenograft near the bone fixation site. Host vessels and fibroblasts invading the interfibrillar septa of the bovine xenograft after a 6-month implantation period.

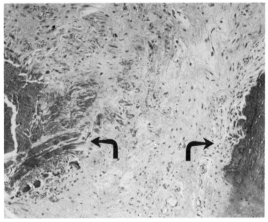

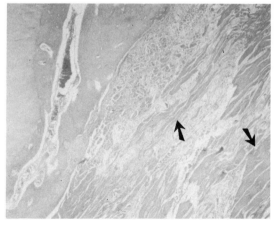

Figure 17–15. Dense collagenous tissue surrounding the graft within or near the intra-articular entrance of the tibial bone tunnel. (See on the left side the graft and on the right side the tunnel wall.)

Figure 17–18. Host tissue ingrowth in the intra-articular region near the bone–graft interface after a 22-month implantation period.

tissue ingrowth in the intra-articular region after 22 months of implantation near the bone–graft interface.

This ingrowth is not nearly as rapid in human beings as in the dog. It is now evident that bovine xenografts perform more like a true prosthesis than like an ingrowth scaffold. Only time will tell if this slow, host-oriented ingrowth will ultimately take over the stress-bearing function of the xenograft, since there is as yet no evidence that the xenografts lose their ability to do so.

CONCLUSIONS

This clinical study demonstrates that certain surgical techniques are important for successful utilization of the bovine xenograft as an ACL replacement. The objective of these techniques is to position the graft isometrically and to avoid any impingement of bone on the graft. Such impingement is most probable at the anterior and superior aspect of the notch, the adjacent femoral condylar surface, and the internal entry ports of the femoral and tibial tunnels. These technical factors, together with an extra-articular iliotibial band rotational stabilization (Lemaire) and, a well-controlled rehabilitation program appear in this study to result in successful correction of ACL deficiencies, with good stability and function retained for a minimum of two years.

The occurrence of synovial reactions was, in all cases, associated with fraying or rupture of the xenograft for technical or traumatic reasons, and appeared to be a typical acute-phase inflammatory response induced by particles of collagen. The presence of effusion, therefore, is strongly indicative of a fraying or ruptured graft, which should be confirmed arthroscopically before surgical correction.

Although uniform, host-oriented tissue ingrowth takes place, this occurs at a rate so slow as to preclude any estimate of the point in time when host collagen might take over the stress-bearing function of the ligament, if and when such should be required.

Finally, ACL reconstruction has been successfully performed with bovine xenografts in patients with chronic ACL insufficiency, and knee stability and function has been maintained for over two years.

REFERENCES

1. Abbink EP, Kramer FJK. Preliminary report on the use of xenografts in knee instability problems. Trans Annu Meeting Eastern Orthop Assoc 1982.
2. Daniel D, Malcam LL, Stone ML, Perth H, Morgan J, Riehl B. Quantification of knee stability and function. Contemp Orthop 1982; 5(1):83.
3. Hey Groves EW. The crucial ligaments of the knee joint: their function, rupture and the operative treatment of the same Br J Surg 1919; 7:505.
4. McMaster W. A histologic assessment of canine anterior cruciate substitution with bovine xenograft. Clin Orthop Relat Res 1985; 196–201.
5. Noyes FR, DeLucas JL, Torvik PJ. Biomechanics of anterior cruciate ligament failure: an analysis of strain-rate sensitivity and mechanisms of failure in primates. J Bone Joint Surg (Am) 1974; 56:236–253.
6. Sidles JA, Larson RV, Garbini JL, Matsen FA III. Ligament length relationships in the moving knee: Interactive Graphics for Orthopaedic Surgeons. Seattle, Wash.: University of Washington Press, 1986.

18

ARTHROSCOPIC ANTERIOR CRUCIATE LIGAMENT RECONSTRUCTION WITH PROCOL XENOGRAFT BIOPROSTHESIS

TERRY L. WHIPPLE, M.D., F.A.C.S.

The ProCol xenograft bioprosthesis was a sterile, ready-to-use product. Its biomechanical properties would seem to make it well suited for reconstruction of the anterior cruciate ligament, and it could be implanted with arthroscopic techniques. The clinical experience with this prosthetic ligament in cruciate reconstruction through open implantation techniques has been promising in limited series in Europe and the United States as reported in Chapters 16 and 17 of this book. Presently, however, the product has been withdrawn and is not commercially available.

Irrespective of the material selected for cruciate reconstruction in an intra-articular procedure, the practical advantages of minimally invasive surgical techniques are indisputable if the procedure can be done at least as effectively as through a conventional arthrotomy. Introduction of a prosthetic graft under arthroscopic control affords excellent visualization, bright illumination, and the advantage of magnification in preparing the points of entrance and exit of the graft through the joint. Additionally, arthroscopic examination of the joint permits thorough evaluation for any associated intra-articular pathology in cruciate-deficient knees. As the arthroscopic procedure is performed in a fluid medium, irrigation of the entire joint is

possible to ensure removal of all particulate matter at the conclusion of the procedure.

Minimally invasive surgical techniques afford the postoperative advantage of decreased bleeding as compared with conventional arthrotomy. Earlier patient mobilization also decreases the risk of postoperative pulmonary and vascular complications. There is also an advantage to surgical approaches that leave secondary stabilizing structures and other soft tissues less disturbed. Theoretically, less extensive surgical exposure reduces the risk of postoperative infection. Reduction of pain and improvement in cosmetic appearance of surgical scars is obvious.

It must be reemphasized, however, that arthroscopic insertion of intra-articular cruciate grafts is only advantageous when it can be done at least as well as through conventional arthrotomy. To maximize these advantages of cruciate reconstruction under arthroscopic control, elaborate surgical planning and meticulous attention to detail is imperative. The surgical team must be coordinated preoperatively through role rehearsal. The patient should be positioned to provide circumferential access to the knee. The operating room is arranged to allow adequate sterile work space for preparation of the graft, easy access to numerous instruments, and a clear view of the arthroscopy video monitor. A complete supply of surgical instruments should be sterilized and ready to use in implanting the graft, as well as to cover every contingency. There is no room in such a technically demanding operation for needless delays or inconveniences.

AUTHOR'S PREFERRED TECHNIQUE

Regardless of the exogenous material or prosthetic device selected for arthroscopic reconstruction of the anterior cruciate ligament, the following procedures have proved efficient and advantageous.

The patient is positioned on the operating table with the back slightly flexed to reduce lumbar strain during the prolonged procedure. The video monitor and other electronic devices are positioned on a table or platform over the patient for easiest viewing by the surgeon. The leg is exsanguinated, and is stabilized by a brace affixed to the side rails of the operating table (Fig. 18–1), exposing at least 8 in. of thigh distally. The foot of the table is lowered, and the leg is prepared and draped as for any other sterile procedure. This way, the knee can be flexed from 0 to 100 degrees in the sterile surgical field.

The surgeon stands at the foot of the table facing the knee, the assistant stands to the lateral side, and the scrub nurse locates the instruments on the non-operative side of the patient. A large-bore inflow cannula is introduced on the medial side of the joint just above the superior pole of the patella. An arthroscope with a 25- to 30-degree foreoblique lens is introduced into the intercondylar notch through the transpatellar tendon, an approach described by Gillquist and Hagberg [1]. The joint is thoroughly inspected for associated articular cartilage or meniscus damage, and appropriate procedures are performed if additional pathology is found.

Through an anteromedial portal, a shaver is used to excise from the intercondylar notch the ligamentum mucosum, excessive fat pad tissue, and any remains of the anterior cruciate ligament that do not completely span the intercondylar notch from tibia to femoral condyle. A powered burr equipped with suction for arthroscopic use is then placed in the anteromedial portal, and 5 to 10 mm of the lateral and anterior walls of the intercondylar notch are resected. These surfaces are tapered gradually to the posterior and superior aspect of the lateral wall of the intercondylar notch. One should note that the orientation of the femoral condyle may be misleading in this position. When the knee is flexed 90 degrees with the patient supine, the most posterior aspect of the femoral condyle is oriented downward, and the anterior aspect is oriented upward.

When the intercondylar notch is widened, the hook portion of an arthroscopic drill guide is placed in the anteromedial portal. It is embedded in the lateral femoral condyle in the superior area of origin of the anterior cruciate ligament. The oblique femoral tunnel to be drilled will enter the lateral wall of the intercondylar notch with an elliptical opening, extending farther distally than the located point (Fig. 18–2).

The drill guide is assembled to the hook probe extra-articularly (Fig. 18–3). The cortex of the femoral metaphysis is exposed through a lateral, 4-cm incision. A guide pin is then drilled through the jig, oriented as close as possible to the axis of the femoral shaft, and enters the joint on the lateral wall of the intercondylar notch at the tip of the hook probe.

The hook probe and drill guide are used next to select the epicenter of attachment of the anterior cruciate graft on the tibia. This point must be posterior enough to avoid impingement of the graft on

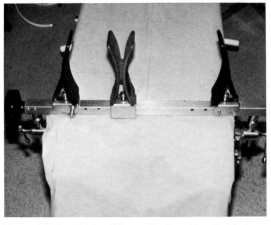

Figure 18–1. Thigh stabilizer affixed to side rails of operating table—Concave plates embrace thigh in pneumatic tourniquet. (Precision Surgical Instruments, Richmond, Va.)

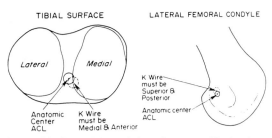

Figure 18–2. Artist's rendering of proper guide-pin placement on tibia and femur. (Courtesy of William Clancy, M.D.)

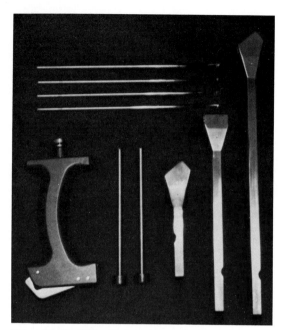

Figure 18–3. Drill guide for arthroscopic cruciate reconstruction. Three guide-arm angles allow convenient placement of incision for guide pin. (Dyonics, Inc., Andover, Mass.)

the intercondylar notch anteriorly when the knee is extended. The ideal point is located along the lateral margin of the articular surface of the medial tibial plateau anterior to the tibial spine. Here again, the opening of an oblique tunnel through the tibia will have an elliptical shape, extending farther posteriorly and laterally from the point se-

lected on the tibia (Fig. 18–2). Through a 3-cm anteromedial incision, a second guide pin is passed to the selected point of insertion on the tibia with the aid of the drill guide.

The guide pins are removed, and a No. 1 silk suture is passed through the pin tracks with aid of a flexible ligature passer. The suture is attached to a tensiometer, which is then anchored in the tibial pin hole. The knee is carried through a range of motion with the tibia externally rotated to monitor the excursion of the suture. If more than 2 mm of excursion are observed, one of the holes must be repositioned.

This exercise is intended to identify the so-called isometric points of attachment for the cruciate graft. In reality, this is a rather fallacious concept, as there is no truly isometric arrangement of the normal anterior cruciate ligament. The normal ligament arises from the femur as a cord-shaped structure and spirals anteriorly and medially across the intercondylar notch to insert on the tibia in a long, flat configuration. The ligament fibers wind about one another through knee flexion to remain tight. Recognizing the complex structure of this ligament, it is naive to consider that single points of origin and insertion would represent the route of an average central fiber, which would remain taut through full range of motion. More-superficial fibers of the graft will assume either longer or shorter courses through the joint more peripherally to the defined center of attachment. Nevertheless, when reconstructing the anterior cruciate ligament with a cord-shaped structure containing linear fi-

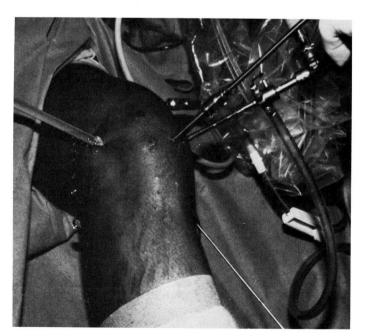

Figure 18–4. Illustration of tunnel placement for arthroscopic reconstruction of anterior cruciate ligament, right knee. Guide wire remains in tibia. Cannulated reamer has been used to create a tunnel in the lateral femoral condyle.

bers, the selected points of origin and insertion should optimally permit a functional range of knee motion without excessive tightening or loosening of the graft.

The silk suture is removed and the guide pins are replaced in their respective holes. Tunnels are then created in the femur and tibia with a cannulated reamer (Fig. 18–4). The reamer should be approximately equal in diameter to that of the ProCol xenograft bioprosthesis. Again, the burr is introduced to chamfer the edges of both femoral and tibial tunnels to remove any sharp bone margins.

The ProCol xenograft bioprosthesis is sufficiently stiff to be pushed easily through the femoral tunnel. Under arthroscopic visualization, it can be grasped intra-articularly with a forceps inserted through the tibial tunnel, and drawn across the intercondylar notch into the tibial tunnel, exiting through the anteromedial skin incision (Fig. 18–5). Again, the knee is carried through a range of motion to observe if excursion of the graft is present. There should be essentially no motion of the graft within the bony tunnels.

The proximal end of the graft is affixed to the lateral femoral cortex with a ligament washer and screw. The knee is held in 0 degrees of extension, the tibia is externally rotated, and the proximal tibia is pressed backward. The graft is then pulled tight through the tibial tunnel, and is attached distally. Staples may be used in the external opening of the tibial tunnel for attachment of the graft in thin individuals if the screw head might be too prominent. The excess graft is excised, the incisions are closed in anatomic layers, and an immobilizing splint is applied with the knee flexed approximately 45 degrees.

POSTOPERATIVE TREATMENT

The ProCol xenograft bioprosthesis does not undergo biologic remodeling as allografts or autogenous tissues do. Therefore immobilization postoperatively is required only to ensure biologic fixation of the graft in bony tunnels. Nevertheless, a conservative postoperative protocol has been used in most cases of arthroscopic anterior cruciate reconstruction with the xenograft bioprosthesis during investigational stages.

The extremity remains splinted, with minimal motion for six weeks. Walking on crutches, putting no weight on the reconstructed knee is continued for three to four months. Range-of-motion exercises without stress are permitted from the sixth week. Hamstring isometrics and quadriceps strengthening between 30 and 60 degrees are begun six to eight weeks after surgery.

CLINICAL SERIES

Arthroscopic reconstruction of cruciate-deficient knees with the ProCol xenograft bioprosthesis has been less successful than anticipated. Failures usually resulted from graft rupture following abrasion against bone surfaces, which occurred

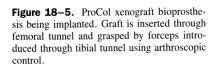
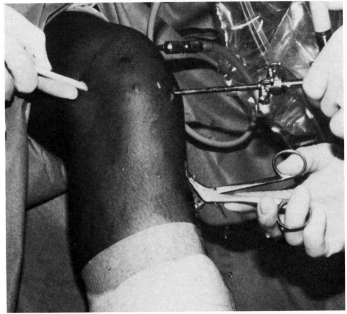

Figure 18–5. ProCol xenograft bioprosthesis being implanted. Graft is inserted through femoral tunnel and grasped by forceps introduced through tibial tunnel using arthroscopic control.

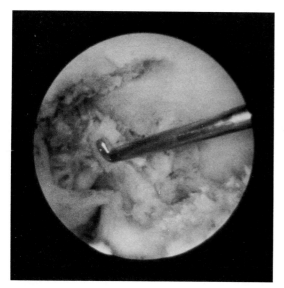

Figure 18—6. Arthroscopic appearance of ruptured stump of ProCol xenograft bioprosthesis 10 months after implantation.

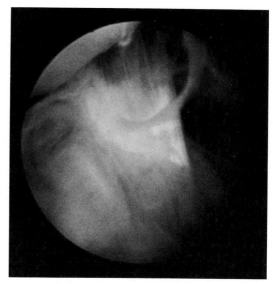

Figure 18—7. Synovial proliferation at the insertion of ProCol xenograft bioprosthesis six months after implantation.

with greater frequency than in similar series performed through a conventional arthrotomy, as described in Chapters 16 and 17 (Fig. 18–6).

The largest series of arthroscopic anterior cruciate ligament (ACL) reconstruction with this prosthesis was compiled by Levitt et al [2]. Seventy cases were reported with similar surgical techniques and postoperative management, with a follow-up range from 15 to 38 months, averaging 23 months. Table 18–1 shows the age distribution of patients in this series. Fifty-two of the 70 procedures were performed for chronic ACL deficiency with instability, and 18 cases represented acute ligament ruptures. Thirty-four patients had undergone previous procedures for knee instability; 28 of the 70 cases had a partial meniscectomy performed concurrently.

The ProCol bioprosthesis reconstruction failed in 31 per cent of the cases in this series. A sterile synovitis (Fig. 18–7) developed in 29 per cent of the cases, and the graft remains were removed in 22 cases at an average of 11 months after implantation. Failure was reported in only 13 per cent of a series in which concurrent extra-articular stabilizing procedures were performed with the ProCol bioprosthesis being implanted through a conventional arthrotomy [3].

From the arthroscopic series, the synovium and graft remains of 12 of the failures were analyzed histologically and with immunofluorescence studies. Eight of the 12 demonstrated particulate graft material in the synovial fluid or villi, but none showed any evidence of infection, activated collagenase, or T- or B-cell response (Fig. 18–8). This suggests strongly that the mode of failure was gradual abrasion and shedding of graft particles into the joint, eliciting a typical foreign-body synovial response but with no associated evidence of immunologic rejection [4]. The specific factors responsible for the difference in results in ProCol cruciate reconstruction performed under arthroscopic control versus those performed through arthrotomy are unclear. Abrasion of the graft in cases performed arthroscopically may be related to rotational motion within the joint where no extra-articular procedure was performed to constrain tibial rotation.

There is conclusive evidence that the ProCol xenograft bioprosthesis is biocompatible in terms of sterility, chemistry, and immunogenicity. Its biomechanical properties appear commendable as an implant for ligament reconstruction in cruciate-deficient knees, and the material is durable with

TABLE 18–1. AGE DISTRIBUTION OF PATIENTS UNDERGOING ARTHROSCOPIC ACL RECONSTRUCTION WITH PROCOL BIOPROSTHESIS.

Under 20	6
20–29	31
30–39	27
40–49	3
Over 50	3
Total	70

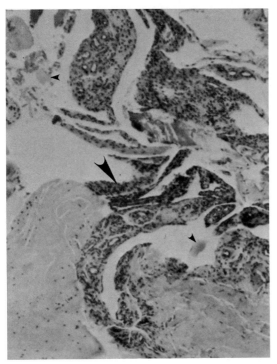

Figure 18—8. Photomicrograph of synovium from a patient with a ruptured ProCol bioprosthesis. Note proliferation of synovial cells (large arrowhead) and wear particles from graft (small arrowheads). (Courtesy of William L. Lanzer, M.D.)

respect to cyclic bending and tensile loading. However, it is clearly not resistant to abrasion against adjacent bone. The ideal procedure for use of the ProCol xenograft bioprosthesis for ACL reconstruction has not been determined. The device may be better tolerated and protected against wear if implanted extra-articularly as a lateral restraint against rotatory knee instability. Although it can be implanted accurately inside the joint, under arthroscopic control, to date this has not been a reliable procedure.

REFERENCES

1. Gillquist J, Hagberg G. A modification of the technique of arthroscopy of the knee joint. Acta Chir Scand 1976; 142:123–130.
2. Levitt L, Whipple TL, Springer I. Anterior cruciate ligament reconstruction utilizing the bovine xenograft. Presented at the Annual Meeting of Arthroscopy of North America, New Orleans, 1986.
3. Abbink P. Prosthetic ligament reconstruction of the knee. Presented at the Third Annual Course for American Academy of Orthopedic Surgeons, Scottsdale, Ariz., 1986.
4. Lanzer WL. Histological testing of failed xenograft ACL implants. Presented at a meeting of the European Society of Knee Surgery and Arthroscopy, Basel, Switzerland, 1986.

Note: On May 7, 1987 the PMA for ProCol Bioprosthesis was voted ''not approvable'' by the FDA orthopedic panel. The panel was concerned about effusions that may have been related to antibody production. Dr. Lanzer felt that the low level of antibodies was not directly related to the synovitis observed.

There was also concern with the ratio of patients per investigator in the United States study. This came as a result of a limitation of the continuing original study and probable excessive number of investigators at the beginning of the study.

The overall explant rate of the ACL prosthesis was 23.5%. Variables to consider regarding this number include the fact that in the beginning it was not apparent that immobilization and aggressive notchplasty were required. In addition, if Dr. Abbink's European data is included, this explant rate falls to 14.7%.

In any event, at the time of writing (11/5/87) there are no further studies regarding the Xenotech ACL prosthesis in the United States.

19

THE LEEDS–KEIO LIGAMENT: BIOMECHANICS

BAHAA B. SEEDHOM, B.SC., PH.D.

INTRODUCTION

The Leeds–Keio ligament is a hybrid-type implant; it is not a prosthesis in the strict sense, although initially the implant carries all of the tensile load, until ingrown tissue matures and becomes well aligned and capable of sharing the load with the implant. Neither is the implant of the stent type; it does not biodegrade and entirely "bow away" to the ingrown tissue. Tests in the laboratory predict that it would retain a considerable fraction of its initial strength for a very long period.

The implant is made of polyester–polyethylene terephthelate—known as Dacron in the United States and terylene in Europe. This material has been used in the human body in the form of arterial grafts for more than 20 years.

The adopted method for anchoring to bone is unique to this implant. It relies on and benefits from both bone and tissue ingrowth. While some see it as a drawback that it takes a finite time for the anchor to be established with this method, one great advantage is that once it has done so, the strength of the anchor increases with time. This is a feature that a pure mechanical fixation does not possess.

The surgical procedure is simple but demands precision. It is facilitated by the design of both implant and the special surgical instruments. The procedure does not interfere with, nor does it require the sacrifice of any autogenous tissue. Furthermore, it requires removal of a minimal amount

of bone, perhaps considerably less than that required in any other reconstructive procedure. The implant and the procedure are the result of the successful collaboration of members from Leeds University (United Kingdom) and Keio University (Japan), hence the name.

This chapter discusses the principles behind the design and anchoring of artificial ligaments in general, and their applications in particular to the development of the Leeds–Keio ligament.

DESIGN CONSIDERATIONS

While it can be argued that similar design principles may be employed when designing a prosthetic ligament or prosthetic knee, the designer would have to give special thought to patients in need of ligament reconstruction. Patients receiving artificial prosthetic ligaments are different in many respects from those receiving artificial knee joints. The latter tend to be older and their conditions of deformity, pain, and instability have developed over many years. For these patients, a knee replacement that removes pain and restores even a modicum of function represents a great boon and effects a welcome and dramatic change in their lives. A reduced range of flexion may not affect their ability to cope with their daily needs. On the other hand, patients receiving a ligament replacement are mostly young and athletic individuals who have become incapacitated in a sudden manner. So (unlike the much older group), the memory of what it is to be fit and competitive has not been diluted with time. They are credulous, hopeful, and on the whole very impatient. To them a mediocre result is totally unsatisfactory and greatly disappointing. Furthermore, a successful result is satisfactory only if it continues to be so. Revisions represent a great disruption to professional athletes. Hence, a reconstructed knee cruciate ligament must allow as near a full range of flexion as possible; it must rectify aberrant movement between the bones and so restore stability to the joint; and it must be strong and durable.

The constraints within which the designer has to work are tight. There are important requirements for long-term success of a cruciate reconstruction procedure. Since all these requirements are essential, failure of the implant is certain if any of them is left unfulfilled. The stage at which failure occurs depends on which of the design requirements have been ignored, since their individual influences come into play at different stages.

The requirements for long-term success are briefly discussed below:

1. The implant must be correctly placed; when a cruciate is reconstructed, it is well recognized that the range of flexion (assuming no adhesions have occurred) is dependent on the anchoring sites of the ligament to the bone. Correct placement is therefore of great importance; the immediate, if not the whole, outcome of the surgical procedure depends on it.
2. The anchor of the implant to the bone must be of sufficient strength.
3. Whether the implant is a true prosthesis or one that acts as a scaffold for tissue ingrowth, it must have adequate strength. A true prosthesis will continue to act as the sole tensile component throughout its useful life; an implant of the stent or scaffold type will still have to act as the main load-carrying component for a period.
4. The load-extension characteristics of the implant are of great importance and the implant stiffness should be carefully chosen so as to "forgive" some inaccuracy in placement. If slightly misplaced, an extremely stiff implant will most likely fail at the anchor or the intra-articular section linking the two bones, whichever is the weaker of the two. Or else, the range of flexion may be restricted if the implant (or anchor) did not fail.

   The stiffness of an implant of the scaffold type is important for another reason. For the ingrown tissue to become mature, well aligned, and capable of sharing load with the implant, it must be subjected over a period to tensile strains. These strains are likely to be extremely small in a stiff implant, and normally the tissue ingrown around such an implant remains fibrotic, amorphous, and immature.
5. A long enough fatigue life is essential. Bear in mind that the period during which the implant will be used may be between 30 and 50 years. Therefore the device must be capable of retaining a substantial residual strength after having been subject to many millions of load cycles.

The above requirements will be discussed further in the context of the reconstruction of the anterior cruciate ligament (ACL).

PLACEMENT OF THE LIGAMENT

The ACL is a complex structure, and none of the implants discussed in this book, including the Leeds–Keio ligament has aimed at anatomical reconstruction of the natural ligament. It has been shown that not all of the fiber bundles in the natural ligament are taut throughout the range of flexion of the knee [1]. Also, it is recognized that placement of the femoral attachment is more critical than the tibial. It is a problem for which more than one solution has been presented; the two most widely adopted are the isometric and over-the-top types of placement.

The solution adopted for the Leeds–Keio ligament was to place it isometrically. It is a pragmatic solution in that it attempts to load all the fibers of the implant equally, but even this is not quite achieved, since the implant is not attached at a single point, but through a bone tunnel of a finite dimension. This means that the filaments of the implant will not be subjected to uniform tension throughout the range of flexion.

The sites of isometric placement on both femur and tibia have been studied on cadaveric knees (Ball WG, et al.: unpublished data). The change in length of the intra-articular portion of the implant was measured for five positions of through-tunnels in the femur for both the anterior and posterior cruciate ligaments. The positions of these tunnels are illustrated in Figure 19–1a. Similar measurements were obtained for the over-the-top method of attachment. Also, two positions for tibial attachment through bone tunnels (shown in Figure 19–1b) were examined. The results are presented in Tables 19–1 and 19–2.

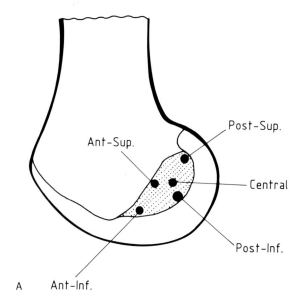

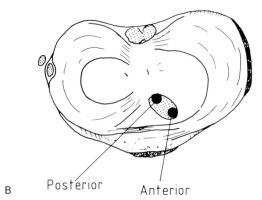

Figure 19–1. (a) Tested sites of anterior cruciate placement on the femur. Ant denotes anterior, Sup. superior, Post posterior, and Inf. inferior. (b) Tested sites of anterior cruciate placement on the tibia.

From Table 19–1 it can be seen that it is possible to achieve a near isometric placement for the ACL on the femur. This site can only be defined as the most superior and posterior position, within the natural area of attachment, avoiding damage to the articular cartilage. The position is defined with the long axis of the femur pointing in the vertical direction. The anterior and superior site is the one that corresponds to the maximum change in length of the ligament. It can also be seen that in the over-the-top position the ACL lengthens as the knee is extended and slackens if it is flexed beyond the angle of flexion at which the device is tightened. (In this experiment the angle was 45 degrees.)

Table 19–2 shows that the location of the attachment to the tibia is not as critical as that to the femur. However, the site we recommend is the more anterior of the two indicated. This site is defined as follows: as far as possible anteriorly and medially within the natural area of attachment, but without damaging or undermining either of the anterior meniscal attachments to the tibia. This anterior position for the tibial attachment is preferred to the posterior one since at the latter the implant would be more inclined to the tibial plateau and so would be less effective in carrying loads in the anteroposterior direction.

ANCHORING METHOD AND DESCRIPTION OF THE IMPLANT

In our method, anchoring is achieved by trapping the implant, which has numerous holes, between two freshly cut bony surfaces, so that as they heal they unite through the holes in the implant and thus secure it by the interlocking bone trabeculae and connective tissue. For the reconstruction of the ACL, the details of both procedure

TABLE 19–1. CHANGES IN LENGTH (IN MILLIMETERS) OF THE ANTERIOR CRUCIATE LIGAMENT (ACL) CORRESPONDING TO THE DIFFERENT PLACEMENT SITES ON THE FEMUR.*

Femoral Position of ACL	Angle of Flexion†									
	0	15	30	45	60	75	90	105	120	135
Posterior–superior	1.0	0.9	0.0	0.0	0.0	0.0	0.4	0.3	0.0	0.5
Posterior–inferior	6.2	3.5	1.2	0.0	−0.3	−2.0	−1.0	−2.0	−1.2	−2.0
Anterior–superior	0.0	−1.0	−0.8	0.0	2.5	5.25	7.8	10.8	12.3	15.8
Anterior–inferior	3.8	1.7	0.0	0.0	1.0	2.8	5.7	7.8	10.3	12.7
Central	2.5	0.5	−0.7	0.0	0.7	2.0	3.2	4.0	5.2	6.2
Over the top	2.3	1.5	0.75	0.0	−0.3	−1.3	−3.0	−4.8	−5.5	−5.5

*Averages of readings from four specimens.
†Negative numbers mean that the distance between the placement sites reduces.

TABLE 19–2. CHANGES IN LENGTH (IN MILLIMETERS) OF THE ANTERIOR CRUCIATE LIGAMENT (ACL): EFFECT OF TIBIAL PLACEMENT SITE.*

Tibial Position of ACL	Angle of Flexion									
	0	15	30	45	60	75	90	105	120	135
Anterior	0	0	0	0	0.5	0.5	0.5	1.0	1.5	2.0
Posterior	1.0	0.5	0	0	0	0	0	0.5	0.5	1.0

*The femoral attachment site was the most superior and posterior but two sites for placement on the tibia (anterior and posterior) have been tested. Averages of results from two specimens.

and implant design had to be worked out. With respect to the procedure, the aims were to increase the area of anchoring above that normally achieved by mechanical methods (knotting, staples, toggles, and bollards), to cause minimal damage to bone and soft tissue, and to carry out the procedure with accuracy and in a short period.

The anchor was achieved here by trapping the implant between a bone tunnel and a bone plug, the difference between whose diameter and that of the tunnel was just enough to accommodate the implant. The bone plug was 9.5 mm in diameter and 20 to 25 mm long, thus affording an anchoring area between 6 and 7.5 sq cm. About half this area would be available for bone and tissue ingrowth through the implant. The bone plugs are removed from the sides of anchoring in both femur and tibia, thus obviating the need for making incisions elsewhere in the body to obtain bone plugs from other sites. A bone plug is obtained by removing a small amount of ''bone dust,'' thus creating an annular space around the plug, which is subsequently removed by a special instrument. On removing a bone plug, a thorough tunnel of a smaller diameter than that of the plug is drilled, emerging at the ligament-anchoring site in the joint space, as illustrated schematically in Figure 19–2.

The device itself was designed with special features to facilitate the implantation procedure. These features are illustrated in Figure 19–3a. The implant is made of pure polyester monofilaments, in an open-weave structure. Although woven in one piece, it consists of two main sections. The first is tubular and seamless; the second is flat. The first section subdivides into a short tubular section 30 to 50 mm long, followed by a closed and densely woven section 7 to 10 mm long, followed by a pouch 35 to 37 mm long formed by a slit in only one side of the tubular section, which extends approximately 55 mm further. For the convenience of threading the implant through the bony tunnels, a cord is attached to the tubular section of the ligament. As will be seen later, the densely woven,

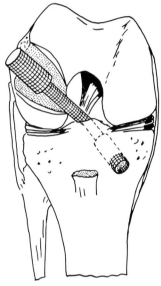

Figure 19–2. Concept of the anchoring method with the Leeds–Keio ligament.

closed section and the pouch are important features that facilitate the procedure.

Since the implant is loosely woven, its structure is likely to be distorted by snagging against bone trabeculae, if not drawn through the bone tunnels with extreme care. While this distortion may have no effect on the strength or function of the implant, it is still undesirable, as it may inconvenience the surgeon during the procedure. For this reason, the implant is placed within a tubular sheath of transparent polyethylene, which prevents this distortion (Fig. 19-3b).

Once the bony tunnels have been prepared, the sheathed ligament is threaded through the tibial tunnel first and a length of 15 cm is drawn into the intra-condylar space. The implant is then drawn through the femoral tunnel. The sheath and cord is cut with scissors above the double knot within the sheath. The ligament is withdrawn from the sheath

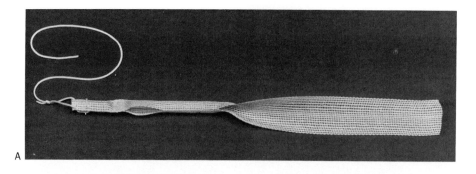

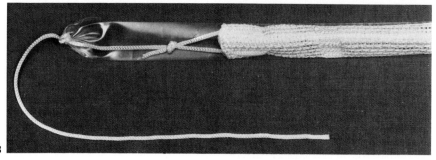

Figure 19–3. (a) The Leeds–Keio ligament. (b) The implant is placed within a flexible polyethylene sheath.

(which should be held fast at its end protruding from the tibial tunnel), so that the pouch protrudes beyond the sheath. The femoral bone plug is introduced within the pouch as near as possible to the closed end. The ligament and sheath are both firmly gripped and pulled so that the femoral bone plug is drawn into its tunnel and is prevented from being drawn into the intercondylar area by the bony shoulder formed because of the smaller through-hole. The ligament is also prevented from slipping around the bone plug by the closed end and densely woven section. The sheath can finally be withdrawn from around the implant, leaving its woven structure perfectly intact.

On introducing the tibial bone plug, the implant is stapled to the bone, folded over itself, and sutured both to itself and to the periosteal tissue, and the remaining section of the ligament is then cut with scissors. The staple is not a primary means of fixation; it is used to ensure that the ligament will not slip around the bone plugs and become loose in the early postoperative stages (or even while handling the limb during the application of a plaster cast). At the femoral end the ligament is cut well above the densely woven section after it has been sutured to the periosteal tissue.

INSTRUMENTATION

Since the dimensions of the bone plug and locations of the ligament attachment sites were ex-

tremely critical for successful implanting of the ligament, special instruments were designed for the procedure. These are shown in Figure 19–4.

The reamer is used to form a bone plug. It has a thin cylindrical section with fluted cutting edges on the side, as well as sharp cutting teeth at the end. By pressing the reamer against the bone and oscillating it about its axis, it removes bone dust, thus creating an annular space around the bone plug. Should the latter become detached, it can be ejected from the reamer using the push rod.

However, the bone plug normally remains attached and it has to be removed by the bone-plug extractor. This is a single component, one end of which is cylindrical, with a thin-walled section. Part of this thin-walled section is machined out so that the remaining part has a cross-section that is a little more than half a circle. The middle section of the instrument has a flat surface on the opposite side of the machined part mentioned above. The other end of the instrument is simply a handle (Fig. 19–5). The thin-walled section has identical dimensions to those of the reamer. To remove the bone plug, the extractor is introduced into the annular space around the bone plug and pushed to its limit. The handle is held firmly and a hammer is used to apply a short, sharp strike on the flat surface of the instrument. One strike may be sufficient to shear the bone plug from where it is attached at the bottom. When the bone plug has been detached it can easily be seen moving within the

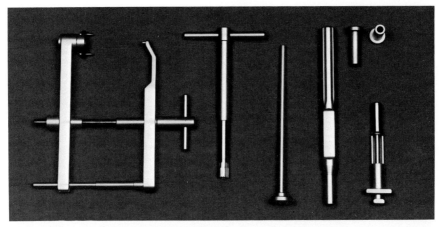

Figure 19–4. The instruments used for implanting the Leeds–Keio ligament, from left to right, are the clamp, reamer, the bone-plug extractor, the bone-plug introducer, the push rod, and the drill-bit guide.

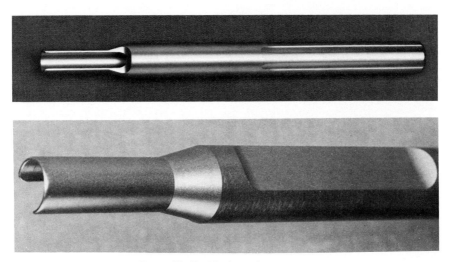

Figure 19–5. The bone-plug extractor.

extractor if the latter is rotated slightly. As the extractor is withdrawn, the trapped bone plug within it can be easily removed. The procedure is illustrated in Figure 19–6.

On removing the bone plug, the drill bit is introduced into the tunnel in order to extend it through to the attachment site of the implant. This is schematically illustrated in Figure 19–7.

As mentioned earlier, placement of the implant within the joint is of great importance. Since removal of the bone plug and subsequent drilling is approached from outside the joint, correct "aiming" is crucial, so that the through-tunnel emerges at the intended site of the implant attachment. To accomplish this successfully the reamer is used only within the guide located within one of the two arms of the clamp. This guide, which has two

sharp pins, can be rotated within the clamp and so adjusted until both pins pierce the bone. The other arm of the clamp has a single pin, which is secured in the intended attachment site of the implant. Figure 19–8 illustrates the use of the clamp on the femur. Before reaming, the clamp should be firmly tightened, thus control of the direction of the common axis of both bone plug and the through-hole may be achieved.

Replacing a bone plug (i.e. tibial side) while keeping the implant taut is an extremely important matter for the success of the procedure; this is facilitated by the use of the bone-plug introducer shown in Figure 19–9. This device has an extremely thin-walled section and a central plunger. The main body of the instrument has an open section in its side for introducing the bone plug into

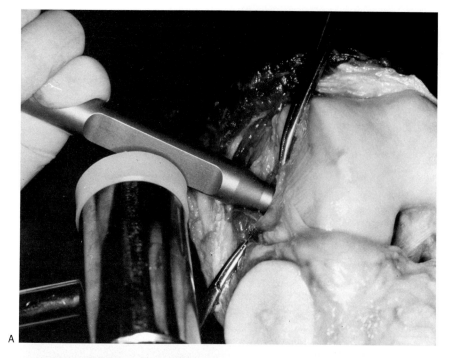

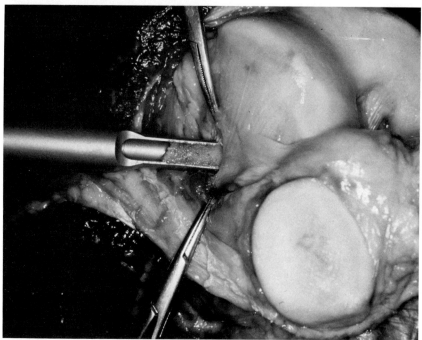

Figure 19–6. Method of using the bone plug extractor to remove a bone plug. (A & B)

the instrument. When replacing the tibial bone plug, the instrument is introduced in the bone tunnel surrounded by the implant, which must be kept taut. The plunger must be in the forward position, as shown in Figure 19–9b when introducing the instrument into the tunnel. This is to protect the

instrument from distortion and the implant from being damaged by the thin-walled section. Once the instrument is fully in the bone, the plunger is retracted so that it clears the opening in the side of the instrument.

The bone plug is introduced within the instru-

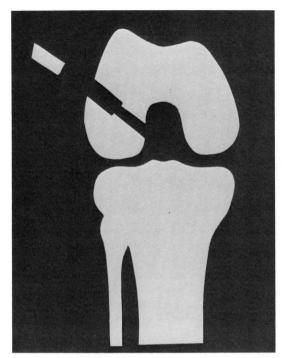

Figure 19—7. Schematic representation of the femur after removing a bone plug and drilling a through-tunnel emerging at the intended site of placement in the femur.

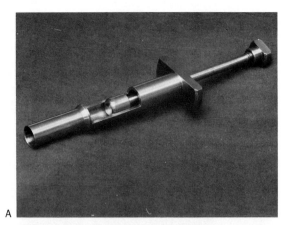

A

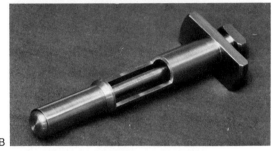

B

Figure 19—9. (a) The bone-plug introducer. (b) The central plunger must always be in the forward position when the instrument is not in use.

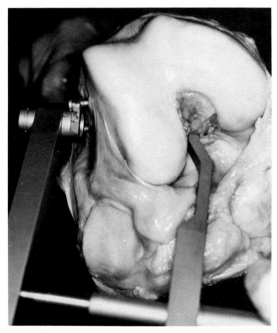

Figure 19—8. Use of the clamp on the femur.

ment through the side opening and pushed with forceps until it disappears into the thin-walled section of the instrument. Pressure is applied on the plunger by the thumb and the body of the instrument is withdrawn from around the bone plug using the index and middle fingers. The procedure is illustrated in Figure 19–10.

TESTING OF THE ANCHORING METHOD AND STRENGTH OF THE ANCHOR IN ANIMALS

The ACL was reconstructed using this implant in five pigs (six to seven months old; weight, 80 to 90 kg). The pig was chosen because the size of its knees allows sufficiently large bone plugs to be obtained. These were 6.5 mm in diameter, and the through-hole was 4.5 mm (as opposed to 9.5 and 6.5 mm, respectively, for the human knee). The tensile strength of the implant used for the animal experiment was 840 to 870 N.

The pigs were killed at 1 mo, 7 mo, 9 mo, and the last two (within one week) at $17\frac{1}{2}$ mo postoperatively.

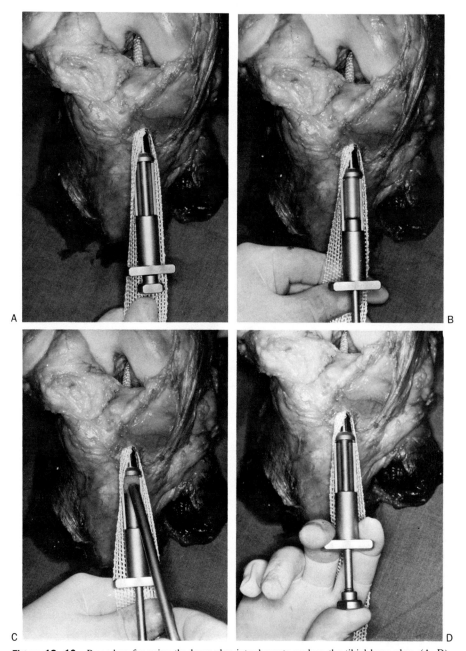

Figure 19—10. Procedure for using the bone-plug introducer to replace the tibial bone plug. (A–D)

Bone histology was studied in the first three animals. Transverse sections were prepared through the femoral plug, thus showing it, the tunnel, and the annular space occupied by the implant. At one month postoperatively, the section showed a few bony spicules bridging this annular space, thus joining the plug and the bone tunnel (Fig. 19–11). The number of bony outgrowths increased at seven and nine months postoperatively, thus increasing the contribution of bony outgrowth to the anchor (Figs. 19–12 and 19–13). It must be noted that where the annular space was not bridged by bone trabeculae uniting the tunnel to the plug, it was filled with fibrous tissue, which would no doubt contribute to the strength of the anchor.

Unaided visual examination of connective tissue ingrowth around the intra-articular section of the implant showed that within one month postopera-

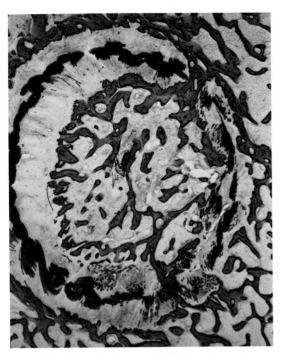

Figure 19–11. A section through the bone plug region one month after implantation in the pig.

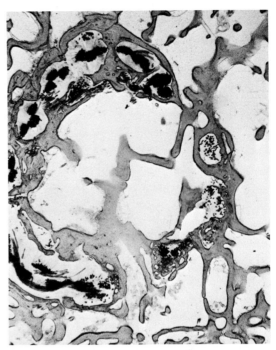

Figure 19–13. A section through the bone-plug region after nine months postoperatively.

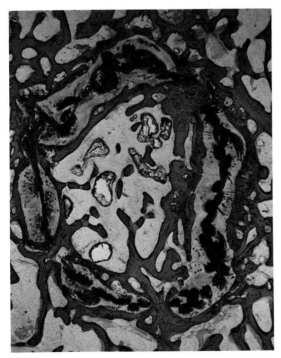

Figure 19–12. A section through the bone-plug region after seven months postoperatively.

tively extensive fibrous growth had occurred around the implant. Seven months postoperatively, the extent of this fibrous reaction appeared to be reduced and taken on a more mature appearance. The "neoligament," composed of the artificial fibers and the invasive connective tissue, compared favorably in appearance with that of the natural ligament of the pig (Fig. 19–14). (It must be noted, however, that there is a considerable difference between the complex structure of the natural ACL of the pig and that of the implant, which is much simpler.) Where the ligament is attached to the femur (Fig. 19–14c), fibrous tissue can be seen to surround the ligament where it emerges from the tunnel through the femur. This observation was not only interesting but extremely encouraging; without this soft-tissue growth around the ligament, its fibers would continuously abrade against bony surfaces and with time, the ligament would fail secondary to abrasion. This tissue ingrowth provides protection for the implant from abrasion. Similar growth was observed where the ligament emerges through the tunnel at its tibial attachment (Fig. 19–15).

In these experiments the greater emphasis was placed on bone ingrowth in the region of the plug; but some experimental work was carried out to establish whether the tissue ingrowth around the implant added to its strength. This was done by

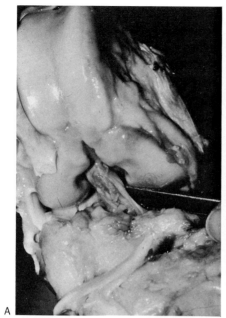
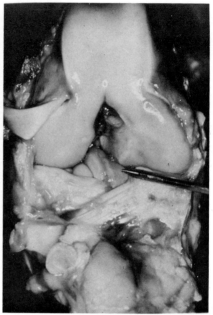

A

B

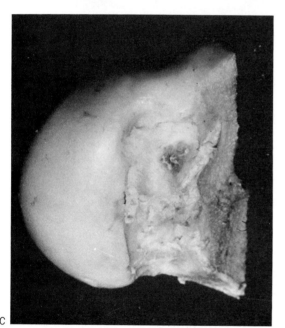

C

nine months postoperatively the implant failed at 950 N. At 17 months postoperatively it failed at 2600 N. As mentioned earlier the prosthetic ligament fabric alone, when tested in the laboratory, failed at 840 to 870 N. Thus the fibrous growth strengthens the implant considerably.

Figure 19—14. (a) The neoligament appearance seven months postoperatively. (b) The natural ACL in the pig; there is a considerable difference in structure between the natural ACL of the pig and that of the implant. (c) Fibrous tissue can be seen to surround the ligament where it emerges from the tunnel through the femur.

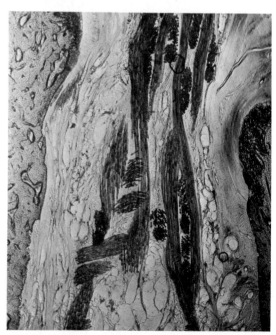

severing all the tissue surrounding the joint except for the implant and the ingrown tissue. The femur and tibia were gripped separately and distracted in a tension-testing machine and the load–displacement curves were recorded. It was found that at

Figure 19—15. A section through the tibial tunnel in the portion which does not contain a bone plug, the implant is shown to be surrounded by fibrous tissue which protects the ligament from abrasion against bone.

MECHANICAL PROPERTIES OF THE IMPLANT

Strength and Stiffness

As mentioned earlier, even though this implant is of the scaffold type, which promotes ingrowth, it was important that its strength be adequate to act as the main tensile load-bearing component for some time, until the neoligament is established. The strength of such a device is a function of both the device material property and the structure of the device itself. The strength of the implant must be measured under similar conditions to those under which the implant will operate in the body. Because the implant material is a polymer, its response to load is time dependent. Its strength as well as its stiffness will be influenced by the rate at which it is strained. The rate of strain varies a great deal in the body and it has been suggested in the guidelines of regulatory bodies for prosthetic ligament devices that the implant should be tested at strain rates of between 1 per cent and 100 per cent per second. Tensile tests were therefore carried out on this implant under the following conditions:

1. After sterilization, to take into account the effect of the process on the mechanical properties.
2. In saline solution at 37°C, since it was shown that the effect of the difference between ambient temperature and body temperature has a small but significant effect on the properties of the device.
3. After preconditioning the device by subjecting it to a tensile sinusoidal load of 50 to 500 N at 25 Hertz for a period of three hours and then allowing it to relax for a period of three hours after unloading it.
4. At three different strain rates: 1 per cent, 50 per cent, and 100 per cent per second.
5. At a gauge length of 40 mm.
6. The implant was gripped between rubber-lined steel clamps. This more closely approximates the operating conditions of the implant in the body (being surrounded by ingrown tissue), than if it were clamped between two hard surfaces.

The results showed that:

1. The strength of the implant is in excess of 2000 N, which is well above the figure of 1750 N published in the literature [2] for the ACL from young adult humans. It can also be noted that the strain rate does have some effect on the maximum breaking strength, so that it is approximately 7.5 per cent and 10 per cent higher at strain rates of 50 per cent and 100 per cent per second, respectively, above its value at the lowest strain rate of 1 per cent per second.
2. The stiffness of the implant within the grips used also varies with the strain rate. It has been calculated from the load-displacement graphs as the maximum breaking tensile load achieved divided by the corresponding elongation. At a strain rate of 1 per cent per second, the stiffness had a mean value of 195 kN/m and it increased to 262 and 279 kN/m at the two higher strain rates. The value of the stiffness quoted by Noyes and Grood [2] is about 180 kN/m, measured for a strain rate of 10 per cent per second. Thus at the lower strain rate the stiffness of this implant within the grip is only a little higher than that of the natural ACL. If we take into account the compliance and slip within the clamps, the stiffness of the device is approximately twice the values quoted.

It must be remembered that the stiffness of this kind of implant is a function of its length. The longer the implant, the smaller its stiffness for the same cross-sectional area. Hence, if we take into account the true lengths of an implant in the joint we should include not only the intra-articular portion linking the bones, but also the two short lengths in the through-hole sections that do not contain the bone plug. These vary from one joint to the other and by including them the stiffness of the implant would reduce. For example, if the effective length of the implant was 50 mm, its stiffness would be 80 per cent of an implant 40 mm in length.

FATIGUE TESTING AND RESULTS

The ACL is normally subjected to cyclic loading during walking, which is the most predominant of the human locomotive activities, and also during strenuous sporting activities such as jogging, running, and sprinting. Therefore fatigue testing is extremely important for an implant that will act as a permanent ligament prosthesis. The reported value of force acting on the ACL is rather low during walking—170 N—but during strenuous activities it is about 450 N and that during a jolt has been estimated at about 650 N. To test the implant in the fatigue mode at a low value of force may become irrelevant if it was first tested and proven to be safe at the higher load. Again, the test conditions must be representative or as close as possible to those under which the implant will operate. The Leeds–Keio ligament has been subjected to cyclic loading under various conditions, which can be summarized as follows:

1. Mostly in saline solution at 37 to 39°C but sometimes in air at room temperature.
2. After sterilizing the ligament either by autoclaving or irradiation.
3. The sinusoidal cyclic loading was between 50 and 500 N, at 25 Hertz, thus representing typical loading of the ligament during strenuous activities.
4. Various kinds of clamping the ligament in the test machine were tried. The first four specimens were between a semisoft grip, which was achieved by gripping the implant between two steel plates lined with a layer of cotton cloth on one side and a layer of rubber on the other. During the rest of the tests the implant was gripped between two steel plates, each of which was lined with a thin layer of rubber. The latter is more representative of the soft tissue surrounding the implant within the bony tunnels and would give it protection from abrasion against bone.

A summary of the results is shown in Table 19–3. The ligament did not fail in any of the above experiments; it was not our intention to establish the fatigue life of the ligament as such, i.e., the number of load cycles at which the ligament fails for a given cyclic load (in this case 500 N). The intention was to find the maximum tensile load at failure, after subjecting the ligament to fatigue by cyclically loading it. So, after applying a different number of load cycles (as indicated in Table 19–3), the ligament was subjected to a tensile load at a strain rate of 50 per cent per second and the residual strength was recorded. It is encouraging that the residual strength of the irradiated ligament can be as high as 65 per cent of its original strength after approximately 63 million cycles. Of particular interest was the seventh test, which was carried out in room temperature air (according to the guidelines of the Food and Drug Administration for fatigue-testing of artificial ligaments). The implant in this particular instance was subjected to approximately 78 million cycles at a sinusoidal load of between 50 and 500 N, followed by 16 million cycles at a sinusoidal load between 50 and 700 N, and the residual strength was 1380 N. It is highly unlikely that any implant will be subjected to jolt loading on millions of occasions. However, if we assume that the implant was subjected to load during running and that the distance covered in a cycle is between 1.7 and 2.2 m, then 94 million cycles corresponds to a distance covered during running between 160,000 to 205,000 km. These correspond to approximately 67 to 85 mi per week for 30 consecutive years. Although the residual strength of the implant measured after this intensive fatigue-testing exceeds the strength of the natural ACL in elderly individuals (400 to 1100 N), the implant might become considerably weaker in 30 years. However, it must be remembered that the additional strength imparted to the implant by the ingrown tissue has not been taken into account.

TABLE 19–3. SUMMARY OF RESULTS OF FATIGUE-TESTING OF THE LEEDS—KEIO LIGAMENT.

Sterilization procedure	Environment	No. of load cycles	Max tensile force (N)	Freq. (Hz)
1 Autoclaved	Air (20°C)	35×10^6	1400	30
2 Autoclaved	Saline (39°C)	23×10^6	1000	30
3 Autoclaved	Saline (39°C)	45×10^6	900	30
4 Irradiated	Saline (39°C)	19.8×10^6	830	30
5 Irradiated*	Saline (39°C)	29.7×10^6	1400	30
6 Irradiated*	Saline (39°C)	62.8×10^6	1280	25
7 Irradiated*	Air (20°C)	78×10^6 plus 16×10^6†	1380	25

*Specimens clamped between two steel plates each lined with a thin layer of rubber. All other specimens were clamped between two steel plates, one lined with a layer of cotton cloth, the other with rubber.
†The load applied here was also sinusoidal with a maximum value of 700N.

SUMMARY

The concept and development of the Leeds–Keio artificial ligament have been described. The implant is anchored by a method that benefits from both bone and tissue ingrowth. Special instruments have been developed to facilitate the operative procedure. Extensive mechanical tests show that the implant has the appropriate mechanical properties in terms of strength, stiffness, and adequate fatigue life. While the implant becomes invaded with connective tissue that increases the strength of the composite (implant fibers and induced tissue), the implant does seem to retain a considerable proportion of its original strength after being subjected to extensive fatigue cyclic loading equivalent to that occurring during a strenuous activity such as running. It therefore seems that although ingrown tissue contributes much to the strength of the implant–ingrown tissue composite, the implant by itself may be capable of coping with load demands in the knee of a sporting individual.

REFERENCES

1. Girgis FG, Marshall JL, Monajen AL. The cruciate ligaments of the knee joint: anatomical, functional and experimental analysis. Clin Orthop 1975; 106:216.
2. Noyes FR, Grood EF. The strength of the anterior cruciate ligament in humans and rhesus monkeys. J Bone Joint Surg (Am) 1976; 58:1074.

20

CLINICAL STUDY OF ANTERIOR CRUCIATE LIGAMENT RECONSTRUCTION WITH THE LEEDS– KEIO ARTIFICIAL LIGAMENT

KYOSUKE FUJIKAWA

INTRODUCTION

The treatment of injuries of the cruciate ligament is the same old, but always new, problem. Although various reports have been made on the primary repair of fresh injuries, as well as on the reconstruction of chronic injuries, there still remain many problems to be solved. For this purpose, extensive efforts have been made in recent years to develop a strong, durable artificial ligament that causes no sacrifice of the autogenous tissue. Efforts have also been made to simplify the operative procedure and to ensure consistently successful operative results.

The type of the artificial ligament for the knee can be broadly divided into the following. The first is a simple prosthesis, an artificial ligament promising to provide life-long support. Its major advantage is that the patient may return to his or her activities of daily living soon after the surgery. However, it seems doubtful whether the prosthesis can and will actually withstand the stress in the long term, such as 30 to 40 years, or more.

The other type of the artificial ligament is the scaffold built by a process known as tissue induction. It takes a little time after the operation until the implant is covered with inducted tissue, but the artificial ligament works as a ligament in the initial stage and at the same time acts as a scaffold onto which natural tissue grows. Finally, it is expected to be completed biologically.

LEEDS–KEIO ARTIFICIAL LIGAMENT

In developing an artificial ligament for the knee, we must face up to two problems to be solved, one is what material and construction we should choose and the other is how to fix the implant to the bone.

The Leeds–Keio artificial ligament (Fig. 20–1), which is a scaffold ligament, is made of polyester and woven to form a mesh structure. It is tubular in the main middle section. One of the ends has a pouch where a bone plug is inserted to anchor the substitute to the bone. The other end is simply split open. The diameter of the tubular part is 11 mm and the length is 55 to 60 cm, which is long enough for the combination technique of intra-articular anterior cruciate ligament (ACL) reconstruction and lateral extra-articular reinforcement for anterolateral rotatory instability.

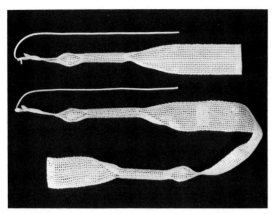

Figure 20–1. Leeds–Keio Artificial Ligaments: Short Type (Upper); Long Type (Lower).

The details of the mechanical properties of the Leeds–Keio artificial ligament are described in Chapter 19.

A novel aspect of the Leeds–Keio artificial ligament is the method of anchoring it to the bone (Fig. 20–2). We call this the biologic anchoring system because the bone plug, which is obtained when the bony tunnel is made, is put into the tubular ligament after introducing the substitute within the tunnels as described later. In subsequent weeks, fixation strength increases with time as the condylar bone outside of the ligament grows through the numerous holes of the mesh construction and unites the bone plug, thus providing a powerful anchor of the ligament to the bone. Furthermore, fibrous tissue grows around the ligament and the new growth increases the strength of the anchor as well. The staples are also used in order to strengthen the anchor in the early stage.

INDICATIONS

Cruciate reconstruction with the Leeds–Keio artificial ligament is indicated to any chronic ACL or posterior cruciate ligament (PCL) tear or both, and even for augmentation of fresh cruciate injuries. The knees with combined ligamentous injuries and knees previously operated on are particularly indicated for this surgery because of the shortage of the sufficient autogenous donors.

OPERATIVE PROCEDURES

Basically, there are two procedures in so-called ACL reconstruction (Fig. 20–3). One is intra-articular ACL reconstruction alone and the other is intra-articular reconstruction plus lateral extra-articular reinforcement. The second procedure should be indicated for the so-called ACL-deficient knee with gross anterolateral rotatory instability.

Currently, I usually perform intra-articular ACL reconstruction and lateral extra-articular reinforcement with one long type of the Leeds–Keio artificial ligament. This is because the ACL-deficient knee is usually associated with anterolateral rotatory instability, which is difficult to control with the intra-articular procedure alone.

The instruments specially designed for this procedure are of a ligament guide, two reamers and pushers, a centering guide, a bone-plug extractor, and a bone-plug introducer, which are shown in Figure 20–4.

The reconstructive surgery was formerly done through a long anteromedial incision with the patella retracted. Now the joint is opened through two small incisions on the upper lateral and lower

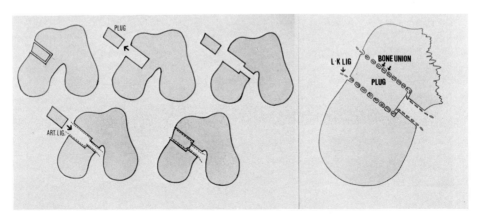

Figure 20–2. Anchoring System of the Substitute.

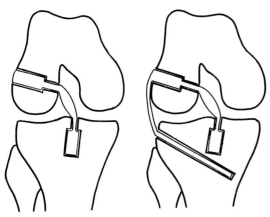

Figure 20–3. Reconstruction of the ACL: Intra-articular Reconstruction (Left) and Intra-articular Reconstruction and Lateral Extra-articular Reinforcement (Right).

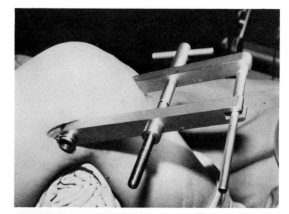

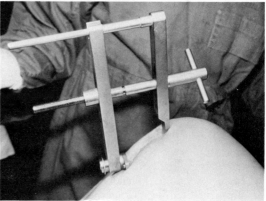

Figure 20–5. Operating Procedure: (1) Setting the Ligament Guide on the Femoral and Tibial Condyle.

anterolateral region of the knee. This is called a semiclosed procedure. The intra-articular and extra-articular operations can be performed under direct vision, as was the previous open procedure.

The ligament guide is first placed on the lateral femoral condyle (Fig. 20–5). The first portion of the bone tunnel, 11 mm in diameter and 20 to 25 mm in length, is made with a reamer, and at the same time a bone plug of the same length is obtained from the tunnel. Then the second portion of the tunnel of a smaller diameter (6 to 6.5 mm) is drilled through, toward the anchoring spot of the substitute. The same procedure is repeated on the medial tibial condyle, and another bone plug is

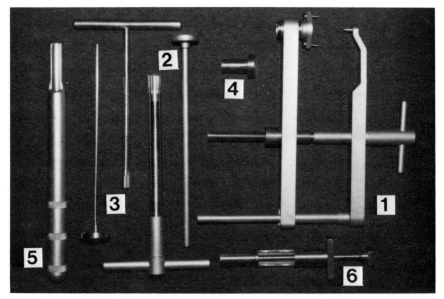

Figure 20–4. Instruments for ACL Reconstruction with Leeds–Keio Artificial Ligament: (1) Ligament Guide; (2) Reamer and Pusher; (3) Reamer and Pusher; (4) Centering Guide; (5) Bone-Plug Extractor; (6) Bone-Plug Introducer.

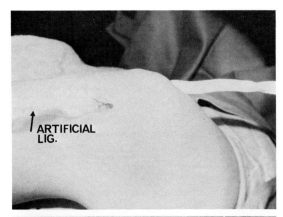

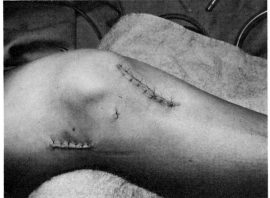

Figure 20—6. Operating Procedure: (2) Passing the Substitute through the Bone Tunnels and Skin Suture.

taken out. The third bone tunnel of 4 to 5 mm in diameter is drilled through from the superolateral corner of Gerdy's tubercle to the medial side of the tibia.

The artificial ligament is passed through the tunnels (Fig. 20–6) and first fixed to the tibial condyle by putting the bone plug exactly back into the cav-ity of the tubular part of the ligament and in the original position on the tibial condyle. The ligament is then pulled so that the bone plug locks it at the mouth of the smaller tunnel. The staple is also used to reinforce the fixation temporally in the initial stage. Then the femoral side of the substitute is fixed at 30 degrees of knee flexion with the bone plug, using the bone-plug introducer under tension. The tibia should be slightly rotated externally. Next, the substitute is passed on the lateral side of the joint toward Gerdy's tubercle, under the iliotibial tract, and outside of the lateral collateral ligament and then passed through the third tunnel keeping the same knee angle. Finally, the substitute is fixed on the medial side of the tibia with the staples under tension.

The incisions are sutured in layers after inserting a suction drainage system. The joint is put on the CPM device.

It is also possible to perform this procedure arthroscopically.

ANCHORING SPOTS AND RUNNING ROUTE OF THE IMPLANT

The positioning of the substitute attachment and its running route are of prime importance for good clinical results. Ideally, the distance between the two anchoring spots should be isometric through the full range of knee motion in order to keep constant tension on the reconstructed substitute.

According to our experiments, on the femur it should be placed as far posteriorly and superiorly as possible in the original attaching area, and anteriorly and medially on the tibia so that the distance between the two anchoring spots becomes nearly isometric through the full range of knee motion (Figs. 20–7 and Graph 20–1). The changes in ten-

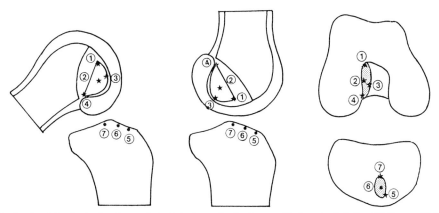

Figure 20—7. Study of the Anchoring Spots of the Substitute. On the Femur: (1) Anterior-Inferior; (2) Center; (3) Posterior-Inferior; (4) Posterior-Superior. On the Tibia: (5) Anteromedial; (6) Center; (7) Posterior.

GRAPH 20–1.

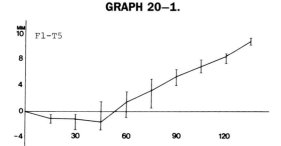

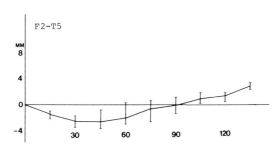

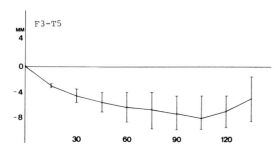

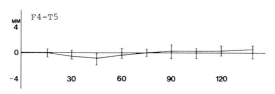

Study of the Anchoring Spots of the Substitute. F4—T5 Is Shown to Be Nearly Isometric.

sion of the intra-articular substitute are 12 to 18 N through the full range of knee motion when it is anchored at these fixation sites. The positioning on the femur is far more influential than that on the tibia.

The outer tunnel mouth of the femoral condyle should be placed at the posterior and superior edge of the condyle, so that running routes of the intra-articular and extra-articular substitute can be parallel and placed on the same plane, which can avoid disturbance of knee motion or slackness of the substitute after surgery.

The distance between the femoral and tibial anchoring spots of the lateral extra-articular substitution cannot be isometric in a strict sense. According to the measurement by the strain gauge (provided by MIE company), the tension of the extra-articular substitute became suddenly high at 20 degrees of knee flexion, increasing up to 60 degrees. After that it became flat to 100 degrees of knee flexion.

The substitute should be passed through the outside of the lateral collateral ligament in the lateral extra-articular reinforcement procedure. If it goes under the lateral collateral ligament, the substitute and the lateral collateral ligament are impinging on each other in the knee motion because the substitute is trapped by the lateral collateral ligament in extension of the knee and released in flexion. Therefore the final fixation of the substitute on the medial side of the tibia should be performed at 30 degrees of knee flexion with the tibia externally rotated.

POSTOPERATIVE CARE

The joint is mobilized on the CPM device immediately after the surgery from 30 to 60 degrees. After one week, the range of knee motion is increased up to 30 to 90° degrees. Partial weight bearing with a brace (20 to 90 degrees ROM) is usually allowed 3 to 4 weeks postoperatively. Jogging short distances, etc., are allowed with a brace 12 weeks after reconstruction. Sports activities are gradually permitted three to five months postoperatively.

We think that three to four weeks of careful postoperative care should be required until the scaffold is protected from friction at the mouths of the bone tunnels with newly formed tissue. It has often been reported that autogenous tissue, as well as artificial ligaments are broken with shear and friction at the mouth of the bone tunnel, which produces significant complications. (Table 20–1)

TABLE 20–1. POSTOPERATIVE PROGRAM.

	Operation
	CPM device with 30–60° movement
1 wk	CPM device with 30–90° movement
2–3 wks	Brace with 30–90° movement
8 wks	Brace with 20–full flexion
12 wks	Jogging etc. with Brace
14–20 wks	Return to Sports activities

RESULTS

More than 350 Leeds–Keio artificial ligaments were inserted into knee joints with torn cruciates since February 1982. These included 264 ACL tears, 23 PCL tears, and 73 both ACL and PCL tears. As much as possible, the associated injuries were treated at the same time. In this survey, only the clinical results of ACL reconstruction are presented, as PCL reconstruction has not a long enough postoperative period to discuss here.

One hundred and forty-six cases with over 24 months of postoperative history were reviewed directly, according to our criteria. The initial 80 joints were the first series, using only intra-articular reconstruction. The next 66 cases were the second series, using a combination technique of intra-articular reconstruction and lateral extra-articular reinforcement. The clinical data obtained indicated that the second series has led to better results.

As shown in Table 20–2, in the first series the

TABLE 20–2. RESULTS OF POSTOPERATIVE INSTABILITY TESTS.

First Series (80 Joints)

Evaluation	Lachman Test %		Anterior Drawer Test %		Jerk Test %	
Excellent (Negative)	60.0		42.5		57.5	
		82.5		75.0		75.0
Good (1+)	22.5		32.5		17.5	
Fair (2+)	10.5		12.5		12.5	
Poor (3+)	7.0		12.5		12.5	

Second Series (66 Joints)

Evaluation	Lachman Test %		Anterior Drawer Test %		Jerk Test %	
Excellent (Negative)	85.7		76.2		85.7	
		95.2		85.7		90.5
Good (1+)	9.5		9.5		4.8	
Fair (2+)	4.8		9.5		9.5	
Poor (3+)	0		4.8		0	

Percentage (%) refers to percentage of patients

TABLE 20–3. POSTOPERATIVE RANGE OF KNEE MOTION.

	1st Series (%)	2nd Series (%)
Full	61.1	61.9
Loss		
Less than 10°	11.1	9.5
10–20°	13.9	19.0
21–30°	8.3	4.8
Over 31°	5.6	4.8

Percentage (%) refers to percentage of patients

Lachman test was improved in 82.5 per cent of the patients, although 40 per cent were still graded 1+ or greater. In the second series, the improvement went further, with approximately 95 per cent of the patients showing a favorable Lachman test.

The straight anterior drawer test was also improved by the operation, with 75 per cent of the patients showing favorable results in the first series, although 57.5 per cent of them were still graded 1+ or greater. On the other hand, about 86 per cent in the second series were excellent. The jerk test was improved so that in the first series 75 per cent of the patients were improved, although only 57.5 per cent had a negative test. In the second series, 85.7 per cent had a negative test and 4.8 per cent trace positive, so that 90.5 per cent of the patients had favorable results.

As shown in Table 20–3, the postoperative range of knee movement was equivalent to the normal range of movement in approximately 60 per cent of the first series patients, with only 5.6 per cent of them losing more than 31 degrees of movement. The results were roughly the same for patients in the second series.

THE POSTOPERATIVE ARTHROSCOPIC STUDY

Postoperative arthroscopy (Fig. 20–8) was undertaken in 42 cases, and showed satisfactory tissue induction around the artificial ligament. The findings at three to four months after the surgery showed that the implant had already been covered with newly formed tissue, although it was still quite immature and fibrotic. An extensive vascular network could be seen criss-crossing its surface.

After six to seven months, it was confirmed by probing that the new tissue was firmly fixed to the implant and the vascular network was still seen running on its surface. Tension of the new liga-

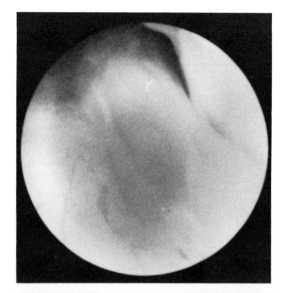

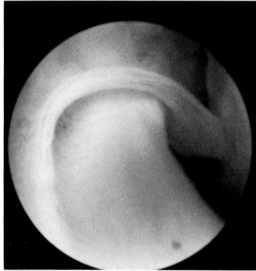

Figure 20–8. Findings of Postoperative Arthroscopy: 3 Months after Operation (Top); 12 Months after Operation (Bottom).

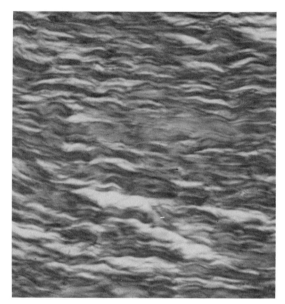

Figure 20–9. Histology of the New Ligament (Biopsy through Arthroscopy).

ment seemed to be maintained throughout a full range of knee motion.

Twelve months after reconstruction, the new ligament developed and matured, looking like a natural one in shape and thickness. The tibial insertion has become fan-shaped, which might be remodeling of the new ligament. The vascular network had already begun to reduce.

The histologic findings on biopsy at this time indicated that, while there were more cells than in the normal ligamentous tissue, new tissue had already developed with the collagen fibers running parallel and longitudinally.

Eighteen months postoperatively, the newly formed ligament could be mistaken on arthroscopic inspection for a normal ligament.

COMPLICATIONS

No patient in this survey had joint effusion, clinical synovitis, thickening of the synovial membrane, or infection. Histologic study of the synovial membrane biopsied at the postoperative arthroscopy showed no more than a slight hint of inflammatory processes. Rupture of the substitute was experienced in five cases. Two of them reinjured their joints after returning to their original sports. All of these ruptures came from the first series. The first two patients underwent reoperation and the combined procedure of intra-articular reconstruction and lateral extra-articular reinforcement was indicated.

COMMENTS

Anterior cruciate reconstruction with the Leeds–Keio artificial ligament has followed a good postoperative course in the clinical trials at Keio University Hospital, particularly in the second series, in which the combination technique of intra-articular ACL reconstruction and lateral extra-articular reinforcement was performed, though the longest follow-up period is still less than six years. Therefore the combination technique should be indicated for ACL-deficient knees with gross anterolateral rotatory instability, and this technique can be performed with one long Leeds–Keio artificial ligament. The most attractive advantages in the procedure are that no autogenous tissue need be sacrificed and that the new ligament is expected to keep its function for as long a period as an original ligament, as it is completed biologically.

Finally it should be strongly emphasized that it is of prime importance to place the implant under good tension through knee motion in order to induce growth of new tissue.

21

FUNCTIONAL BIOMECHANICS OF THE GORE-TEX CRUCIATE-LIGAMENT PROSTHESIS: EFFECTS OF IMPLANT TENSIONING

SCOTT N. STONEBROOK, B.S.E.
ANDREW B. BERMAN, B.S.M.E.
WILLIAM C. BRUCHMAN, B.S.M.E.
JAMES R. BAIN, M.S.

THE DEVICE

The Gore-Tex (W. L. Gore and Associates, Flagstaff, Arizona.) cruciate ligament prosthesis is intended to serve as a permanent replacement for the anterior cruciate ligament (ACL). Unlike other devices that rely on intra-articular healing to augment strength, it is a true prosthesis. The device is fabricated from expanded polytetrafluoroethylene (PTFE). This material has a unique combination of biocompatibility, strength, flexibility, and porosity [1–3]. The device is constructed from a single long fiber of the material wound into loops. Integral fixation eyelets are formed at each end of these loops, and the strands are plaited into a three-bundle braid. The device is placed through a tibial drill hole, routed over the top of the posterior intercondylar fossa of the femur (as in a modified MacIntosh procedure), and through a femoral drill hole. The eyelets are secured to bone with cortical screws to provide the initial fixation. Permanent fixation is provided by tissue ingrowth among and into the strands in the intraosseous segments.

Prior to the initiation of clinical use, we subjected the prosthesis to a battery of tests in an animal model and a variety of mechanical simulators to assess its biocompatibility and mechanical properties [1, 4]. Several recent attempts at permanent replacement of the anterior cruciate ligament of the knee with prosthetic materials met with failure because the devices had inadequate resistance to creep or flexural fatigue to survive in this demanding application [1]. Given this history, our design work and preclinical studies focused on avoiding these failures. We conducted static and cyclic creep tests modeling the in vivo loading conditions to determine the necessary tensile strength for a PTFE ACL prosthesis. These tests indicated that a strength of 1000 lb (4448 N) was sufficient to prevent clinically meaningful elongation in vivo. [1, 2]. Accordingly, each device is tested to 4448 N during manufacture. (By comparison, the natural ACL of young human beings breaks at approximately 1730 N. [5])

We performed bending tests under load to the equivalent of 20 years in vivo to demonstrate resistance to fatigue [1]. Implants in sheep demonstrated maintenance of stability, good tolerance of the device by the synovial environment, and excellent tissue fixation in the bone tunnels. Although the device is somewhat stiffer than the natural ACL, biomechanical tests in these animals showed that the stiffness of the femur–prosthesis–tibia system is similar to that of the natural bone–ligament–bone system.

CLINICAL USE

Clinical trials of the device were initiated in the United States in October 1982, under the provisions of an investigational device exemption. During the course of this study, 1021 ACL implants were performed (see Chapter 23). Based on data gleaned from these patients, the U.S. Food and Drug Administration approved the device for commercial distribution in October 1986. Use was limited to patients with a previous failed intraarticular reconstruction. As long-term data accrue, broader indications will be considered by the FDA.

All devices in this series were implanted with the over-the-top routing described above. Initial tensioning was accomplished as follows: With the device and the femoral screw in place, the knee was placed in 20 degrees of flexion, firm tension was applied to the tibial eyelet, and the tibial screw site was marked. Following placement of the tibial screw and prior to closure, the surgeon confirmed full range of motion and obliteration of Lachman and pivot-shift signs.

The results of this study were encouraging, with only 5 per cent of the patients showing more than a trace pivot shift at any postoperative time. (See the detailed discussion of clinical results in Chapter 23.) Although these results were encouraging, one troublesome trend emerged when Lachman scores at 3 months after operation were compared with those at 12 to 18 months. A slight increase in laxity had occurred in approximately one third of the patients over this period with apparent stabilization thereafter (Graph 21–1). In this group of patients, the laxity increase was substantial enough to allow a shift of one grade in Lachman score. At three months postoperative, 98 per cent of knees had Lachman scores of 0 or 1+. By 18 months, this had decreased to 88 per cent. Results at two years were essentially identical to those at 18 months.

This increase in laxity was further described by Strum et al. [7] through a quantitative study of anteroposterior stability conducted on 11 patients. At one year after operation, the instrumented

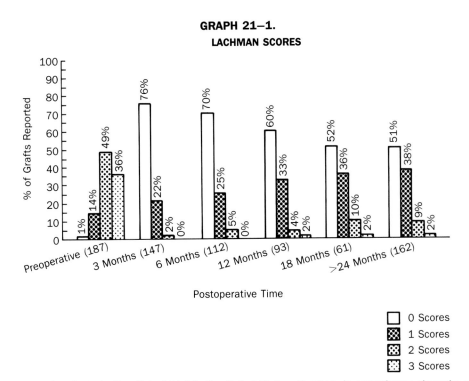

GRAPH 21–1.
LACHMAN SCORES

Postoperative Time

☐ 0 Scores
▨ 1 Scores
▤ 2 Scores
▦ 3 Scores

Lachman scores of patients in the clinical trial in the United States. Numbers in parentheses show the number of patients reporting at each interval.

Lachman test at 200 N showed that 55 per cent of patients had an anterior laxity greater than 8 mm and an involved–noninvolved laxity difference greater than 2 mm. Knees had firm Lachman end points, but they exhibited more anterior tibial laxity than expected.

We recognized that this shift in scores was not due to breakage of the device or failure of its fixations, since patients continued to report satisfactory functional stability (Chap. 23), and since essentially all of the reported pivot-shift scores (Graph 21–2) in the study as a whole remained in the stable region (scores of 0 to 1+). Moreover, knees did not develop extreme anterior laxity—at no postoperative interval were more than 2 per cent of the involved knees in the 3+ categories (>10 mm displacement) for the Lachman or pivot-shift tests.

Given the preclinical creep studies that predicted only negligible elongation of the device with time [1], this early increase in laxity was perplexing. This unexpected finding prompted a series of experiments that elucidated the mechanism of laxity increase and ultimately led to a method of surgical preconditioning and tensioning designed to prevent recurrent laxity.

STUDIES IN VITRO

The phenomena allowing increased laxity were first demonstrated in a study conducted at the University of California at Los Angeles [Markolf K: personal communication]. In reproducing these findings, the device was implanted in instrumented cadaver knees, and anterior drawer forces were applied to the joint. With the method of implantation used in the clinical study (marking the tibial screw site with the device under firm manual tension, joint flexed to 20 degrees), the knee demonstrated a mean 5-mm increase in laxity after just a few applications of a 200-N drawer force (Graph 21–3), with only negligible increase thereafter. A 5-mm increase in translation of the tibia on the femur will allow an increase of 1 in the Lachman score. Subsequent research focused on the effects of graft tensioning on the resulting mechanics of the bone–prosthesis–bone system.

We determined the magnitude of the increase in anterior tibial laxity by implanting 18-cm devices over the top in cadaver knees. With the femoral screw in place, we preloaded the prosthesis to 44, 89, 133, and 178 N (10, 20, 30, and 40 lb), and fixed the tibial eyelet. With the knees at 20 degrees

GRAPH 21–2.

PIVOT SHIFT SCORES

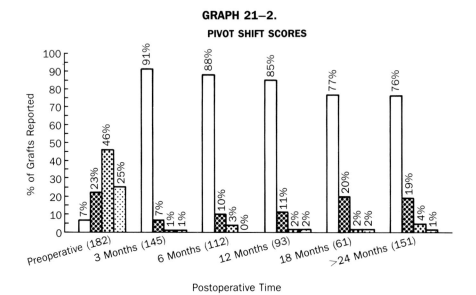

Postoperative Time

☐ 0 Scores
▨ 1 Scores
▨ 2 Scores
▨ 3 Scores

Pivot-shift scores of patients in the clinical trial in the United States. Numbers in parentheses show the number of patients reporting at each interval.

GRAPH 21–3.

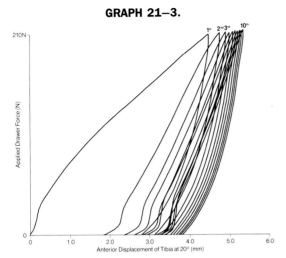

Postoperative development of recurrent laxity in a cadaver knee implanted with an ACL prosthesis, using the original tensioning technique. The first 1021 ACL implants in the United States followed this method. The tibial fixation site was selected with the knee flexed 20 degrees and the graft under "firm manual tension." Just 10 applications of a 210-N (45-lb) anterior drawer force at 20 degrees produced 5.4 mm of anterior displacement of the tibia, increasing the Lachman score from 0 to 2+.

(Fig. 21–1) showed that a length change of the device ($\triangle$) theoretically increases the anterior tibial laxity (*d*) as follows:

$$[d + 2]^2 = \triangle^2 + 10 \triangle + 4.0,$$

where $\triangle$ and *d* are expressed in centimeters, and the assumption is made that all elongation that takes place in the device contributes to increased anteroposterior laxity of the joint. (I.e., the initial elongation in the femur–prosthesis–tibia system takes place before significant tissue ingrowth has occurred in the bone tunnels. Rigid fixation of the device to the bones via ingrowth would tend to shorten the effective length of the device subject to elongation.)

Using this relation, we compared the results of the two preloading studies. With both methods, increases in the preload reduced the subsequent lengthening of the graft, but the observed laxity was consistently greater in the cadaver studies than that predicted by mechanical simulation (Graph 21–4).

A subsequent series of experiments in cadavers was directed at intraoperative methods of eliminating the sources of laxity. Keith Markolf [personal communication] suggested that one method of preventing the early recurrence of laxity would be to route the device in place, fix the femoral screw, perform multiple knee flexions/extensions with manual tension on the tibial eyelet, then fix the tibial screw. He called this procedure "preconditioning." To develop a practical implant technique, we performed flexion/extension under manual tension at various loads on the tibial eyelet, and studied the subsequent recurrence of laxity under cyclic anterior drawer loads applied at 20 degrees. Empirically, we found that firm manual tension applied to the device with a bone punch generates up to approximately 89 N (20 lb) of tension in the device. Preconditioning studies showed that 20 knee flexions/extensions 0 degrees–45 degrees–0 degrees under an 89-N load, followed by fixation at 20 degrees under 89 N of tension, are sufficient to eliminate the initial elongation component from the device and fit the artificial ligament to the patient's bone and soft-tissue anatomy, thus minimizing the postoperative development of laxity.

The recommendation to fix the tibial screw site at 20 degrees at 89 N was derived from tensioning studies that showed this method to result in a bone–prosthesis–bone system that mimics the load-displacement characteristics of the ACL-competent knee (Graph 21–6). Initially, the femur–prosthesis–tibia system is somewhat stiffer than the natural femur–ACL–tibia system, but after 100 load applications in situ, the stiffness of the

of flexion, we imposed cyclic anterior drawer forces of 0 to 285 N at 1 cycle per second. A 285-N load is an estimate of the mean force applied to the young human ACL, weighted for activities [3]. Increasing the preload force reduced the subsequent development of anterior tibial laxity (Graph 21–4).

To isolate the sources of this laxity, we studied the effects of preloading on mechanical simulators. We performed these tests with the device loaded in a straight configuration and over a 12.7-mm radius and two 1.5-mm radius pins to simulate placement over the top of the posterior intercondylar fossa of the femur and through a tibial bone tunnel. As in the previous experiment, the prosthesis was preloaded to 0 to 178 N, and cyclic drawer loads of 0 to 285 N were applied. The resulting strains, measured as per cent elongation at the 100th load cycle (Graph 21–5), show a marked reduction in elongation with increasing preload. Grafts loaded over a radius consistently showed more elongation than those pulled straight.

To compare the results of these two tests, it was necessary to determine the relation between a length change in the device and the resultant increase in anterior translation of the tibia on the femur. Examination of the geometry of the femur–prosthesis–tibia system in representative cadavers

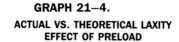

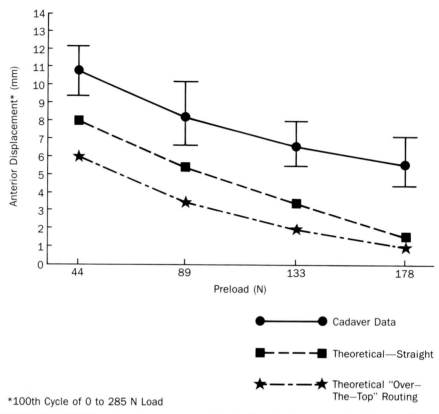

*100th Cycle of 0 to 285 N Load

Anterior tibial laxity generated in cadaver knees compared to the theoretical values derived from studies on mechanical simulators (Graph 21–5). Laxity is expressed as the anterior tibial translation observed at the 100th 0 to 285-N anterior drawer load applied at 20 degrees. Increasing the preload decreases the subsequent development of laxity, as expected, but initial creep and compression of the prosthesis do not account for all of the observed laxity.

implanted knee approaches normal values (Graph 21–6).

DISCUSSION

Prior to the initiation of this study, we recognized several mechanisms that could allow postoperative increases in laxity in knees reconstructed with this prosthesis. One of these results from improper preparation of the route through the posterior capsule: capsular tethering and soft-tissue entrapment. This occurs when the point where the device pierces the capsule is not on a direct line between the posterolateral portion of the intercondylar notch and the inferior exit of the femoral drill hole. As the patient becomes active and places cyclic loads on the device, the graft assumes a straight path, and laxity results. Soft-tissue entrap-

ment can also occur when a mass of capsular tissue is captured between the device and posterior femur. In vivo loading of the device compresses these tissues, they resorb, and laxity results. These soft-tissue problems can be mitigated if the surgeon exposes the posterior femur during implantation, allowing examination of the relation of the soft tissues and bone to the device. Improper reduction of a globally unstable joint or redundant graft material in the bone tunnels can also lead to immediate postoperative instability of the knee. These mechanisms, however, cannot account for the observed frequency of recurrent laxity in the clinical series (Graph 21–1).

The present study addresses additional mechanisms of postoperative increases in anterior tibial laxity. These studies demonstrate that postoperative laxity in some patients can result from insufficient tension applied at implant, even though all

GRAPH 21–5.
GRAPH PRELOAD VS. ELONGATION

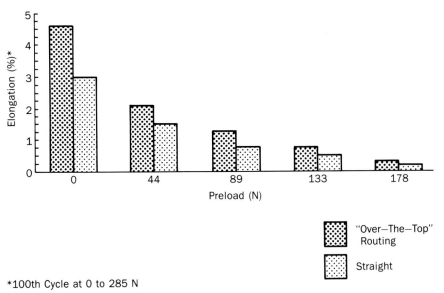

*100th Cycle at 0 to 285 N

Effect of simple tensile preloads on subsequent elongation under cyclic loads. This study on a tensile-test apparatus predicts that grafts implanted with higher preloads will allow less anterior tibial laxity in vivo.

knees were stable at surgery. Comparing the cadaver studies to those in mechanical simulators (Graphs 21–4 and 21–5) shows that the laxity that occurs with patient activity can arise from a reorientation of strands due to the passage of the prosthesis around curved bony contours and the resulting compression of the prosthesis against bone, an initial "slack" in the macrostructure due to bundle-to-bundle compression in the tripartite braid, and compression of soft tissues restraining the device from an unimpeded course between the femoral and tibial bone tunnels.

To eliminate laxity originating from these mechanisms, improvements in implantation technique were evaluated. From studies of the effects of simple preloads on subsequent laxity of the system (Graphs 21–4 and 21–5), we knew that a preload of 178 N (40 lb) or greater would minimize post-

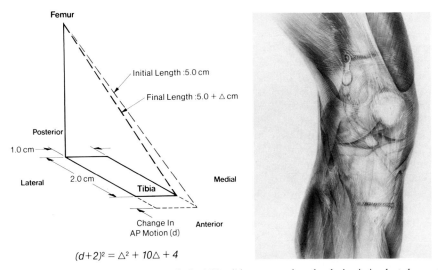

$$(d+2)^2 = \Delta^2 + 10\Delta + 4$$

Figure 21–1. Typical geometry of the femur–prosthetic ACL–tibia system when the device is implanted over the top of the posterior intercondylar fossa of the femur, showing the effect of a given elongation of the device (Δ) on increased tibial translation (d). (Anatomic figure, copyright 1985, Frederic Harwin, used with permission.)

GRAPH 21–6.

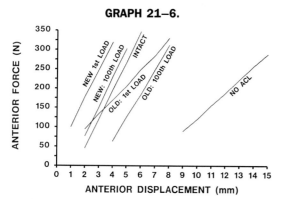

Load-displacement relations of cadaver knees with the ACL intact, the ACL excised, and the ACL replaced with the PTFE prosthesis. The knee is flexed 20 degrees. The prosthetic ligaments are implanted by the original technique (firm manual tension at 20 degrees) and the new technique (20 preconditioning cycles 0 degrees–45 degrees–0 degrees under 89 N of tension; final tensioning 89 N at 20 degrees). Using the old technique, the system becomes loose on the first load application (Graph 21–3). By the 100th load, knee stiffness and anterior laxity are intermediate between normal and ACL-deficient knees. Strum et al. [7] saw this in clinical cases. With the new preconditioning and tensioning technique, the knee is initially stiffer than normal, but exhibits the force-elongation characteristics of a normal knee after 100 load applications.

operative increases in anterior tibial laxity, but such high loads cannot be consistently applied with the existing instrumentation. We therefore consider preconditioning (flexion/extension under manual tension), followed by final tensioning at a specific moderate load, to be a practical alternative to the application of heavy preloads.

We recommend that the device be preconditioned and tensioned as follows: Once the device has been drawn in place and the femoral screw has been set, engage the tibial eyelet with the bone punch and apply an inferiorly directed manual load of 89 N (20 lb). Maintaining this load and holding the eyelet free of the tibial cortex, flex and extend the knee 0 degrees–45 degrees–0 degrees 20 times. After preconditioning the device, the tibial screw site is selected with the knee flexed 20 degrees and the device held under a manual load of 89 N. After selecting the appropriate site for the tibial screw, the knee is flexed to 90 degrees, which unloads the device and facilitates placement of the screw. (A more detailed, practical description of the improved technique is given in Chapter 23.)

The advantage of this technique is that it allows an accurate match of laxity and stiffness of the implanted joint to those of the natural knee (Graph 21–6). The disadvantage of this method is

that knee-to-knee variability is not entirely eliminated by placing the final tension on the system at 20 degrees of flexion. Though identical loads are placed on seemingly similar knees at 20 degrees of flexion, the resultant loads generated at full extension vary substantially. Knee-to-knee differences in geometry may thus lead to overloading or underloading the prosthesis at full extension.

To produce uniform in vivo loads at full extension, surgical tensioning must be performed with the joint at full extension. As of this writing (December 1986), we are developing an implant method with improved instrumentation that will allow the application of greater loads during the preconditioning phase and the application of a known final tension at full extension. Tensioning the device with the knee at full extension will reduce the possibility of overtensioning or undertensioning the prosthesis. Standardization of these loads will reduce variability in technique.

The preconditioning and tensioning methods proposed here will reduce the early recurrence of anterior laxity in patients receiving this expanded PTFE prosthesis in the ACL position. Since creep elongation is a logarithmic function of time (or, more properly, the number of load applications), additional increases in laxity are expected to be minimal over the lifetime of the patient (Graph 21–7).

To the orthopedic surgeon skilled in replacement of the ACL with autogenous tissue grafts, it may not seem reasonable to tension a strong, stiff prosthetic ACL to a point where the affected joint is tighter than the contralateral knee. However, this must be done to ensure the long-term maintenance of stability. Intraoperative attempts to match the load-displacement characteristics of the bone–prosthesis–bone system to those of the normal knee will result in recurrent laxity of the affected knee.

It must be noted that although the cadaver studies reproduced the mechanism of laxity increase, the magnitude and rate of increase were accelerated in comparison to that seen in the living knee. Instrumented cadaver knees implanted with the prosthesis using the original technique (no preconditioning; device fixed at 20 degrees under an 89-N load) developed a 1+ or greater increase in Lachman scores after relatively few load cycles (Graphs 21–3, 21–4, and 21–6), while many patients in the clinical study did not demonstrate the 0 to 1+ shift until one year or more after operation (Graph 21–1), and some continue to have 0 scores at more than three years after operation.

These differences in rate and extent may be due to several factors. First, this study clearly demonstrates that implant tensioning at surgery has a

GRAPH 21–7.

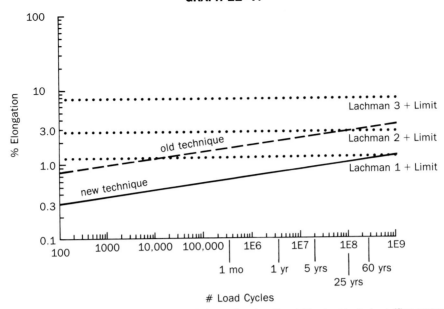

Projected development of anterior tibial laxity through time, showing the old implant technique (firm manual tension at 20 degrees) and the new preconditioning/tensioning technique (20 cycles of 0 degrees–45 degrees–0 degrees at 89 N; final set, 89 N at 20 degrees). Creep elongation of prosthetic ligaments in vivo is a logarithmic function of the number of load cycles applied to the knee [1]. This projection assumes a constant rate of 4.2 million knee loads per year at a weighted mean load of 285 N [1]. Increases or decreases in patient activity will affect the rate at which anterior laxity develops. The relation of device elongation to increases in the knee's Lachman score assumes the femur–prosthetic ACL–tibia geometry shown in Graph 21–5, and a Lachman increment of 5 mm.

With the old technique an active patient with moderately heavy ACL loading progresses to a Lachman score of 1+ or even 2+ within the first year. With the new technique, preconditioning the prosthesis minimizes the initial postoperative laxity.

major effect on the degree of laxity that develops postoperatively. Variability in surgical tensioning probably accounts for much of the difference between the predicted and observed Lachman scores (Graphs 21–7 and 21–1, respectively). Furthermore, cadaver knees are rarely as tight as living knees. We have never documented a true 0 Lachman score in a fresh specimen. This may be a subtle effect of autolysis on the ACL and collateral passive restraints. This is supported by the observation that while living ligaments generally undergo only slight, recoverable elongation due to creep with vigorous exercise [6], in our laboratory, fresh bone–ACL–bone preparations display irreversible deformation with cyclically applied loads approximating those generated in vivo. Age may also be a factor—the patients in the clinical study had a mean age at implant of 27.6 years (Chap. 23), while the cadaver knees used in our simulators were generally from older donors. Variations in patient-activity level undoubtedly also contributed to the relatively slow return of 1+ laxity in some knees in the clinical study in the United States (Graph 21–1).

SUMMARY AND CONCLUSIONS

Critical evaluation of the results of use of the Gore-Tex Cruciate Ligament Prosthesis in the United States indicated a slight decay in Lachman scores in the early postoperative period. This shift was primarily a conversion of 0 scores to 1+ scores.

Although scores of 1+ (0 to 5 mm of anterior tibial displacement) are within the range of normal knee stability, the progression from a taut condition at 3 months to slight laxity at 12 months or more raised concerns about the source of this increased anteroposterior movement. This unexpected finding stimulated a series of experiments in cadavers and mechanical simulators. The laxity increase was found to be related to the tensioning technique used to implant the prosthesis. Inadequate tensioning leads to laxity, due to an initial elongation of the prosthesis, reorientation of the device to fit the patient's individual bone structure, and compression of soft tissues. These findings led us to propose several modifications to the original implantation technique that will greatly reduce the occurrence of postoperative laxity. The improved technique also provides a more accurate approximation of normal knee stiffness values, thus improving the functional biomechanics of the reconstruction.

REFERENCES

1. Bolton CW, Bruchman WC. The Gore-Tex™ expanded polytetrafluoroethylene prosthetic ligament: an *in vitro* and *in vivo* evaluation. Clin Orthop 1985; 196:202–213.
2. Bruchman WC, Bain JR, Bolton CW. Prosthetic replacement of the cruciate ligaments with expanded polytetrafluoroethylene. In: Feagin JA Jr, ed. The crucial ligaments. New York: Churchill Livingstone (in press).
3. Bruchman WC, Bolton CW, Bain JR. Design considerations for cruciate ligament prostheses. In: Jackson DW, Drez D Jr, eds. The anterior cruciate deficient knee: new concepts in ligament repair. Saint Louis: CV Mosby 1987.
4. Collins HR. Experimentelle und erste klinische Erfahrunger mit der Gore-Tex^R-Prosthese des Ligamentum cruciatum anterius [Experimental and early clinical experience with the Gore-Tex^R Cruciate Ligament Prosthesis]. Prakt Sport-Traum Sportmed 1985; 4:33–38.
5. Noyes FR, Grood ES. The strength of the anterior cruciate ligament in humans and rhesus monkeys: age-related and species-related changes. J Bone Joint Surg (Am) 1976; 58:1074–1082.
6. Steiner ME, Grana WA, Chillag K, Schelberg-Karnes E. The effect of exercise on anterior-posterior knee laxity. Am J Sports Med 1986; 14:24–29.
7. Strum G, Markolf K, Ferkel R, et al. *In vivo* AP stability measurements of patients with synthetic anterior cruciate ligaments. Orthop Trans 1986; 10:253.

22

CLINICAL AND LABORATORY STUDIES WITH THE GORE-TEX LIGAMENT AT UCLA

KEITH L. MARKOLF, PH.D.

INTRODUCTION

The choice of treatment for the anterior cruciate ligament (ACL)-deficient knee continues to be a source of controversy. One surgical approach for the chronically unstable knee is replacement of the ACL with a synthetic substitute. The Gore-Tex prosthetic ligament is a multistranded polytetrafluoroethylene (PTFE) device intended as a permanent load-carrying implant. In this chapter, I will be reporting instrumented test results and clinical findings of a group of patients undergoing Gore-Tex ligament replacement at the Center for Disorders of the Knee in Van Nuys, Calif. All patients were tested before and after surgery at the UCLA Biomechanics Laboratory. Our laboratory preconditioning studies of this ligament in fresh cadaver specimens will also be discussed, and my recommendation for proper surgical implantation presented.

THE UCLA INSTRUMENTED CLINICAL TEST APPARATUS

The most recent model of the UCLA instrumented clinical test apparatus has been mentioned in Chapter 3 and is again shown in Figure 22–1. The patient is seated on the floor with the back supported by a reclining chair and the knee is flexed to 20 degrees. The foot is strapped to a plate that can be locked into positions of neutral (foot straight up) and 15 degrees of internal and external rotation. The femur is "grounded" to the base of the apparatus by a clamping device, which contains sand-filled leather pads to support and rigidly fix the femur. Anterior displacement of the femur is blocked by a sand pad that contacts the patella. This patellofemoral clamping force must be directed perpendicularly to the articulating surfaces of the patella and femoral condyles as clamping pressure is applied, or the patella will sublux distally on the femur. This motion can be sensed if the margin between patella and sand pad is palpated during femoral clamping. If the patella is not stable as the knee is clamped, the anterior sand pad must be repositioned to eliminate this problem. The sand pads at the base of the apparatus contact the posterior femoral condyles; care must be taken to ensure that the joint line is anterior to these pads, or posterior tibial translation will be blocked. An instrumented force handle is connected to a strap wrapped around the calf just below the tibial tubercle. A spring-loaded plunger connected to a displacement transducer senses motion of the tubercle as anteroposterior (AP) force is applied.

Thus, in our test system, the femur is assumed to be rigidly fixed to the base and tibial motion is

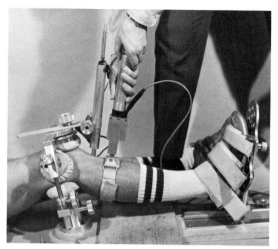

Figure 22–1. The UCLA instrumented clinical test apparatus. A response curve of force versus displacement of the tibia with respect to the femur is recorded at 20 degrees of knee flexion. Anterior laxity is calculated at 200 N of tibial force, and anterior stiffness at 100 N.

measured with respect to the framework. However, in practical terms, absolute rigid femoral fixation is impossible to achieve and some femoral motion must always occur. The assumption is made that femoral motion will be equal for both knees, emphasizing the importance of bilateral testing. A continuous x–y recording of anterior–posterior force versus displacement is obtained for each foot rotation position. Laxity (the tibial displacement for a given level of applied force) and stiffness (the slope of the force versus displacement curve) are calculated from the test curve.

Prior studies on patients with ACL-deficient knees have shown that increased laxity of an ACL-deficient knee is best demonstrated at 20 degrees of knee flexion. Injured–normal differences in anterior laxity are greatest at 200 N of anterior tibial force, and injured–normal differences in anterior stiffness are best sensed at 100 N of applied anterior force [7]. We have also reported on the use of this device in testing normal subjects [1, 6–8], ACL-deficient subjects [2, 5, 7, 8], and patients before and after autogenous-tissue ACL reconstructions [4, 5].

THE GORE-TEX PATIENT GROUP

The patient group we studied consists of 11 men and 8 women who underwent arthroscopic Gore-Tex implantation, with an over-the-top femoral placement. The indications for ligament reconstruction included frequent buckling with activities of daily living (which could not be controlled by bracing and vigorous rehabilitation), 2+ or greater Lachman score, and a positive pivot shift. The mean age was 33 (19 to 42). The time from injury to surgery averaged 56 mo (6 to 234). All patients but one had had prior surgery: six had one prior operation, six had two, four had three, and two had four. All 19 patients underwent preoperative and postoperative testing on the UCLA instrumented clinical testing apparatus. The length of follow-up (surgery to postoperative testing) in this preliminary report ranged from 12 to 17 mo (mean, 13.6).

CLINICAL RESULTS

Clinical results were determined by analysis of the James–Larson knee-rating forms. In this system, a total score of 200 points is awarded; 100 points are subjective and 100 are objective. In the subjective category, points are given for pain, range of motion, swelling, laxity, walking, running, climbing stairs, jumping, and working. The objective points include atrophy, effusion, flexion/extension, varus–valgus laxity, pivot shift, AP drawer sign, Lachman score, and functional activities.

All patients showed significant improvement in both subjective and objective scores. In the subjective category, the mean preoperative score was 50 and the postoperative score was 81. Objectively, the mean score improved from 67 to 87. Table 22–1 summarizes preoperative and postoperative symptoms of giving way. Preoperatively, the patients were almost equally divided among the mild, moderate, and severe categories, while postoperatively, 95 per cent of the patients were in the none or slight categories. The grades of pivot shift are tabulated before and after surgery in Table 22–2. Preoperatively, 84 per cent fell into the 2+ and 3+ categories, while 84 per cent were in the 0 and 1+

TABLE 22–1. GIVING-WAY SYMPTOMS

	None	Slight	Mild	Moderate	Severe
Preoperative	0	0	7	6	6
Postoperative	14	4	0	1	0

TABLE 22–2. PIVOT-SHIFT SIGN

	[0]	[1+]	[2+]	[3+]
Preoperative	0	3	10	6
Postoperative	2	14	3	0

categories postoperatively. All pivot-shift tests reported here were performed with the patient awake.

INSTRUMENTED TEST RESULTS

The mean changes in anterior laxity and stiffness resulting from Gore-Tex implantation in these patients are illustrated in Graph 22–1. Panel A shows that the mean anterior laxity of the normal knees (5 mm) was unchanged between the two test periods, and agrees well with prior measurements in normal subjects [8]. This also illustrates the consistency and reproducibility of our test procedure. Preoperatively, the laxity of the injured knees averaged 10 mm, which also agrees with prior measurements of ACL-deficient knees [8]. Postopera-

GRAPH 22–1.

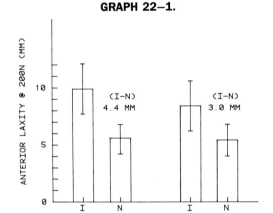

A

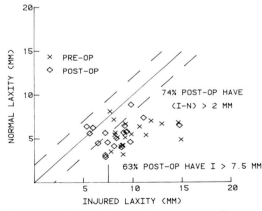

B

(a) Anterior laxity before and after surgery. The mean improvement in side-to-side difference was 1.4 mm. Mean laxity of the unoperated knees did not change, demonstrating the reproducibility of the test apparatus. I–N denotes injured–normal. (b) Injured–normal scattergram of anterior laxity at 200 N of tibial force. Postoperatively, only 26 per cent of the patients fell within the normal range for side-to-side difference in anterior laxity.

tively, the mean laxity of the injured knees was 8.6 mm. Although the mean 1.4-mm reduction in side-to-side anterior-laxity difference was statistically significant, Gore-Tex implantation clearly did not return these patients' injured knees to normal. Panel B shows the injured–normal scattergram of anterior laxity. This method of presentation is useful because a data point for each patient is shown. Prior studies with this device have established the 95 per cent confidence intervals for normal laxity and side-to-side differences in normal laxity [8]. The vertical bar on the horizontal axis (at 7.5 mm) indicates the cut-off limit for anterior laxity: 95 per cent of normal individuals will have an anterior laxity less than 7.5 mm. The limits for normal side-to-side differences in anterior laxity are indicated by the two 45-degree dashed lines: 95 per cent of normal knees will have a side-to-side difference of 2 mm or less. Ideally, one would like to see all the postoperative data points to the left of the 7.5-mm line, and between the two 45-degree dashed lines. In this series, only 26 per cent of the patients fell within the normal range for side-to-side difference, while 37 per cent had an anterior laxity of 7.5 mm or less.

Anterior stiffness before and after Gore-Tex implantation is shown in Graph 22–2. Panel A shows that there was no significant change in anterior stiffness of the normal knee between the two tests. The mean injured-knee stiffness, which was 42 per cent of normal preoperatively, was restored to 63 per cent of normal postoperatively. This is especially interesting since the stiffness of the isolated Gore-Tex ligament is approximately 2.5 times greater than that of the human ACL. This emphasizes the importance of soft tissues and fixation geometry in determining the final structural stiffness of the device after it has been implanted in the knee. The mean injured–normal difference in anterior stiffness was slightly more than halved by the Gore-Tex procedure, but did not return to zero. The stiffness scattergram of Graph 22–2B shows that 63 per cent of the patients were within the normal range for side-to-side difference in anterior stiffness postoperatively, while 42 per cent still had an injured knee stiffness greater than the lower cut-off limit of the normal range.

Graph 22–3 illustrates changes in anterior laxity and stiffness with rotation of the foot. Panel A shows that mean anterior laxity of the normal knee increases slightly as the foot is externally rotated. This pattern also holds true for the injured knee before and after surgery. The injured–normal laxity difference was relatively constant for the three foot rotation positions. The patterns of anterior stiffness change with foot rotation (Graph 22–3B) are more interesting. The normal knee demon-

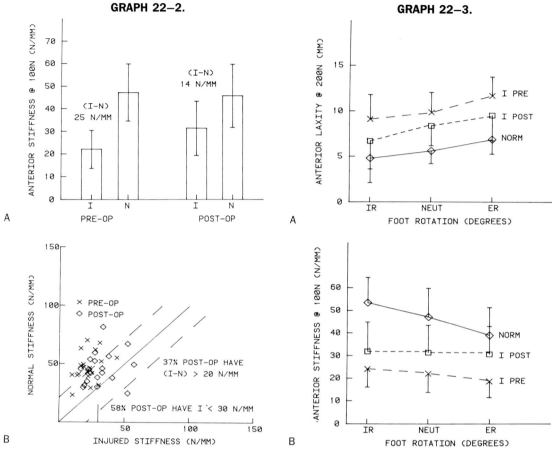

GRAPH 22–2.

GRAPH 22–3.

(a) Anterior stiffness before and after surgery. Stiffness postoperatively was 63 per cent of normal, even though the stiffness of the Gore-Tex ligament itself is approximately 2.5 times that of the natural ACL. I–N denotes injured–normal. (b) Injured–normal scattergram of anterior stiffness at 100 N of anterior force. Postoperatively, 63 per cent of the patients fell within the normal range for side-to-side stiffness difference.

(a) Variation in anterior laxity with foot rotation. The normal pattern of increased laxity with foot rotation is also evident for injured knees before and after surgery. IR denotes internal rotation, NEUT neutral, ER external rotation, PRE preoperative, POST postoperative, and NORM normal. (b) Variation of anterior stiffness with foot rotation. Normal knees demonstrate decreased stiffness with external rotation of the foot. This pattern was also evident for the injured knees preoperatively. Postoperatively, stiffness was unchanged with foot rotation.

strates a 27 per cent reduction in stiffness from 15 degrees internal to 15 degrees external foot rotation. Preoperatively, the injured knees also showed this pattern, but to a lesser degree (22 per cent reduction). Postoperatively, anterior stiffness did not change with foot rotation, and the postoperative injured–normal stiffness difference was greater with internal foot rotation than with external rotation. This could be related to the over-the-top placement of the Gore-Tex ligament.

Graph 22–4 illustrates what we believe to be the *major* argument for instrumented AP laxity testing. Here, the machine laxity measurements are plotted for various clinical grades of the Lachman sign, recorded by the physician before and after surgery. There is no statistically significant difference in mean machine laxity values between clinical Lach-

man grades preoperatively and postoperatively. It is interesting to note the large laxity variations within in each clinical grading group. For example, in knees graded by the examiner as 3+ preoperatively, the machine injured–normal laxity differences ranged from 0.8 to 10.0 mm. Similarly, in knees rated 1+ postoperatively, the side-to-side difference ranged from 0 to 8 mm. This clearly illustrates the imprecision and basic inconsistency of the clinical examination, and establishes the need for a more objective instrumented test evaluation.

Associations between the pivot-shift sign and anterior laxity are suggested in Graph 22–5, in which the mean anterior laxity values are tabulated in the various pivot-shift categories. Preopera-

GRAPH 22—4.

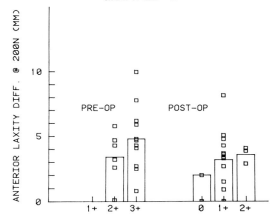

Machine measurements of anterior laxity grouped according to clinical Lachman grades as determined by the examining physician before and after surgery. There is a general trend of increased mean machine laxity with increased Lachman scores. There is a wide variation of laxity measurements within a given Lachman grade, illustrating the variability encountered with the manual laxity examination.

tively, the anterior laxity averaged 10 mm for all categories, as all patients had a positive pivot-shift sign. Postoperatively, patients with no pivot shift had a mean anterior laxity of 7.5 mm, while those who still had a 1+ or 2+ pivot shift had slightly greater laxity (9.5 mm). This 2-mm difference in anterior laxity was significant only at the $P < 0.09$ level, and can be considered suggestive of a statistical difference. This finding implies that there may be a laxity cut-off limit that separates knees

GRAPH 22—5.

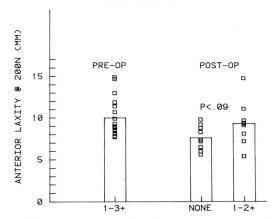

Machine measurements of anterior laxity grouped into various categories of pivot shift. Postoperatively, a difference in mean laxity was suggested between patients with no pivot shift and those graded 1+ to 2+. There was considerable scatter in values within a given grade.

with a positive pivot shift from those with no pivot shift. Larger patient groups would be required to substantiate or disprove this hypothesis.

One might expect that select clinical variables such as functional scores or patient symptoms may be correlated with the stiffness and laxity variables measured on the test apparatus. Correlations were sought between all clinical variables and all machine variables, but none were found. The question then remains: Why are these patients improved clinically and functionally, when the objective machine measurements have improved only marginally? One possible explanation may be a more vigorous and persistent muscle rehabilitation program following surgery. Another possibility could be related to the elimination of the pivot-shift sign after surgery, an improvement that may not be directly related to the straight AP tibial translation recorded with our test device. Finally, a placebo effect can never be discounted in surgery of this type since both patient and physician desire a positive outcome for the surgical procedure.

Perhaps a more important question is Why do 79 per cent of the patients still have a side-to-side difference in anterior laxity greater than 2 mm two years after the procedure? One possible explanation relates to potential stretching of the Gore-Tex ligament fibers due to cyclic in vivo loading. Published laboratory test results from the manufacturer [3] indicate that in a tension mode of loading, cyclic creep of the device is minimal and cannot account for the magnitude of laxity increases necessary to produce 5 mm of right–left laxity difference. Other possible factors include errors in the placement of the tibial tunnel holes, the over-the-top femoral placement, and proper tensioning of the device within the knee at surgery.

CADAVER STUDIES WITH THE GORE-TEX LIGAMENT

We have recently completed a series of laboratory loading tests with Gore-Tex ligaments, which were inserted into fresh frozen cadaver knees. To begin, we mounted fresh specimens into a material-testing machine that has special fixtures to record AP force versus displacement response curves before and after ligament implantation. For the intact knee, the response curve usually stabilized (i.e., repeated test curves would overlie one another) after a few AP loading cycles with 200 N of applied tibial force. However, when the Gore-Tex ligament was implanted and the specimen again loaded, we observed that AP laxity continued to increase with repeated cycles, even after 50 load cycles or more. We believe that this apparent ligament stretch-out is related to a number of physical factors.

The first is a reorientation of the Gore-Tex ligament fiber strands. As the ligament passes over the top of the femoral condyle and through the tibial tunnel hole, the PTFE fibers must change orientation and work in to a new configuration. This includes changes from an initial braided configuration to a more "flattened-tape" shape as it passes around bony contours and over tunnel-hole edges. A second effect is the entrapment of soft tissues (i.e., cartilage and capsular tissue near the femoral insertion) between the ligament and bone. Compression of these soft tissues with repeated cycles can produce an increase in AP laxity.

Based upon our laboratory experiments, we have developed (and strongly recommend) a manual *preconditioning* procedure at the time of surgery to eliminate this apparent initial stretch-out. In this procedure, the femoral eyelet is first secured into bone with a screw. An assistant then places an appropriately sized Steinman pin through the tibial eyelet, grasps the pin transversely with the fingers, and pulls on the eyelet with approximately 200 N (45 lb) of tension as the surgeon takes the knee through a series of flexion/extension cycles. It is important for the assistant to maintain ligament tension along the long axis of the tibia as the knee is flexed and extended between 0 and 90 degrees. This requires "following" the tibia with the tension force as the knee is worked through a range of motion.

Table 22–3 summarizes our laboratory experience with this technique on six fresh-frozen cadaver knees. In these tests, AP laxities of the intact knees were first recorded, and averaged 11.4 mm. The Gore-Tex ligament was then implanted ac-

cording to the manufacturer's recommended guidelines. This involved flexing the knee to 30 degrees and applying some tension to the tibial eyelet after the femoral eyelet had been screwed into bone. When we followed this procedure and then performed the first 200-N AP load cycle at 20 degrees of flexion, the knees were an average of 3.3 mm more lax than the intact specimens. However, with two additional specimens in which the tibial eyelet was pulled with greater force prior to screw fixation, the laxity of the intact knee at 20 degrees of flexion was more closely approximated. After the first reference AP load cycle with the Gore-Tex ligament was recorded, the knee was removed from the fixtures and 10 cycles of manual flexion/extension were performed with a constant tibial eyelet pull of 200 N (45 lb). The knee was then remounted in the test fixtures and a new AP test curve was recorded. As can be seen in Table 22–3, the mean laxity increase after the first 10 flexion/extension cycles was 4.3 mm; 10 more flexion/extension preconditioning cycles increased the laxity an additional 0.5 mm, as did a third group of 10 cycles. Therefore, with 30 cycles of preconditioning total, a mean laxity increase of 5.3 mm was observed. Subsequent application of 50 straight AP load cycles on the material-testing machine produced an additional 0.7 mm laxity increase, until the response curve finally stabilized.

Table 22–3 emphasizes the importance of the first 10 cycles in preconditioning the ligament *in situ*. The next 20 cycles will take out another 1 mm of AP laxity. The total AP laxity increase after load cycling was complete ranged from 5.2 to 7.0 mm for these six specimens. Our prior in vivo test results have shown that this amount of AP lax-

TABLE 22–3. SUMMARY OF ANTEROPOSTERIOR (AP) CYCLIC TESTING WITH 200 N OF TIBIAL FORCE (SIX FRESH CADAVER SPECIMENS)

		AP Laxity at 200 N (mm)		
		Mean	*SD*	*Range*
Total AP laxity of the intact knee at 20 degrees		11.4	1.8	9.3–14.3
Increase in laxity after repeated manual preconditioning cycles of the Gore-Tex ligament (knee flexion/extension under a constant 200-N ligament tension)	0–10 Cycles	+4.3	0.9	3.2–5.4
	10–20 Cycles	+0.5	0.3	0.1–0.9
	20–30 Cycles	+0.5	0.3	0.2–1.0
Additional laxity increase due to 50 AP load repetitions (after manual preconditioning)		+0.7	0.3	0.3–1.0
Total laxity increase		+5.9	0.7	5.2–7.0

ity represents the difference between a normal knee and an ACL-deficient knee. Hence, even if the ligaments in the 19 patients tested on our in vivo apparatus were properly tensioned at surgery, the lack of preconditioning at implantation could well account for the large observed right–left differences two years after surgery.

It is therefore important that this apparent stretch-out be removed with proper preconditioning techniques prior to tibial eyelet fixation. The question then remains: After proper preconditioning, how much tension should be applied and at what angle of knee flexion? Based upon tests in our laboratory during which Gore-Tex ligament tension was recorded during knee flexion and extension, we recommend tensioning the tibial eyelet to 200 N at full extension, making a mark on the tibia with a center punch to mark the screw-hole position, flexing the knee to slacken the ligament and finally inserting the tibial eyelet screw. In this way, the knee will be certain to attain full extension, and flexion contractures will be avoided. Some reduction in ligament tension at extension may be anticipated during in vivo cyclic use. We believe that if this protocol is followed, patient improvements in AP laxity should be substantial with this device. We are presently preoperatively testing a new group of patients whose ligaments have been inserted using these new techniques. We plan to test these patients postoperatively in order to verify the effectiveness of the new preconditioning protocol.

REFERENCES

1. Bargar WL, Moreland JR, Markolf KL, Shoemaker SC. The effect of tibia-foot rotatory position on the anterior drawer test. Clin Orthop 1983; 173:200–203.
2. Bargar WL, Moreland JR, Markolf KL, Shoemaker SS, Amstutz HC, Grant TT. In-vivo stability testing of postmeniscectomy knees. Clin Orthop 1980; 150:247–252.
3. Bolton CW, Bruchman WC. The Gore-Tex expanded polytetrafluoroethylene prosthetic ligament—an in vitro and in vivo evaluation. Clin Orthop 1985; 186:202–213.
4. Ferkel R, Goodfellow D, Markolf K, Zager S, Weibel W. The ACL deficient knee—substitute or follow along? Annu Meeting Orthop Res Soc 1984; 9:132.
5. Kochan A, Markolf KL, More RC. Anterior-posterior stiffness and laxity of the knee after major ligamentous reconstruction. J Bone Joint Surg (Am) 1984; 66:1460–1466.
6. Markolf K, Graff-Radford A, Amstutz H. In vivo knee stability—a quantitative assessment using an instrumented clinical testing apparatus. J Bone Joint Surg (Am) 1978; 60:664–674.
7. Markolf K, Kochan A, Amstutz H. Measurement of knee stiffness and laxity in patients with documented absence of the anterior cruciate ligament. J Bone Joint Surg (Am) 1984; 66:242–253.
8. Sherman OH, Markolf KL, Ferkel RF. Measurements of anterior laxity in normal and anterior cruciate absent knees with two instrumented test devices. Clin Orthop Relat Res 215:156–161, 1987.

23

U.S. EXPERIENCE WITH GORE-TEX RECONSTRUCTION OF THE ANTERIOR CRUCIATE LIGAMENT

H. ROYER COLLINS, M.D.

Reconstruction of the chronically unstable knee continues to be a problem for the orthopedic surgeon. More than 65 methods using autogenous materials, allografts, and prosthetic materials have been reported, with varying degrees of success [1, 2, 6-16, 19, 21-24, 27-29, 31, 33]. Portions of the patellar tendon, the iliotibial tract, the semitendinosus and gracilis tendons, and menisci have been used as autogenous grafts. Various prosthetic materials have been used as stents, augmentation devices, and biodegradable scaffolds [17, 18, 20, 30, 32]. Biologic tissues such as bovine or human allografts have been used as substitutes for the cruciate ligaments [10, 25, 26]. Despite some good results with autogenous material and with some of the prosthetic materials, and promising early results with allografts, failures have occurred, particularly in persons with poor collagen tissue. These procedures have also required long periods of immobilization, followed by bracing and extensive rehabilitation, often taking a year before the patient can return to work or normal activities.

After seeing several patients whose multiple attempts at reconstruction of their unstable knee had failed, we realized that there was a need for a prosthetic ligament. Although the ideal solution would seem to be a graft that gives immediate strength so that immobilization is not required, and yet is bio-

degradable, so that it could be replaced by the host's own collagen tissue over a period of time, we were concerned that the collagen tissue formed in most of these patients was of poor quality and with time would tend to stretch.

Therefore we decided a better solution was to implant a prosthetic ligament that gave immediate strength, so that cast immobilization was not necessary; would allow the ingrowth of the host tissue, particularly in the bony fixation holes; but would not necessarily rely upon the intra-articular ingrowth of collagen tissue and would last for the lifetime of the individual—a permanent prosthetic replacement.

The Gore-Tex, expanded polytetrafluoroethylene (PTFE) prosthetic ligament (W.L. Gore and Associates, Inc. Flagstaff, AZ.), which has a multifilament looped configuration composed of essentially pure PTFE that has been expanded to form a structure consisting of solid nodes of PTFE interconnected by fine, strong, highly oriented PTFE fibrils, was decided upon. The material possessed a very high tensile strength. The resultant microstructure contains more than 70 per cent air by volume and is characterized by fibrils averaging at least 60 μm in length. PTFE is inert and not subject to biochemical degradation. Thus its mechanical properties do not degrade with time. The porosity of the material is sufficient to allow ingrowth from surrounding fibrous and osseous tissue.

Biomechanical and biologic studies performed on animals by Bolton and Bruchman [4, 5] were extremely encouraging. In November 1982, clinical studies were begun.

MATERIALS AND METHODS

In this multicenter study, involving 20 investigators, 1021 total patients had the Gore-Tex ligament implanted for anterior cruciate insufficiency. Seven hundred twenty-two of these patients were men and 299 were women, with a mean age of 27.6 years. All surgeons used an over-the-top technique, although some of the prosthetic ligaments were implanted with an open technique and others using arthroscopic control. A prospective study was carried out, with patients evaluated at three-month intervals for the first year, and then at six-month intervals for subsequent years. This chapter is a computer analysis of 187 patients with a two-year or longer follow-up as of January 31, 1986. Complications that occurred in all 1021 patients will be discussed.

OPERATIVE PROCEDURE

In all patients, examination was carried out on the unanesthetized patient and then after anesthesia had been administered. Preoperative antibiotics were administered and the incision depended upon whether an open procedure or an arthroscopic procedure was being done and whether associated ligamentous instabilities needed to be corrected at the same time. In patients with only anterior cruciate insufficiency a medial parapatellar incision was made, with the open technique, exposing the knee and the intercondylar notch. If there was impingement on the intercondylar notch, a notchplasty was carried out using an osteotome or dental burr, making certain that there were no rough edges or impingement sites laterally, anteriorly, or posteriorly in the notch (Fig. 23–1).

A tibial drill hole was then made with a 2.4-mm Kirschner wire starting 2 to 3 cm distal to the tibial plateau, and 1 cm medial to the patellar tendon, exiting within the knee at the center of the anatomic insertion of the anterior cruciate ligament. Palpation of the J-mark on the tibial plateau facilitated placement. Care was taken to be sure that this point was just anterior and lateral to the medial tibial spine and correct position of the K-wire was determined by fully extending the knee and noting

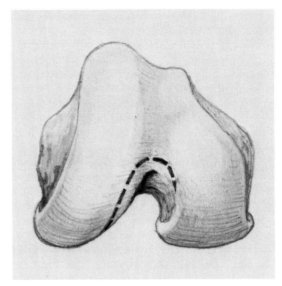

Figure 23–1. Notchplasty performed to avoid impingement.

that the Kirschner wire was pointing directly at the posterior aspect of the intercondylar notch, just medial to the lateral femoral condyle (Fig. 23–2). The Kirschner wire was then over-drilled with a 7.9-mm ($\frac{5}{16}$-in.) cannulated drill bit, taking care to avoid thermal necrosis. The entry and exit holes were chamfered, using a dental burr and appropriate rasps so that no sharp edges remained.

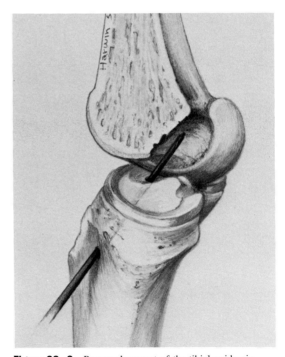

Figure 23–2. Proper placement of the tibial guide pin.

Following this a lateral incision was made starting at the lateral femoral condyle, proceeding proximally in line with the iliotibial band for approximately 2 in. The iliotibial band was exposed and split 2 cm anterior to the intermuscular septum exposing the vastus lateralis. The vastus lateralis was retracted anteriorly and branches of the lateral superior geniculate artery were cauterized as they were met. The lateral shaft of the femur was thus exposed.

A second incision was then made just posterior to the intermuscular septum in the interval between the iliotibial band and the biceps femoris and blunt subperiosteal dissection was carried out, staying close to the posterior cortex of the femur, retracting the fat pad and neurovascular structures posteriorly and exposing the popliteal area and posterior capsule. The intercondylar notch was thus exposed. A 2.4-mm ($\frac{3}{32}$-in.) Kirschner wire was then inserted, starting at a point 4 to 5 cm proximal to the lateral epicondyle. This Kirschner wire was angled posteriorly, distally, and medially to exit on the popliteal surface of the distal femur, approximately 1 cm proximal to the capsular attachment and 1 cm lateral to the midline, thus pointing toward the intercondylar notch. This guide wire was likewise over-drilled with a 7.9-mm ($\frac{5}{16}$-in.) cannulated drill (Fig. 23–3). The entry and exit holes were likewise chamfered, using a dental burr and

appropriate rasps. Neurovascular structures in the popliteal space were protected during this procedure.

A large curve passer was directed into the anterior joint space, passing posteriorly through the intercondylar notch, perforating posterior joint capsule, and exiting through the lateral incision. The joint capsule was perforated at its femoral attachment directly inferior to the posterior femoral bone tunnel exit (Fig. 23–4). A 100-cm (36-in.) length of umbilical tape, which had previously been marked for measuring, was attached to this passer and brought back through the posterior capsule, into the joint and then passed down through the tibial drill hole.

The other end of the umbilical tape was then passed up through the femoral drill hole, using either a malleable Parham band or folded 20-gauge wire. The umbilical tape leader was then used to determine the correct length of ligament to implant. The marked looped end was positioned about 2 cm distal to the edge of the exit hole on the medial tibial crest. The tape was pulled taut and a mark selected that was at least 2 cm from the proximal edge of the exit hole on the lateral femoral cortex. The prosthetic device was then attached to the umbilical tape and pulled up through the tibial drill hole, through the joint and posterior capsule and then up through the femoral drill hole. This was frequently done in two stages, first passing through the joint, posterior capsule, and out through the lateral incision, sliding the prosthetic ligament back and forth several times to make sure that all slack was removed from the system and then passing the prosthesis up through the femoral drill hole. Following this, the prosthetic ligament

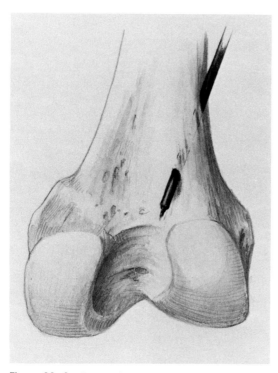

Figure 23–3. Proper placement of the femoral drill hole.

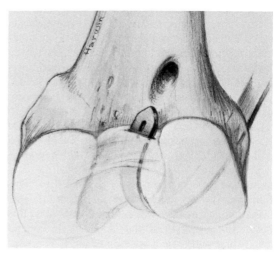

Figure 23–4. Proper position for perforation of posterior capsule with Strover hook.

was attached to the femur with a cortical screw, which was placed 2 cm proximal to the femoral exit hole, making sure that both cortices were contacted. The depth of the drill hole was measured with a depth gauge and then 3 mm was added to this measurement to make up for the thickness of the device.

The tibial screw site was selected with the device under firm manual tension. After completion of the 1,021 investigational implants described in this chapter, an improved tensioning procedure was developed (site Chapter 21). Once the femoral eyelet was attached to the femur, proper tensioning was achieved by pulling the ligament taut with approximately 20 lb of force, while the knee was brought through a range of motion from 0 to 90 degrees approximately 20 times. This was done to make sure that all slack had been completely removed. Once this was accomplished the knee was brought to 20 degrees of flexion and 20 lb of force was placed on the eyelet and a marking hole made on the tibia with a punch. A 3.2-mm drill bit was used to drill the hole in the tibia, which was then tapped and the device fixed with a 4.5-mm AO screw. The knee was then brought through a full range of motion to be sure that the motion was complete and the knee was then tested to be certain that all instability had been completely obliterated (Fig. 23–5).

If the device was implanted arthroscopically, arthroscopic evaluation was first carried out and intra-articular pathology was corrected at that time. A synovial resector was inserted into the joint to clear out the intercondylar notch area for better visualization and then the arthroplasty abraider was inserted to perform a notchplasty as indicated. If necessary, a small osteotome and a small rasp were used, passing them through the small stab wounds to accomplish this notchplasty. Once the joint was prepared for the ligament, a small incision was made starting 2 cm distal to the tibial brim and approximately 1 cm medial to the tibial tuberosity, extending for a distance of approximately 1 to $1\frac{1}{2}$ in. A ligament guide was inserted through the medial stab wound and the guide placed in the appropriate anatomical center of the anterior cruciate ligament insertion. A 2.4-mm ($\frac{3}{32}$-in.) Kirschner wire was then inserted.

Next, the previously described lateral incision was made and the Strover hook with the umbilical tape was passed through the posterior capsule. This was easily visualized using the arthroscope camera. Following this, the tibial guide pin was over-drilled with a 7.9-mm ($\frac{5}{16}$-in.) drill bit and the entry and exit holes were radiused, using the appropriate dental burrs and rasps. A grasper was then inserted through the tibial drill hole and the

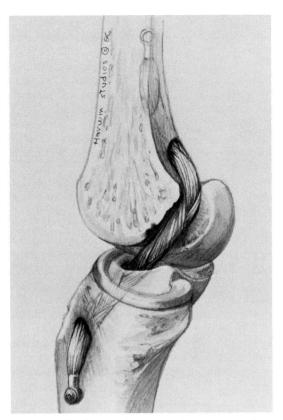

Figure 23–5. Cross-sectional view, showing proper placement of the graft to avoid impingement.

umbilical tape was grasped and pulled out through the joint and through the tibial drill hole. The prosthetic ligament was then attached to the umbilical tape and pulled up through the tibial drill hole through the joint, on through the posterior capsule, and then up through the femur, using the arthroscope for visual control. Fixation of the device was then carried out as previously described.

The wounds were closed and a modified compression dressing was used postoperatively with no immobilization necessary in patients who did not have any other ligamentous procedures carried out. The patient was encouraged to start motion as soon as he or she was comfortable.

POSTOPERATIVE REHABILITATION

The amount of postoperative immobilization depended upon the other procedures that had to be done at the same time. If there were other procedures done that required bracing or cast bracing, this was carried out. In patients who had only intra-articular procedures and implantation of the prosthetic ligament, motion was allowed without any brace as soon as the patient was capable of doing so. The patient generally used crutches for a two-week period and at the time of removal of the sutures, were capable of going without them. Rehabilitation in these instances was started immediately, allowing full range of motion and allowing exercises for the quadriceps and hamstring group of muscles as able. Quadriceps setting and straight-leg raising were started and as soon as sutures were removed and there was no evidence of synovial irritation, progressive resistance exercises were started. The patient was permitted to bear weight as his or her symptoms allowed. As soon as full strength was achieved usual activities were permitted.

In patients who had procedures performed that required cast immobilization or bracing for protection, the rehabilitation was carried out as for autogenous reconstruction. After the immobilizing devices were removed, range of motion was gradually increased, followed by the introduction of a progressive resistance exercise program. Because the prosthetic ligament gave immediate strength, it was not necessary to protect this graft with a restricted range of motion and therefore the quadriceps could be rehabilitated immediately.

RESULTS

As of January 31, 1986, 187 patients had been followed for longer than two years. Of these, 128 were male and 59 were female, with a mean age of 27.5 years. Of these patients, 62 per cent had been injured in sports (Graph 23–1). American football, skiing, and basketball accounted for the greatest number of sports injuries (Graph 23–2). Of the patients, 76 per cent had had a previous surgical procedure, including meniscectomy and extraarticular and intra-articular attempts at reconstruction. Seventy-four per cent required additional procedures at the time of the Gore-Tex implantation (Graph 23–3). Of the 326 additional surgical procedures carried out at the time of implantation, 81 patients required notchplasty, 74 had extra-articu-

lar reinforcement or repair, 71 had meniscectomy, and 34 had capsular tightening, with other procedures such as adhesion removal, osteophyte removal, and lateral release also being performed (Graph 23–4).

Preoperatively, 85 per cent of the patients had an anterior drawer score of 2+ or greater; postoperatively, only 15 per cent exhibited a 2+ or greater anterior drawer score (Graph 23–5). Of these patients, 93 per cent had a positive pivot-shift sign preoperatively and postoperatively this sign was obliterated in 76 per cent of the patients, with 19 per cent showing only a minimal pivot

GRAPH 23–2.

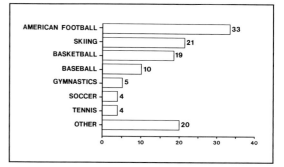

Sports as cause of original injury (total: **116** injuries).

GRAPH 23–3.

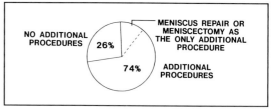

Summary of patients with additional surgical procedures at implantation.

GRAPH 23–1.

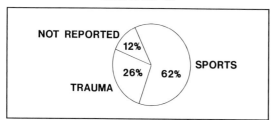

All causes of original injury.

GRAPH 23–4.

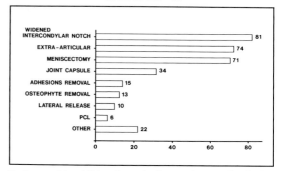

Patients with additional surgical procedures at implantation. The total number of patients was **139** and the total number of procedures was **326**.

GRAPH 23–5.

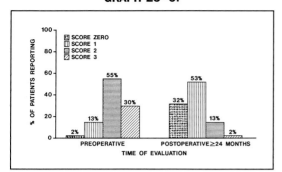

Anterior drawer scores in 184 patients reporting preoperatively and in 161 reporting postoperatively.

GRAPH 23–6.

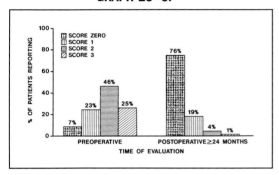

Pivot-shift score in 182 patients reporting preoperatively and in 161 reporting postoperatively.

shift (Graph 23–6). Preoperatively, 85 per cent of the patients had a 2+ or greater Lachman's score (Graph 23–7).

Before Gore-Tex ligament implantation, 78 per cent of the patients had difficulty with activities of daily living. Of these patients, 88 per cent reported that they no longer had difficulty with the activities of daily living after surgery (Graph 23–8). Of our

GRAPH 23–8.

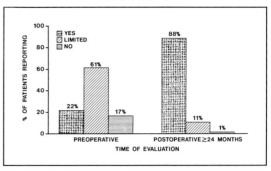

Activities of daily living of 183 patients reporting preoperatively and of 161 reporting postoperatively.

patients, 90 per cent complained of giving way or had the sensation of giving way preoperatively; postoperatively, the giving way was obliterated in 75 per cent of the patients, with only 8 per cent of the patients reporting actual episodes of giving way (Graph 23–9).

Only 6 per cent of the patients did not have pain preoperatively, with 49 per cent having moderately severe pain and 12 per cent severe pain. Postoperatively, this improved to the point that 45 per cent of the patients reported having no pain, with 36 per cent noting mild pain, 16 per cent moderate pain and 3 per cent still having severe pain (Graph 23–10). Swelling was present in 76 per cent of patients preoperatively; postoperatively it was only noted in 24 per cent of our patients (Graph 23–11). Marked improvement was noted in the ability to ascend and descend stairs. Range of motion compared favorably with the contralateral limb without significant loss of motion occurring as a result of this procedure. As might be anticipated, the thigh-girth measurements remained quite good throughout the postoperative course, since the patients were able to be mobilized immediately.

GRAPH 23–7.

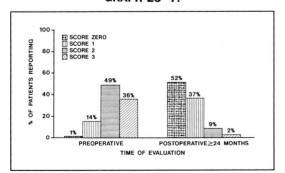

Lachman scores in 187 patients reporting preoperatively and in 161 reporting postoperatively.

GRAPH 23–9.

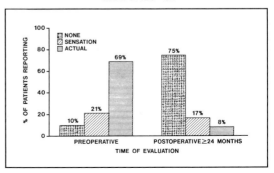

Symptoms of giving way in 185 patients reporting preoperatively and in 161 reporting postoperatively.

GRAPH 23–10.

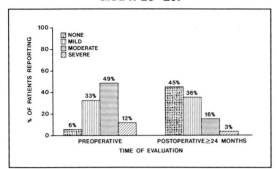

Pain in **186** patients reporting preoperatively and **160** postoperatively. The total number of patients was **187** (**128** men and **59** women) and the mean age was **27.5** years.

GRAPH 23–11.

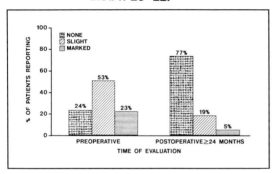

Swelling in **186** patients reporting preoperatively and in **162** reporting postoperatively.

GRAPH 23–12.

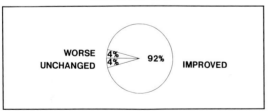

Knee status in **157** patients reporting postoperatively (**24** mo). The total number of patients was **187** (**128** men and **59** women) and the mean age was **27.5** years.

Subjectively, 92 per cent of the patients felt that they were improved. Four per cent of the patients stated that they felt their condition was unchanged and 4 per cent felt that the knee was worse (Graph 23–12).

COMPLICATIONS

Of the 1021 patients operated upon from November 1982 through January 31, 1986, the total

TABLE 23–1. COMPLICATIONS*

	Incidence	Grafts Removed	Grafts Replaced
Device Failures	1.8%	1.8%	1.3%
Instability	2.9%	0.8%	0.5%
Infections	1.3%	1.0%	—
Effusions	4.7%	0.2%	—
Screw Revisions	2.6%	—	—
Others	1.0%	—	—
Total	14.3%	3.8%	1.8%

*Total patients: 1021 (722 men and 299 women); mean age: 27.6 years.

incidence of complications was 14.3 per cent (Table 23–1). Grafts were removed in 38 patients (3.8 per cent).

Grafts were removed because of device failure in 18 patients (1.8 per cent), persistent instability in 8 patients (0.8 per cent), infection in 10 patients (1.0 per cent), and persistent effusions in 2 patients (0.2 per cent). Of the 18 device failures, 13 patients (1.3 per cent) had their graft replaced and of those with instability, 5 (0.5 per cent) had their graft replaced. Three of the 13 patients with infection were treated with systemic antibiotics, aspiration, and local measures and did not need to have their graft removed. Either the tibial or the femoral screw was bothersome in 26 patients (2.6 per cent), generally due to the prominence of the initial screw used for fixation and the screw was removed after the graft had been in place for one year.

DISCUSSION

In this series of 187 patients followed for longer than two years after Gore-Tex anterior cruciate ligament substitution, 60 per cent received their original injury as a result of sport activity, with the highest numbers of injuries occurring in American football, followed by skiing, basketball, and other sports. Seventy-six per cent had had previous surgery performed on their knees, with a large number having previously had attempts to stabilize the knee. After Gore-Tex stabilization, a large percentage of patients were able to return to their preoperative activities, including contact sports.

Although it is noted in evaluating these patients preoperatively that some of them had a 0 anterior drawer score or a 0 pivot-shift score or a 0 Lachman's score, it should be emphasized that all of the patients had an absent anterior cruciate ligament and felt that they were functionally disabled. A possible explanation for these findings was the fact that the scores listed in the graphs reflected the preanesthesia examinations and it was noted that many of the patients demonstrated more instability in the anesthetized state, when they were able to relax completely, with the scores often increasing by 1 or 2 grades. This was particularly true in patients who had had instability for some time and were schooled in techniques for preventing the knee from slipping out of place. It was also noted that the patients may have two positive signs but the third one may be absent, particularly in patients who had had a previous extra-articular repair. In these instances, a pivot shift might be difficult to demonstrate without anesthesia, but the patients felt that the knee was still unstable and that they were functionally disabled.

Initially the procedure was used as a salvage one on the failed knee that had been operated on many times; in many of the early cases there was a considerable amount of arthrosis already present. Although stability was achieved in these cases, many of the patients continue to have pain and some swelling, which was felt to be secondary to the arthrosis. However, many of the patients felt that although there was some pain with a great deal of activity, the degree of pain had been lessened by the procedure.

Device failure is a concern when studying prosthetic implants. In this series, the device failed in 18 patients (1.8 per cent). The failure generally occurred early in this series and if it was going to occur, it generally did within the first six months after implantation. Upon analyzing these cases, it was apparent that abrasion occurred in the notch area in most of the cases, finally causing a guillotine effect, weakening the ligament, with ultimate failure. The anterior notch was the culprit in most cases but in some cases impingement was in the posterior notch area as well. Because of this, notchplasty has become almost a routine procedure in order to be certain that there is no evidence of impingement upon the graft when it is in flexion and in complete extension. Since notchplasty has been performed, the incidence of failure of the prosthetic component has decreased. Also of interest is the fact that 13 of the patients in the group with device failure requested the implantation of another Gore-Tex prosthetic implant. To date, none of these second implants have broken after notchplasty was performed.

A 2.9 per cent incidence of instability has led to some modifications of the procedure described, to make certain that all of the slack is out of the prosthetic material and to be sure that there is no soft-tissue interposition before final fixation. Although the patients demonstrated some slight laxity when testing the anterior drawers at 90 degrees, there was excellent stability through the functional range of motion. The over-the-top method of insertion accounts for the slight anterior drawer sign, which is present with the knee in 90 degrees of flexion, but from a biomechanical point of view, was felt to be indicated to avoid the stress risers that have occurred at the femoral drill hole in previous attempts to use artificial material, with ultimate breakage and failure occurring at that point. Thus far there appears to be no evidence of damage to the prosthetic device at the point of fixation, and good ingrowth of material in the bony tunnels has been shown by Arnosczky in his animal studies [3].

The effusions that occurred in 47 patients (4.7 per cent) have been of some concern. These have generally occurred after heavy exercise or activity, sometimes occurring six months after the implantation and subsiding spontaneously with conservative measures such as rest and antiinflammatory agents. Aspiration of the fluid from the joints and biopsy of the synovial lining has not consistently revealed a cause for this effusion and arthroscopic evaluation has also failed to demonstrate any intra-articular problem.

Thus far, there is no indication of infection in these patients and no particles of PTFE have been consistently demonstrated.

SUMMARY

One thousand twenty-one Gore-Tex prosthetic ligament grafts had been inserted since November 1982, for anterior cruciate ligament instability. The two-year follow-up results are quite encouraging. There are potential advantages to the use of this material. Prolonged immobilization is not necessary because of the immediate strength of the system, allowing immediate motion, with its beneficial effect on the articular cartilage. Rehabilitation can be started as soon as soft-tissue healing allows it, thus preventing the atrophy that prolongs recovery time with other techniques. The use of this device does not burn any bridges. It is not necessary to ''rob Peter to pay Paul'' as with other procedures using autogenous materials, thus maintaining more normal physiologic knee function. The prosthetic ligament can be used when no autogenous tissue is available and if failure does occur another implant can be reinserted or other reconstructive procedures can still be done.

Attention to detail in implanting the device with proper radiusing of the holes to avoid sharp bony impingement areas and notchplasty where indicated to prevent any sharp edges are mandatory to prevent mechanical problems.

In patients who already have significant degenerative change in their joint, with previous meniscectomies having been performed, stability can be achieved, but patients may still continue to have pain and swelling. In most instances this pain has been markedly decreased and the incidence of swelling has also been markedly decreased.

Patients who have participated in athletics preoperatively have been capable of returning to athletics postoperatively, including contact sports and skiing.

It must be stressed that this study represents a group of patients with chronic ligamentous instability, in whom a permanent prosthetic device has been implanted. Continued long-term studies are anticipated to determine if this device will stand the test of time.

REFERENCES

1. Alm A, Gillquist J, Strombers B. The medial third of the patellar ligament in reconstruction of the anterior cruciate ligament. Acta Chir Scand [Suppl] 1974; 445:5–13.
2. Andrews JR, Sander R. A "mini-reconstruction" technique in treating anterolateral rotatory instability (ALRI). Clin Orthop 1983; 172:93–97.
3. Arnoczky SP, Torzilli PH, Warren RF, Allen AA, Spivak J. Biologic fixation of ligament prostheses and augmentations—an evaluation of bone ingrowth in the dog. Orthop Trans 1986; 10(2):280.
4. Bolton CW, Bruchman B. Mechanical and biological properties of Gore-Tex expanded polytetrafluoroethylene (PTFE) prosthetic ligament. Akt Prob Chir Orthop 1983; 26:40.
5. Bolton CW, Bruchman B. The Gore-Tex expanded polytetrafluoroethylene prosthetic ligament: an in vitro and in vivo evaluation. Clin Orthop Relat Res 1985; 196:202–213.
6. Cabaud HE, Feagin JA, Rodkey WG. Acute anterior cruciate ligament injury and augmented repair. Am J Sports Med 1980; 8:395.
7. Clancy WG. Anterior cruciate ligament functional instability: a static intra-articular and dynamic extra-articular procedure. Clin Orthop 1983; 172:102–107.
8. Clancy WG, Narechania RG, Rosenberg D, Gmeiner J, Wisnefske DD, Lange A. Anterior and posterior cruciate ligament reconstruction in rhesus monkeys. J Bone Joint Surg (Am) 1981; 63:1270–1284.
9. Clancy WG, Nelson DA, Reider B, Narechania RG. Reconstruction using one-third of the patellar ligament, augmented by extra-articular tendon transfers. J Bone Joint Surg (Am) 1982; 64:352.
10. Collins HR, Hughston JC, DeHaven KE, Bergfeld JA, Evarts CM. The cruciate ligament substitute. J Sports Med 1974; 2:11.
11. DuToit GT. Knee joint ligament substitution: the Lindemann Heidelberg operation. S Afr J Surg 1967; 5:25.
12. Ellison AE. Distal iliotibial-band transfer for anterolateral rotatory instability of the knee. J Bone Joint Surg (Am) 1979; 61:330–337.
13. Eriksson E. Reconstruction of the anterior cruciate ligament. Orthop Clin North Am 1976; 7:167–179.
14. Friedman MJ, Sherman OH, Fox JM, DelPizzo W, Snyder SJ, Ferkel RJ. Autogeneic anterior cruciate ligament (ACL) anterior reconstruction of the knee: a review. Clin Orthop 1985; 197:9–14.
15. Insall JN, Joseph DM, Aglietti P, Campbell RD. Bone block iliotibial band transfer for anterior cruciate insufficiency. J Bone Joint Surg (Am) 1981; 63:560–569.
16. Ireland J, Trickey EL. MacIntosh tenodeses for anterolateral instability of the knee. J Bone Joint Surg (Br) 1980; 62:340.
17. James SL, Kellam JF, Slocum DB, Larson RL. The proplast prosthetic ligament stent as a replacement for the cruciate ligaments of the knee. Akt Prob Chir Orthop 1983; 26:116–120.
18. Jenkins DHR, McKibbin B. The role of flexible carbon-fibre implants as tendon and ligament substitutes in clinical practice. J Bone Joint Surg (Br) 1980; 62:497–499.
19. Jones KG. Results of use of the central one-third of the patellar ligament to compensate for anterior cruciate ligament deficiency. Clin Orthop 1980; 147:39–44.
20. Kennedy JC. Application of prosthetics to anterior cruciate ligament reconstruction and repair. Clin Orthop 1983; 172:125–128.
21. Kennedy JC, Roth JH, Mendenhall HV, Sanford JB. Intra-articular replacement in the anterior cruciate ligament deficient knee. Am J Sports Med 1980; 8:1–14.
22. Lipscomb AB, Johnston RK, Snyder RB, Brothers JC. Secondary reconstruction of anterior cruciate ligament in athletes by using a semitendinosus tendon. Am J Sports Med 1979; 7:81–84.
23. Losee RE, Johnson TR, Southwick WD. Anterior subluxation of the lateral tibial plateau. J Bone Joint Surg (Am) 1978; 60:115–130.
24. Marshall JL, Warren RF. Reconstruction of functioning anterior cruciate ligament: preliminary report using quadriceps tendon. Orthop Rev 1979; 6:49–55.
25. McMaster WC. A histologic assessment of canine anterior cruciate substitution with bovine xenograft. Clin Orthop 1985; 196:196–202.
26. McMaster JH, Weinert CR, Scranton P. Diagnosis and management of isolated anterior cruciate ligament tears: a preliminary report on reconstruction with the gracilis tendon. J Trauma 1974; 14:230.
27. Mott HW. Semitendinosus anatomic reconstruction for cruciate ligament insufficiency. Clin Orthop 1983; 172:90–93.
28. Nicholas JA, Minkoff J. Iliotibial-band transfer through the intercondylar notch for combined anterior instability (ITBT procedure). Am J Sports Med 1978; 6:341–353.
29. O'Donoghue DH. A method for replacement of the ACL of the knee. J Bone Joint Surg (Am) 1963; 45:905–924.
30. Park JP, Grana WA, Chetwood JS. A high-strength Dacron augmentation for cruciate ligament reconstruction: a two-year canine study. Clin Orthop 1985; 196:175–186.
31. Scott WN, Schosheim PM. Intra-articular transfer of the iliotibial muscle-tendon unit. Clin Orthop 1983; 172:97–102.
32. Weiss AB, Blazina ME, Goldstein AR, Alexander H. Ligament replacement with an absorbable copolymer carbon fiber scaffold—early clinical experience. Clin Orthop 1985; 196:77–86.
33. Zarins B, Rowe CR. Combined anterior cruciate ligament reconstruction using semitendinosus tendon and iliotibial tract. J Bone Joint Surg (Am) 1986; 68:160–178.

24

ARTHROSCOPIC INSERTION OF THE PROSTHETIC GORE-TEX LIGAMENT

JAMES M. FOX, M.D.

Before contemplating arthroscopic insertion of a prosthetic anterior cruciate ligament versus an open procedure, the orthopedic surgeon must determine who are the appropriate patients for this technique. The factors to be considered are the associated extra-articular stabilization procedure, and the overall rationale for arthroscopic versus open arthrotomy.

To determine the appropriateness of isolated anterior cruciate ligament reconstruction, a long-term review of 127 cases of reconstruction performed for chronic anterior instability was performed in 1984 [2]. Forty-three patients underwent the reconstructive technique, including intra-articular substitution for the anterior cruciate ligament, plus associated extra-articular procedures. These were compared with 84 patients who had an isolated anterior cruciate ligament intra-articular substitution performed.

These comparison groups were equivalent in age, sex, duration of symptoms, prior surgical procedures, chronicity of complaints, preoperative subjective symptoms, and preoperative objective examination. Long-term comparison of these two groups demonstrated no significant difference in their ultimate results, measured on the James 200-point rating scale. Group 1 consisted of the combined intra-articular substitution plus extra-articular procedures and averaged 166.2 points, while those in Group 2, with an isolated anterior cruciate reconstruction, scored 169.1. These results encouraged us to continue our efforts at arthroscopic

reconstruction of the anterior cruciate ligament with various materials, including autogenous tissues, allografts, and prosthetic devices.

The first disadvantage to arthroscopic insertion is that it does not allow for the additional extra-articular stabilizations; in particular, capsular reefings, tenodesis of the iliotibial band, or advancement of the posterior lateral complex for posterior lateral instability. We have found that these procedures appeared to be necessary only for the most severe components of rotatory instability.

In Chapter 23, Collins reviewed the initial 1000 Gore-Tex ligament substitutions and reported on a two-year follow-up study. Objective measurements of stability, including Lachman score (Graph 24–1), and pivot-shift score (Graph 24–2), demonstrated that there were no significant overall differences between arthrotomy and arthroscopy. Similar results were obtained with the anterior drawer sign, thigh girth, flexion and extension measurements. In a similar fashion, comparison of subjective parameters, such as episodes of giving way (Graph 24–3), ability to engage in activities of daily living, ascending stairs, descending stairs, pain, and swelling were equivalent between arthrotomy and arthroscopy. Also, the incidence of complications (Table 24–1) was equivalent, except for slightly increased incidences of removal of tibial screws and symptomatic effusions.

The second disadvantage of arthroscopic insertion is the experience necessary to perform these techniques, both for the surgeon and the assistants.

GRAPH 24–1.

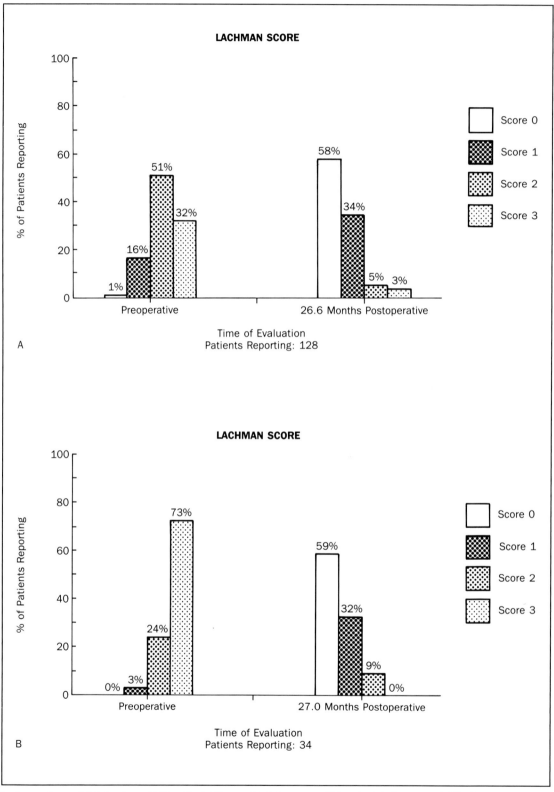

Lachman Score: (a) Arthrotomy (128 patients) Versus (b) Arthroscopy (34 patients). Courtesy of W.L. Gore and Associates, Inc.

GRAPH 24–2.

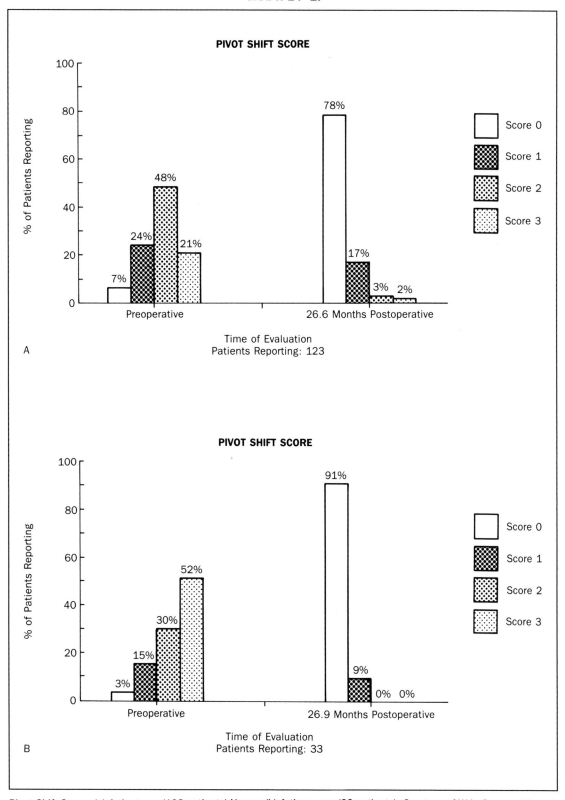

Pivot-Shift Score: (a) Arthrotomy (123 patients) Versus (b) Arthroscopy (33 patients). Courtesy of W.L. Gore and Associates, Inc.

GRAPH 24–3.

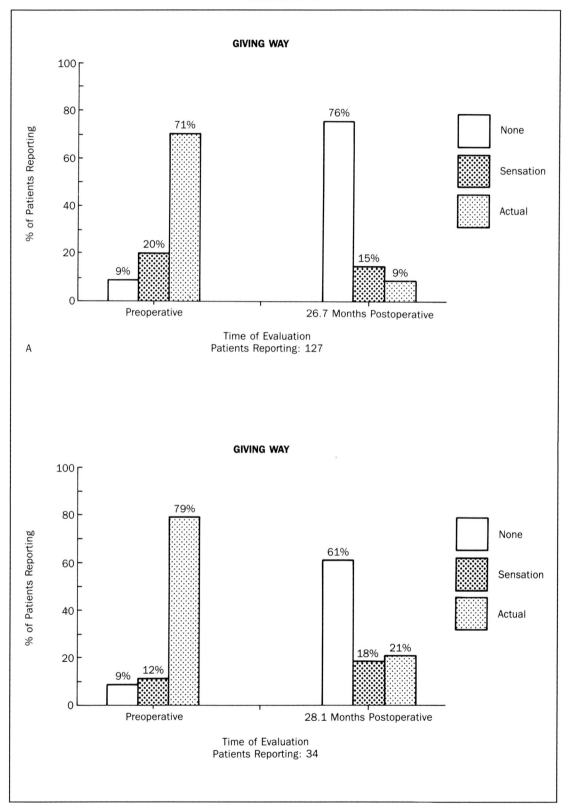

Giving Way: (a) Arthrotomy (**127** patients) Versus (b) Arthroscopy (**34** patients).

TABLE 24–1. COMPLICATIONS

Arthrotomy (146 Patients)

	Incidence	Grafts Removed	Grafts Replaced
Device failures	5 (3.4%)	5 (3.4%)	4 (2.7%)
Instability	10 (6.8%)	2 (1.4%)	2 (1.4%)
Infections	2 (1.4%)	2 (1.4%)	1 (0.7%)
Effusions	8 (5.4%)	—	—
Screw revisions	12 (8.2%)	—	—
Others	3 (2.1%)	—	—

Arthroscopy (34 Patients)

	Incidence	Grafts Removed	Grafts Replaced
Device failures	1 (2.9%)	2.9%	2.9%
Instability	1 (2.9%)	—	—
Infections	—	—	—
Effusions	4 (11.8%)	—	—
Screw revisions	6 (17.6%)	—	—

Confidence in one's ability to maneuver expeditiously through these small areas is gained with practice.

The advantages of the arthroscopic technique as opposed to arthrotomy are equivalent to the advantages recognized in arthroscopic meniscectomy versus arthrotomy: decreased postoperative pain, decreased hospital stay, and increased patient mobility [1]. These advantages have been illustrated in our initial group of 95 patients who underwent arthroscopic insertion of the Gore-Tex ligament. The mean hospital stay was 2.4 days; 95 per cent of the patients were controlled with a schedule III (acetaminophen with codeine) or schedule IV (propoxyphene napsylate with acetaminophen) pain medication, and 90 per cent of the patients had discontinued their use of crutches within 10 days of the surgical procedure.

Another advantage of arthroscopic insertion is the excellent illumination and magnification provided by the viewing system. The ability to maneuver the arthroscope into the recesses of the intercondylar notch area allows inspection of the passage of the prosthetic graft, confirming adequate opening of the intercondylar notch, and the ability to visualize any small osteophytic spurs or sharp bony edges that may impinge on the graft.

SURGICAL TECHNIQUE

The standard operative environment is a laminar-flow operating room. Prophylactic antibiotics are used routinely—specifically, the cephalosporins—for the first 24 hours. One gram intravenously at the time of surgery and 250 mg by mouth every 6 hr for 36 hr is the recommended dosage. Equipment used for the procedure includes a 4.5-mm 30 oblique wide angle arthroscope; a video system, including a CCD (chip) camera and three-quarter-inch video recorder, draped for sterility; standard hand arthroscopy equipment, including scalpel blades and straight and upbiting basket forceps; a motorized intra-articular shaver (Dyonics Manufacturing, Andover, MA.); a motorized abrader system (Dyonics); suction rasps (Arthrofile; Dyonics); Vector II system (Dyonics), ligament guide, internal and external chamfering, silicone plug; the Gore-Tex graft system (W.L. Gore & Associates, Inc. Medical Products Division, Flagstaff, AZ)—specifically, the ligament lengths of 14, 16, and 18—and rasps; a standard arthrotomy set, including self-retaining retractors, assorted clamps, needle holders, etc.; and appropriate cannulated drill bits, and a battery power source (Dyonics).

After completing a thorough arthroscopic evaluation and performing indicated intra-articular procedures, including removal of loose bodies, intra-articular shaving, and treatment of meniscal tears, careful attention is given to the intercondylar notch area. In chronic instability this is always narrowed (Fig. 24–1). A thorough notchplasty is performed, utilizing appropriate gouges, then the motorized abrasion system (Fig. 24–2).

A 5-cm medial tibial incision is now made, paralleling and 1 cm medial to the patellar tendon and from a point originating 3 cm below the medial tibial plateau (Fig. 24–3). Utilizing the Vector drill-guide system, a $\frac{3}{32}$-in. guide pin is now placed (Fig. 24–4), making sure that the intra-articular point is localized in the anatomical center of the anterior cruciate ligament area (Fig. 24–5). Sequential cannulated drill bits are used, enlarging the hole to $\frac{5}{16}$ in. (Fig. 24–6).

At the time of drilling, the tip of the intra-articular guide pin is covered with a small curette, to prevent the guide pin from being inadvertently driven across the joint and puncturing the articular surface or the posterior capsular area (Fig. 24–7). Drilling is performed under battery power, which is a low-speed type, to prevent increased heat generation and thermal necrosis from retarding bone growth into the bony tunnels.

Following the drilling of the hole, it is important to chamfer (i.e., radius) the internal and external surfaces in order to remove any sharp bony edges, and make sure that these have been appropriately smoothed; any sharp edges will cause damage to the prosthesis (Figs. 24–8 and 24–9). The tibial

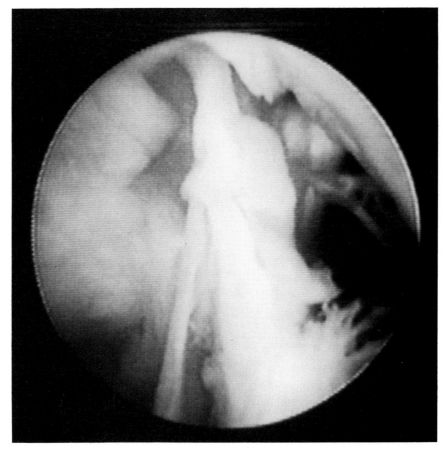

Figure 24—1. Arthroscopic view of narrowed intercondylar notch.

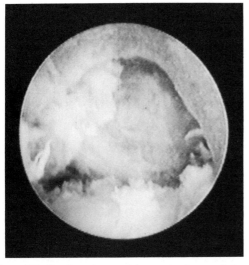

Figure 24—2. Open intercondylar notch after notchplasty.

hole is now plugged with a silicone stopper, to prevent leakage of fluid and maintain joint distention (Fig. 24–10).

Attention is now directed to preparation of the femoral tunnel. A 7-cm lateral incision (Fig. 24–11) is made, beginning at the lateral femoral epicondyle and extending proximally. Fascia lata is incised, paralleling its fibers. One incision is made centrally, and soft tissue is dissected down to the lateral femoral shaft. A second incision is made approximately 2 cm posteriorly, at the posterior edge of the iliotibial band, and again soft tissue is dissected onto the posterior surface of the lateral intercondylar area (Figs. 24–12).

Using the Vector® drill-guide system, a $\frac{3}{32}$-in. guide pin is placed from the lateral femoral shaft approximately 4 cm above the lateral femoral epicondyle. The pin is then directed inferiorly, posteriorly, and medially in a long oblique fashion, exiting 1 cm medial to the lateral gastrocnemius origin and 1 cm proximal to the posterior capsular insertion (Figs. 24–13 and 24–14). As with the tibial tunnel, this is drilled with cannulated drill bits to

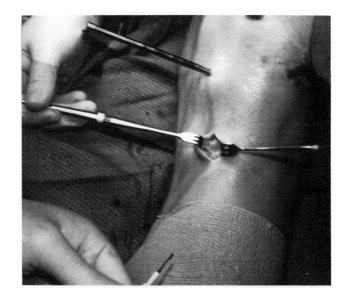

Figure 24–3. Surgical incision on the tibia.

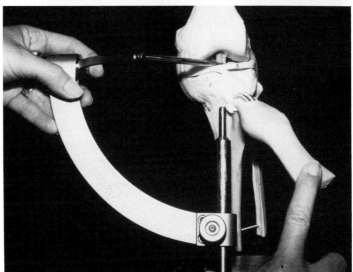

Figure 24–4. Vector® system (Vector II®) guide wire on tibia.

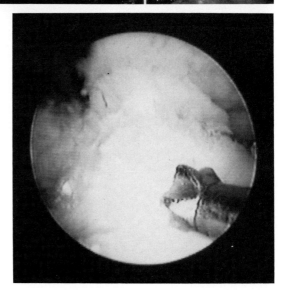

Figure 24–5. Anterior arthroscopic point of guide on tibial attachment, anterior cruciate ligament.

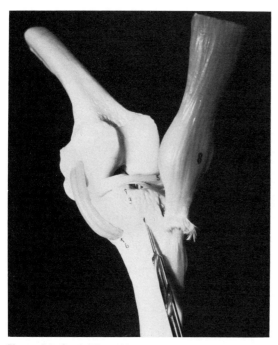

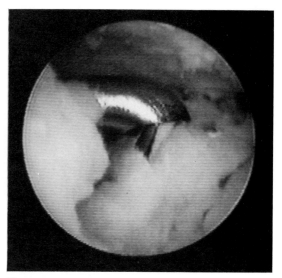

Figure 24–7. Intra-articular view through the arthroscope, showing curette on guide pin.

Figure 24–6. Drilling with cannulated drill bits.

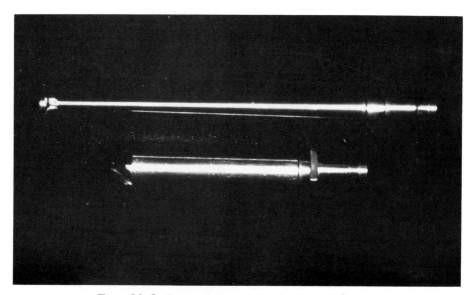

Figure 24–8. Intra- and extra-articular chamfering devices.

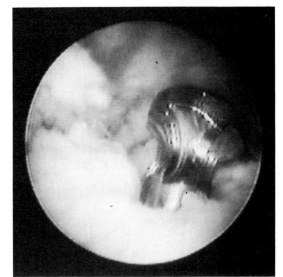

Figure 24—9. Chamfering device, intra-articular.

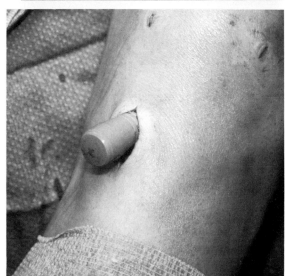

Figure 24—10. Plugging tibial hole with silicone plug.

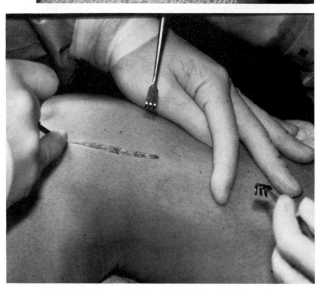

Figure 24—11. Superior lateral incision on the femur.

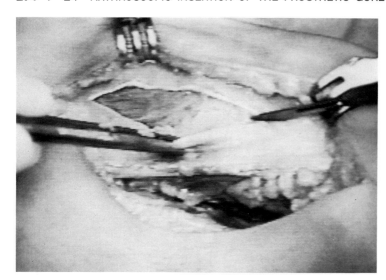

Figure 24–12. Two incisions on the iliotibial band.

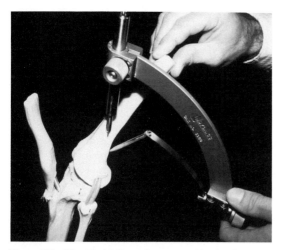

Figure 24–13. Model Vector® system guide pin, femur.

$\frac{5}{16}$ in., and then internal and external chamfering (i.e., radiusing) is performed to remove any sharp bony edges. As previously discussed, drilling is performed with a battery system. An umbilical tape measuring 100 cm in length is looped upon itself to equal a length of 50 cm in both limbs of this loop, and then the loop portion is marked at 14, 16, and 18 cm for subsequent passage and measurement (Fig. 24–15). The arthroscope is reinserted into the joint, and from an anterior medial portal an up-biting long rongeur is passed through the intercondylar notch area, puncturing the posterior lateral capsule at the superior edge. Opening the jaws of the rongeur stretches the capsule further.

The capsular hole is freed accordingly, to make sure that there is no soft tissue restricting passage of the ligament. It is also important to confirm that there are no bony osteophytes in this area. Using a curved rasp (Gore Manufacturing), then remove any sharp edges to free the soft tissues.

The free ends of the umbilical tape are then grasped with the rongeur posteriorly (Fig. 24–16),

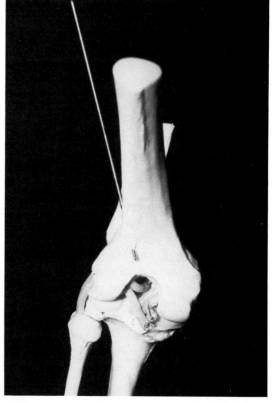

Figure 24–14. Model with guide pin, femoral hole.

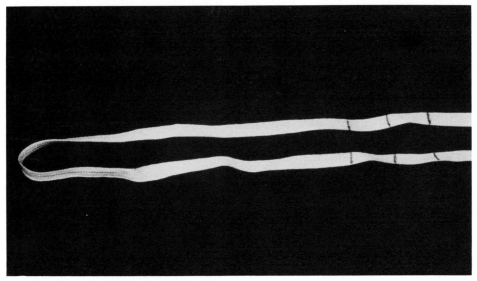

Figure 24–15. Umbilical tape marked at 14, 16, 18 cm.

then drawn through the intra-articular space, grasped through the tibial tunnel, and pulled through the tibial hole (Fig. 24–17). In a similar fashion, the proximal end of the umbilical tape is grasped with an instrument through the femoral tunnel and brought onto the femoral shaft. This marked umbilical tape is now held in place from a point 3 cm above the external femoral hole, and 3 cm distal to the tibial hole, and the appropriate length of 14, 16, or 18 cm is determined for selection of the length of Gore-Tex ligament (Fig. 24–18). The umbilical tape is now repositioned at the posterior capsule and is passed through the eyelet of the selected ligament and then brought with traction through the posterior capsular hole (Fig. 24–19).

After drawing the ligament through the posterior capsular hole, inspection with the arthroscope is performed again to make sure that the intercondylar notch has been appropriately widened to accommodate the ligament, and that there are no sharp or bony edges that would interfere with or affect the mechanical integrity of the prosthesis (Fig. 24–20). If any impingement is noted, the motorized abrasion instruments are now reinserted for further smoothing of these femoral surfaces (Fig. 24–21). The Gore-Tex ligament is now brought through the tibial tunnel, and also through

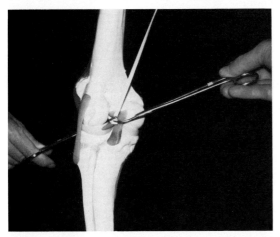

Figure 24–16. Rongeur passed through the intercondylar notch area and grasping umbilical tape.

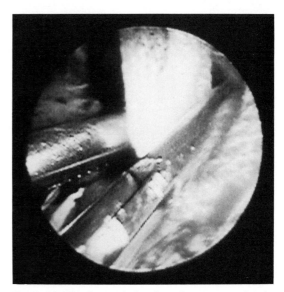

Figure 24–17. Intra-articular view of rongeur grasping the umbilical tape from the tibial hole.

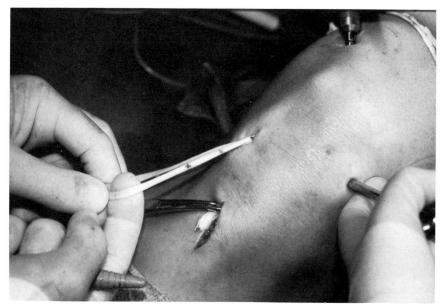

Figure 24—18. Measuring length of ligament with marked umbilical tape.

the femoral tunnel. It is sawed back and forth to make sure that there is free movement, and then positioned equidistant from its femoral and tibial ends. A point 3 cm above the external femoral hole is selected, drilled with the supplied drill bits, tapped, and the appropriate screw length is selected. It is fixed with the bicortical screws supplied by the Gore-Tex Manufacturing Company. It is important to obtain a firm compression fixation.

At this point the femoral end has been fixed, and with 20 lb of distal pull (approximately 90 N of force), the knee is placed through repetitive range-of-motion exercises from 0 to 90 degrees. This is to prestress this multifilamented continuous weave to its maximum length prior to fixation, in order to achieve maximum length of the prosthesis. In ca-

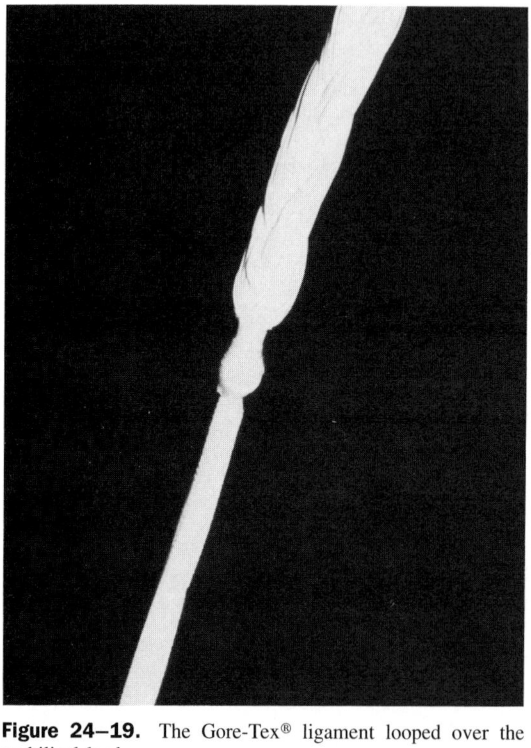

Figure 24—19. The Gore-Tex® ligament looped over the umbilical leader.

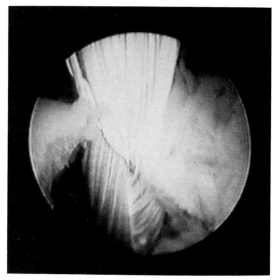

Figure 24—20. Impingement of osteophyte on anterior notch.

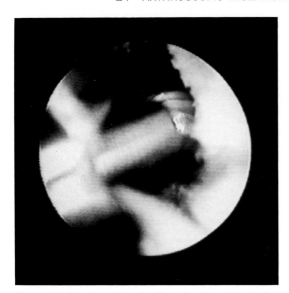

Figure 24–21. Smoothing the femoral surface with abrader.

daver specimens it has been noted that by performing this repetitive range-of-motion exercise with tension, approximately 5 to 10 mm of additional length of the ligament is obtained [22]. At a point 3 cm distal to the external tibial hole, after the appropriate position has been noted, the ligament is fixed to the tibial surface with a smooth Steinman pin for a trial position. Complete range of motion and extension is confirmed to make sure that the knee has not been captured, eliminating complete extension of the joint. Confirmation of stability with correction is done with the Lachman test and pivot-shift test. The ligament is reinspected with

the arthroscope to make sure there is adequate clearance with no bony impingement (Fig. 24–22).

After confirmation of the position, integrity, stability, and complete extension of the knee, the tibial screw hole is now drilled, tapped, and measured, and the biocortical compression screw is used to fix the prosthesis to the tibial surface (Fig. 24–23). A stable fixation is most easily obtained with the knee in 90 degrees of flexion, to alleviate tension across the Gore-Tex prosthesis. The nonisometric over-the-top position of the ligament creates mild laxity when the knee is flexed 90 degrees.

Standard closure is now performed, with a suction drainage system placed in the posterior lateral compartment to prevent hematoma accumulation. Incisions within the fascia lata are closed with interrupted No. 1 absorbable suture. Subcutaneous tissue is reapproximated distally with No. 3 clear absorbable suture, and skin incisions are closed with subcuticular 4.0 clear nylon suture. Adhesive sterile strips are applied for additional protection of the incisions, and then a sterile dressing is applied and held in place with a long, premeasured elastic stocking.

CRITICAL ASPECTS OF INSERTION TECHNIQUE

When performing the surgical insertion procedure, there are a few critical points that must be kept in mind. First, it is important to ensure that the tibial intra-articular hole is made in the joint at

Figure 24–22. Intra-articular view of the Gore-Tex® ligament through the arthroscope.

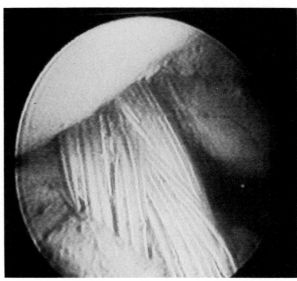

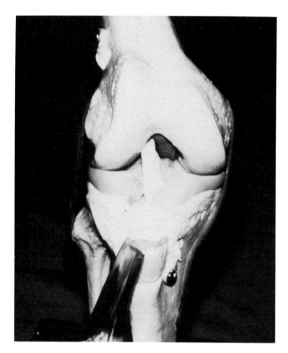

Figure 24—23. Screws and ligament in place.

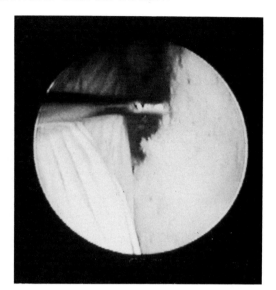

Figure 24—25. Adequate clearance of the removed osteophyte.

the central portion of the anterior cruciate ligament, and that the arthroscope is directed posteriorly to prevent impingement on the anterior portion of the intercondylar notch. Also, it is also critical to free the soft tissue at the posterior capsule. If this is not done, this tissue will separate because of the pressure of the ligament over time, and can cause increasing length with increasing laxity. Use of a low-speed battery system diminishes the risk of thermal necrosis within the bony tunnels, as this may retard ingrowth into the interosseous portion of the prosthesis. Careful chamferring (i.e., radiusing) of the internal and external bony tunnels must be done to eliminate any sharp bony edges that would cause abrasion of the prosthetic ligament and diminish its mechanical strength (Fig. 24–24 and 24–25). Preconditioning the ligament with tension through 20 repetitions of an arc of movement will ensure that maximum length of the prosthesis has been obtained prior to

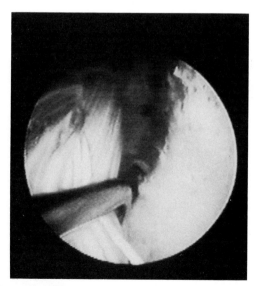

Figure 24—24. View of bony impingement at the posterior femoral notch.

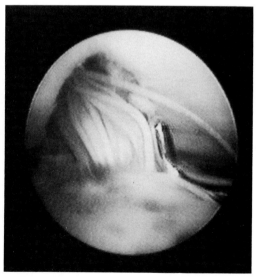

Figure 24—26. Second look, impingement on the ligament with broken strands.

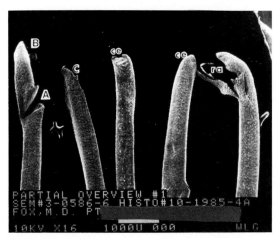

Figure 24–27. Electron microscopy of broken ligament.

insertion, therefore preventing increased laxity that can occur later after repetitive use.

Finally, it is critical to perform a complete and adequately confirmed notchplasty, as any sharp bony edges will cause trauma to the prosthesis (Fig. 24–26), or cause eventual disruption and breakage of the filaments, as demonstrated in the electron microscopy of a broken ligament shown in Figure 24–27.

SUMMARY

The advantages of using the arthroscope to insert the Gore-Tex ligament included decreased postoperative pain, decreased hospital stay, and increased functional mobility. Perhaps more importantly, it allowed the surgeon to take advantage of the technology of the arthroscope to illuminate and magnify the placement, to visualize better and maximize the critical details of insertion. These include confirming position of the ligament, providing adequate clearance within the intercondylar notch area, and removing impinging bony tissue. If attention to these details is not complete, there is an increased risk of diminishing the longevity of

the ligament through progressive pressure necrosis secondary to abrasion on the prosthesis. As experience was gained in using this technique in our initial 95 cases, actual operative time in an uncomplicated case was reduced to approximately 45 minutes.

What has been learned in this four-year experience using the arthroscope for surgical control is the critical importance of attention to detail, not only with the prosthetic Gore-Tex ligament, but also with other anterior cruciate substitutes. Important details include placement of drill holes, chamfering (i.e., radiusing) of bony tunnels, and adequate clearance within the intercondylar notch area, which would, if not tended to, cause pressure across the substituted structure, affecting both its biomechanical capabilities and its longevity. The arthroscopic techniques allow for improved visualization into areas inaccessible to routine arthrotomy techniques.

Finally, it must be emphasized that in this preliminary analysis of the use of a permanent prosthetic device, the results have been extremely satisfactory to the patient and to the treating physician, both subjectively and objectively. The surgical technique of arthroscopic insertion has afforded definite advantages to the patient and to the surgeon. Our confidence in arthroscopy is directly related to the technical facility of the entire arthroscopic team. Continued long-term evaluation is necessary to elucidate additional technical factors, to further perfect surgical techniques, and to explore the ultimate capabilities of this permanent prosthesis.

REFERENCES

1. Northmore-Ball MD, Dandy DJ, Jackson RW. Arthroscopic, open partial and total meniscectomy: a comparative study. J Bone Joint Surg (Br) 1983; 65:400–404.
2. Strum GM, Fox JM, Ferkel RD, et al. Intra-articular versus intra- and extra-articular reconstruction for chronic anterior cruciate ligament instability. Presented at the annual meeting of the American Academy for Orthopedic Surgery, New Orleans, Feb. 20–25, 1986.

25

THE BIOMECHANICS OF ANTERIOR CRUCIATE ALLOGRAFTS

E. PAUL FRANCE, PH.D.
LONNIE E. PAULOS, M.D.
THOMAS D. ROSENBERG, M.D.
CHRISTOPHER D. HARNER, M.D.

INTRODUCTION

Successful replacement of injured knee ligaments with collagenous allografts depends upon the initial and long-term biomechanical integrity of implanted tissues. In vivo, an allograft should provide the strength and elasticity necessary for maintenance of joint stability and juxtaposition, while supplying a natural scaffold for tissue ingrowth, healing, and eventual replacement. These requirements are met if the basic biomechanical properties of the allograft are similar to the stress, strain, and elastic characteristics of the ligaments being replaced and are maintained at appropriate levels during tissue healing. In the case of anterior cruciate ligament (ACL) replacement, the allograft tissue should provide stability at about two times the total tensile strength of the ACL because at least 50 per cent of the initial strength is lost during healing.

As the use of allografts in knee ligament surgery has gained acceptance, the demand for tissue has grown. To accommodate this demand, the variety of collagenous tissue types used as allografts has increased. Originally, fascia lata provided the main source of knee ligament allograft tissue. Now, other collagenous tissues such as Achilles and patellar tendons are being utilized. Initially,

allografts were harvested under sterile conditions and preserved fresh frozen. In an effort to reduce costs and increase tissue supply, gas and cobalt irradiation sterilization techniques and freeze-dried preservation methods have been adopted. However, before these tissue-preparation techniques can be totally accepted, a complete understanding of their effects on the biomechanical properties of allograft tissue is critical. This chapter reports the results of laboratory research with the objective of quantifying and comparing the material properties of and determining the effects of preservation techniques and sterilization procedures on human collagenous allografts prior to their implantation.

Review of Literature

Research to date on the biomechanics of allografts falls into two basic categories: determination of the initial (preoperative) material properties and evaluation of in vivo effectiveness of retention of material properties. Studies on the initial material properties of tissues have concentrated on quantifying the strengths of collagenous allografts [1–4] and have only recently been directed toward evaluating the effects of tissue sterilization and preservation [3, 5]. Most of the research on the material characteristics of fresh-frozen ACL grafts has been accomplished by Noyes, Butler, Grood, and co-

180

workers [1, 2, 4], who recently compared maximum (ultimate) load, stress, and stiffness between several collagenous grafts and the ACL. They found that only the patellar tendon-type grafts were stronger (1.6 to 1.7 times) and stiffer (3.8 times) than normal ACLs. Of the other tissues analyzed, semitendinosus was the closest to ACL maximum load at 0.7 time; 18-mm-wide gracilis, iliotibial tract, and 16-mm-wide fascia lata were much weaker (0.4 to 0.5 time). The data on stiffness followed the same trend. By increasing the width of harvested iliotibial tract and fascia lata tissues, they were able to increase the strength of the graft to be equal to ACL levels. Noyes et al. concluded that grafts with strengths greater than the ACL, such as patellar tendon, are preferable because of the potential for weaker grafts to fail prematurely in vivo [1].

Prior to the recent work of Paulos et al. [3] and Butler et al. [5], very little research addressed the biomechanical effects of sterilization and preservation on allograft tissues. Results of the few studies in this area [6–8] were contradictory. Barad and coworkers [6] demonstrated that deep-freezing at −80°C had no effect on the properties of rhesus monkey anterior cruciate bone-ligament-bone preparations. Thomas and Gresham [7] studied the effects of freeze drying on allograft tissues and found no adverse effect in human fascia lata, whereas Webster and Werner [9] showed a significant decrease in the strength of canine flexor tendons. These conflicting findings are related to differences between laboratories in tissue-preparation methods, freeze-drying techniques, and tissue-reconstitution procedures and highlight the need for controlled studies.

Information pertaining to the retention of the biomechanical properties of collagenous allografts in vivo have come mainly from research using a dog model [10–15]. Generally, the results of these studies have been encouraging. They indicate that the allograft loses approximately half its initial strength during the first 6 to 12 weeks of implantation, followed by a progressive increase in strength up to about one year. Preliminary clinical findings in human beings tend to show less success than that observed in animal experimentation. However, because of the brief clinical experience and the lack of adequate follow-up, these results appear unreliable.

MATERIALS AND METHODS

For the past two years, we have concentrated our efforts in three areas. First, we have examined and compared the basic material properties of un-

sterilized patellar-tendon, fascia-lata, and Achilles-tendon allografts. Second, we have analyzed the effects of standard five-day freeze-drying methods and tissue-reconstitution procedures on the preoperative biomechanical properties of collagenous allografts. Third, we have evaluated the effects of 24- to 36-hour freeze drying, of cold ethylene oxide (ETO) gas sterilization, and of high-dose cobalt irradiation sterilization on the initial biomechanical properties of patellar-tendon allografts. The discussion below provides a general overview of the tissue type, preparation methods, and biomechanical-strength-testing techniques employed.

Allograft Specimens

A total of 92 human allograft samples were obtained from 17 pairs of fresh and fresh-frozen human cadaver legs for use in these studies. Tissues (64 samples) obtained from 10 pairs of cadaver legs (mean age, 44 yr; range, 24 to 62 yr) were used for basic material-property testing and freeze-drying/reconstitution effect analysis. When possible, tissues harvested from each leg included patellar tendon with accompanying tibial and femoral bone fragments, fascia lata, and Achilles tendon with attached calcaneal bone fragment. Two samples lateral and medial, were obtained by dividing each patellar tendon in half. After removing fatty and muscular tissue, the allografts were preserved either by fresh freezing at −20°C or by freeze drying using techniques described below. Tissues harvested from a single leg of each cadaver were preserved in a like manner, so that each preservation technique would be tested on the allografts of one leg in each pair. Table 25–1 shows the number of specimens for each allograft tissue type preserved by fresh freezing and/or freeze drying.

The effects of freeze drying and sterilization were tested using a total of 28 patellar-tendon samples from the legs of the remaining seven human cadavers (mean age, 27 yr; range, 16 to 46 yr). After harvesting and extraneous-tissue removal,

TABLE 25–1. EFFORTS 1 AND 2—SAMPLE NUMBER

	Fresh Frozen	Freeze Dried
Patellar tendon (two samples/leg)	15	16
Achilles tendon	9	7
Fascia lata (One sample/leg)	10	7

each tendon was divided to obtain two patellar-tendon specimens, one medial, the other lateral. One patellar-tendon sample from each donor was then subjected to one of four treatments: (1) fresh freezing without sterilization, (2) freeze drying without sterilization, (3) freeze drying and cold ETO sterilization, and (4) freeze drying and cobalt irradiation sterilization.

Preservation and Sterilization Techniques

In preparation for freeze drying, tissues were cleaned of all fatty tissue and frozen at $-70°C$. Selected allograft tissues harvested from the first 10 cadavers were freeze dried for a five-day cycle in a standard freeze-drying system (Virtis, Gardner, N.Y.). Designated patellar-tendon samples from the remaining seven cadavers were freeze dried using 24- to 36-hour cycles in a system consisting of a Virtis Unitop 600 SL connected to a freeze model 12. The specimens were then stored in airtight containers.

Selected freeze-dried patellar-tendon samples were sterilized by 8-hour cold exposure to ethylene oxide gas in a 3M gas sterilizer and then mechanically aerated for approximately 8 to 12 hours. Sterilization by irradiation was done by exposing freeze-dried patellar-tendon samples to approximately $2\frac{1}{2}$ to $3\frac{1}{2}$ mrads of cobalt-60 gamma radiation.

Biomechanical Test Methods

In preparation for testing, frozen samples were quick thawed in warm water; freeze-dried samples were reconstituted in sterile water. Of the specimens obtained from the first cadaver group, approximately one third of the samples of patellar tendon and fascia lata were reconstituted for only two hours and the rest for 24 hours prior to testing. Each allograft was divided into one to three specimens of approximately equal thickness and each specimen tested separately. Special fixtures were designed to firmly grip both soft tissue and bone. Before testing, the total test length and cross-sectional area of each allograft tissue strip were measured. Once each specimen was gripped and aligned within the test fixtures, and a preload of approximately 10 N was applied. The allograft sample was then tension tested at a constant displacement rate equivalent to 100 per cent strain per second using an Instron 1331 material-testing machine. During each test, a force-displacement curve was generated. Normal saline was used to keep the tissues moist during their preparation for mechanical testing.

Final analysis included only data collected from tests showing in-substance ligament failure. Ultimate load and displacement data were obtained from the Instron force-displacement curves and normalized to ultimate strength (stress) and ultimate strain and modulus of elasticity using cross-sectional area and length measurements. Moduli of elasticity were not determined for tissues tested for basic material properties and five-day freeze-drying effort because of measurement difficulties. Student's statistics ($p = 0.01$) were used to determine significant differences between tissue types, preservation methods, and sterilization techniques. For all statistical comparisons, mechanical data from fresh-frozen allografts provided control values.

RESULTS AND DISCUSSION

Allograft Material Properties

Test results on the material properties of different allograft types are presented in Table 25–2. Comparisons of all three types of allografts, i.e., patellar tendon, Achilles tendon, and fascia lata, indicated that the Achilles tendon possessed the highest ultimate stress followed by the patellar tendon and fascia lata. However, only the fascia lata was found to be significantly weaker than the Achilles and patellar tendons. There were no statistically significant differences in ultimate strain for all comparisons of tissue type. The results we obtained for ultimate strength of patellar tendon and fascia lata are similar to those obtained by Noyes and coworkers, with one exception. They indicated a much higher maximum stress for fascia lata [2]. The difference may be attributed to normal variations in material thickness within fascia lata. For our testing, we chose the portion of fascia having a relatively consistent thickness (usually the thinner areas). The location from which Noyes and coworkers obtained their fascia lata specimen is not specified. Based on our assessment of initial mechanical properties, the tissues of choice would include patellar and Achilles tendons. However, our observations of allograft tension bearing and

TABLE 25–2. ALLOGRAFT MATERIAL PROPERTIES—FRESH FROZEN

	Ultimate Strength (MPa)			Ultimate Strain (CM/CM)		
	Mean	*Standard Deviation*	*N*	*Mean*	*Standard Deviation*	*N*
Patellar tendon	47.44	16.33	15	0.17	0.15	15
Achilles tendon	61.42	25.57	9	0.24	0.19	9
Fascia lata	32.38	13.93	10	0.29	0.11	10

failure modes dictate some caution regarding the Achilles tendon. Unlike patellar tendons and fascia lata, which have parallel collagen fibers, the Achilles tendon exhibits a great deal of fiber crossing and interdigitation. This arrangement of fibers affects the way in which tension is carried and how the tendon fails. The ramifications of such arrangement for in vivo function are still unclear.

Freeze-Drying Effects

The results of analysis on fresh-frozen versus freeze-dried 24-hour reconstituted allografts are presented in Table 25–3. Statistical comparisons between fresh-frozen and freeze-dried allografts showed no significant difference in mechanical strength or strain for all three tissue types. Graph 25–1 graphically portrays the effects of varying reconstitution time for freeze-dried allograft tissues. For both patellar tendon and fascia lata freeze-dried allografts, ultimate strengths were significantly decreased after 2-hour reconstitution, in contrast to strengths after 24-hour reconstitution. Analysis of ultimate strain data indicated no significant differences. These results may help to explain in part the discrepancy between data obtained by us and that obtained by Butler et al. [5]. They reported significant differences in maximum stress and modulus between ethylene oxide freeze-dried specimens and fresh-frozen patellar tendon and fascia lata allografts. However, they rehydrated the freeze-dried specimens for approximately two hours in normal saline. The results of this study indicated that a reconstitution time of 24 hours is sufficient, whereas 2 hours is insufficient to return freeze-dried collagenous allografts to normal strength. Further investigations are needed to de-

GRAPH 25–1.

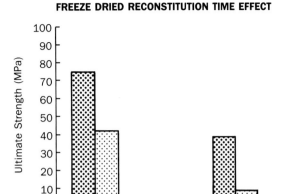

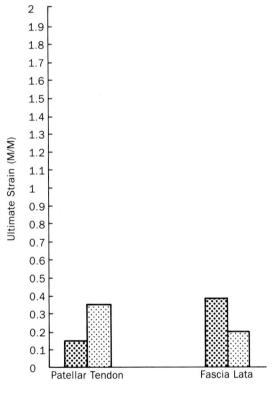

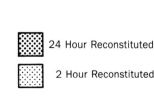

Effects of reconstitution time of the material properties of freeze-dried specimens.

TABLE 25–3. ALLOGRAFT MATERIAL PROPERTIES FRESH FROZEN (FF) VERSUS FREEZE DRIED (FD)

		Ultimate Strength (MPa)		Ultimate Strain (CM/CM)	
		FF	*FD*	*FF*	*FD*
Patellar tendon	Mean	47.44	62.46	0.17	0.18
	Standard deviation	16.33	23.30	0.05	0.09
	N	15	16	15	16
Achilles tendon	Mean	61.42	36.63	0.24	0.23
	Standard deviation	25.57	5.41	0.19	0.06
	N	9	9	9	9
Fascia lata	Mean	32.38	38.60	0.29	0.36
	Standard deviation	13.93	9.87	0.11	0.02
	N	10	7	10	7

termine whether shorter reconstitution times (between 24 and 2 hours) are adequate.

Preservation and Sterilization Effects

Changes in patellar-tendon allografts related to longer duration of freeze-drying procedures and different sterilization treatments are presented in Table 25–4. Analyses of the effect of long-duration freeze drying versus fresh freezing revealed no significant changes in ultimate strength, ultimate strain, or modulus of patellar-tendon allografts. These results coupled with those reported above would indicate that alternate methods of freeze drying (5-day versus 24- to 36-hour) have no significant effect on the retention of material properties.

The analysis of sterilization effect on allograft biomechanics revealed contrasting results. No significant differences in properties were obtained for comparison between fresh-frozen nonsterilized and freeze-dried ethylene-oxide–sterilized patellar-tendon allografts. It should be noted that the ethylene oxide gas sterilization method we selected required a cold rather than a hot cycle. This difference is noteworthy, because not all tissue banks use the cold cycle, and preliminary results indicate that the high temperature of a hot cycle may decrease the strength of allografts. The aeration time after the gas exposure cycle may also be an important factor. Although it probably has little effect on preoperative biomechanical properties of allografts, any remaining ethylene oxide may adversely affect the long-term success and acceptance of the tissue in vivo. Freeze-dried, high-dose cobalt irradiation treatment did result in a significant loss in ultimate strength in comparison to fresh-frozen nonsterilization, freeze-dried nonsterilization, and freeze-dried gas sterilization treatments. No statistically significant changes in ultimate strain and modulus were found with irradiation treatment. However, the trends were

TABLE 25–4. ALLOGRAFT STERILIZATION EFFECTS IN PATELLAR TENDONS

	Ultimate Strength (MPa)		Ultimate Strain (CM/CM)		Modulus (MPa)	
No sterilization; fresh frozen ($n = 8$)	39.15	5.59	0.25	0.10	121.1	37.4
No sterilization; freeze dried ($n = 13$)	32.66	9.51	0.35	0.19	92.2	36.7
Ethylene oxide gas sterilization; freeze dried ($n = 13$)	35.24	11.42	0.26	0.09	109.4	40.2
Cobalt-irradiated; freeze-dried ($n = 14$)	17.52	5.30	0.22	0.10	77.5	31.5

toward decreased values. Butler et al. [5] found that a 1.95-Mrad-dose radiation sterilization did not significantly affect the biomechanical properties of allografts, but the dosage was substantially lower than that given the tissues we tested. With high-dose irradiation treatment, it is probable that bonding within and between collagen molecules is altered either as a result of direct interaction with the gamma radiation or as a secondary effect related to warming of the tissue. Combining our results and those of Butler et al., we propose that there be a prescribed level of radiation dosage to ensure retention of the allograft's material properties. The exact level has yet to be determined.

CONCLUSIONS

Based upon our results and other published studies on the biomechanical properties of fresh preserved and sterilized collagenous allografts, the following conclusions can be drawn.

Patellar-tendon segments appear to be best suited for ACL replacement for two reasons. First, the initial maximum stress of patellar-tendon allografts is approximately 1.5 to 2.0 times greater than for the ACL and therefore compensates for the 50 per cent loss in allograft strength as healing occurs. Second, patellar tendons are usually harvested with bone attached to each end, so implantation is easier.

Collagenous tissues with maximum stress below the ACL level are usable as allografts if the cross-sectional area of the implant is increased to provide the necessary strength. However, the increased size of allograft complicates implantation and may actually be detrimental to function.

Freeze-drying does not appear to alter the initial material properties of collagenous allografts if sufficient reconstitution time is allowed before implantation. Rehydration times of 2 hours or less are insufficient, but 24 hours or more are sufficient to restore biomechanical strength.

Cold ethylene oxide gas sterilization does not affect the biomechanical properties of allografts, whereas high-dose cobalt irradiation decreases ultimate strength. A lower dose of radiation sterilization may result in no compromise to tissue mechanical properties.

A note of caution is in order relative to the extrapolation of our data to clinical success or failure. The strength and integrity of allografts at implantation, although important, may not play as large a part in clinical success as other factors affecting the long-term presence of the allograft in the joint.

REFERENCES

1. Butler DL, Noyes FR, Grood ES, Miller EH, Malek M. Mechanical properties of transplants for the anterior cruciate ligament. Trans Orthop Res Soc 1979; 4:81.
2. Noyes FR, Butler DL, Grood ES, Zernicke RF, Hefzy MS. Biomechanical analysis of human ligament grafts used in knee-ligament repairs and reconstructions. J Bone Joint Surg (Am) 1984; 66:344–352.
3. Paulos LE, France EP, Rosenberg TD, et al. Comparative material properties of allograft tissues for ligament replacement: effects of type, age, sterilization and preservation. Trans Orthop Res Soc 1987; 12:129.
4. Sheh M, Butler DL, Stouffer DC. Mechanical and structural properties of the human cruciate ligament and patellar tendon. Trans Orthop Res Soc 1986; 11:236.
5. Butler DL, Noyes FR, Waltz KA, Gibbons MJ. Biomechanics of human knee ligament allograft treatment. Trans Orthop Res Soc 1987; 12:128.
6. Barad S, Cabaud HE, Rodrigo JJ. Effects of storage at −80°C as compared to 4°C on the strength of rhesus monkey anterior cruciate ligaments. Trans Orthop Res Soc 1982; 7:378.
7. Thomas ED, Gresham RB. Comparative tensile strength study of fresh-frozen and freeze-dried human fascia lata. Surg Forum 1963; 14:442–443.
8. Webster DA, Werner FW. Mechanical and functional properties of implanted freeze-dried flexor tendons. Clin Orthop Rel Res 1983; 180:301–309.
9. Idem. Freeze-dried flexor tendons in anterior cruciate ligament reconstruction. Clin Orthop Relat Res 1983; 181:238–243.
10. Clancy WG, Narechania RG, Rosenberg TD, et al. Anterior and posterior cruciate ligament reconstruction in rhesus monkeys: a histological, microangiographic and biomechanical analysis. J Bone Joint Surg (Am) 1981; 63:1270–1284.
11. Curtis RJ, DeLee JC, Drez DJ. Reconstruction of the anterior cruciate ligament with freeze-dried fascia lata allografts in dogs. Am J Sports Med 1985; 13(6):408–414.
12. McMaster WC. Bovine xenograft collateral ligament replacement in the dog. J Orthop Res 1985; 3:492–498.
13. Nikolaou PK, Seaber AV, Glisson RR, Ribbeck BM, Bassett FH. Anterior cruciate ligament allograft transplantation: long-term function, histology, revascularization and operative technique. Am J Sports Med 1986; 14(5):348–360.
14. Ryan JR, Drompp BW. Evaluation of tensile strength of reconstructions of the anterior cruciate ligament using the patellar tendon in dogs: a preliminary report. South Med J 1966; 59:129–134.
15. Shino K, Kawasaki T, Hirose H, et al. Replacement of the anterior cruciate ligament by an allogeneic tendon graft: an experimental study in the dog. J Bone Joint Surg (Br) 1984; 66:672–681.

26

ANTERIOR CRUCIATE LIGAMENT ALLOGRAFTS

LONNIE E. PAULOS, M.D.
THOMAS D. ROSENBERG, M.D.
WILLIAM DOUG GURLEY, M.D.

The idea of replacing the cruciate ligaments without sacrificing other tissues is very appealing. The ideal graft must have several characteristics, including histocompatibility, sufficient initial strength, continued strength during incorporation, the ability to be stored, and ability to induce the proper cellular response from the host. While animal studies using preserved tendons and ligaments have been encouraging, experience with human intra-articular allografts is limited to only one reported study [31].

OSSEOUS VERSUS LIGAMENTOUS TISSUE TRANSPLANTATION

Much research has been published concerning the transplantation of allograft bone and cartilage [4, 6, 12, 29, 35, 36]. By contrast, far fewer studies are available on ligament and tendon allografts, and the majority of these concern flexor tendon allografts in the hand [8, 14, 19, 25, 27]. Experience with bone may be used as a rough guide; however, it must be emphasized that the transplantation of dense collagen fiber bundles is significantly different from that of porous, cancellous bone. Bone allograft principles cannot and should not be directly applied to ligament allografts, as there are many inherent differences be-

tween osseous and ligamentous tissues, including surface area that is exposed to the host, density of the tissues, the tissue's reaction to freezing, lyophilization and sterilization, completeness of revascularization, responses to motion and stress, and healing response within the intra-articular synovial environment. Whereas osseous proteins that induce the formation of new bone have been identified, no such fibrous or ligamentous morphogenic protein has been found [37].

There is considerable potential for making incorrect inferences if one relies on the fairly extensive data on osteoallografts, instead of realizing that there is a marked lack of basic scientific data on collagenous-tissue transplant.

IMMUNOGENICITY OF TISSUE ALLOGRAFTS

A major concern in transplanting allogeneic tissues has been the immunogenicity of the allograft. Studies of bone allograft show that both freezing and freeze drying reduce the antigenicity of bone grafts [4, 13, 33]. No superiority of freeze drying over fresh-frozen treatment of allograft bone has been shown with respect to antigenicity. Fresh, nonmatched bone does evoke a rejection response [4, 13].

In like manner, fresh tendinous tissue has been found to evoke an immune response in the host [3, 20, 26]. Some of the earliest soft-tissue allograft transplantation work was conducted with flexor tendons in the hand. In the first edition of his textbook, Bunnell casually referred to his experience with tendon allografts, expressing his discouragement at finding adhesions, necrosis, and a marked foreign-body reaction in the surrounding tissues [7]. But Bunnell failed to detail his method of graft preservation. Later, researchers found much more favorable responses with tendon grafts that has been exposed to a variety of preservation techniques, including refrigeration, freezing, merthiolate, ethanol, paraformaldehyde, freeze drying, glutaraldehyde, and radiation [1, 10, 16, 18, 19, 27]. Peacock, who compared fresh, refrigerated, and frozen tendon implants, obtained good results with composite flexor-tendon and tendon-sheath grafts. None of these showed evidence of rejection. Peacock also observed no significant differences in the antigenic potential of tendon grafts as compared with purified collagen grafts, but he used a somewhat crude assay of ''second set'' skin-graft reactions [25, 26].

More recently, Minami et al. [20] used a cytotoxic assay and an antibody absorption test to show that major histocompatibility antigens do exist in the fresh rat tendon tissue, but that the collagen itself does not express them. They concluded that the cellular elements of fresh tendon carried the major histocompatibility antigens, which were lost when the cells were killed by freezing and paraformaldehyde. On the other hand, rat tendons retained their antigenicity when treated by radiation, mitomycin C, and glutaraldehyde [20]. These findings supported prior observations that freezing and paraformaldehyde fixation could change or denature the immunologic potential of tissues [16, 23].

Numerous experiments using preserved tendons for ligamentous and tendon allografts in multiple animal models consistently show no evidence of rejection. Preservation methods included deep freezing, freeze drying, refrigeration, merthiolate, and ethanol [1, 3, 8, 10, 11, 16, 18, 21, 27, 30, 38]. Arnoczky did evoke a rejection phenomenon by transplanting fresh allografts into dog leukocyte antigen (DLA)-mismatched recipients. The rejection was characterized by synovial inflammation, lymphocyte infiltration and perivascular cuffing—characteristics not present in deep frozen allografts [3]. These tendon data parallel other findings that demonstrate better results with histocompatibility matching of frozen bone allografts [4].

No data concerning rejection of allograft tendon or ligaments in human beings can be found. Bright and Green have reported on a mixed series of human, freeze-dried fascia lata allografts used for extra-articular procedures in a population of paralytics. Rejection phenomena were absent [5]. No reports of intra-articular rejections in human beings have yet been published.

COMPARABLE STRENGTH OF FRESH-FROZEN AND FREEZE-DRIED TISSUE ALLOGRAFTS

Any substitute cruciate ligament should have adequate strength initially, since at the time of implantation a cruciate ligament allograft acts as a prosthesis. Research has demonstrated that fresh tissues have adequate strength [22, 24]. Is this strength maintained after processing, freezing, lyophilization, and sterilization? This question was addressed by Thomas and Gresham, who, using a crude hanging-weight method, found no significant difference in the strengths of frozen, freeze-dried, and fresh fascia lata. They did find a significant difference in strengths of fascia lata, relative to age, sex, and cause of death [34]. The consequence of freezing tendons were also investigated by Matthews and Ellis, who examined the changes in the shape of stress–strain curves and changes in the modulus of elasticity of frozen versus fresh cat tendons. They demonstrated a significant decrease in the apparent elastic modulus of the frozen tendons, whereas the shape of the stress–strain curves showed no change [19].

Gibbons et al. recently reported studies on fascia lata grafts that were fresh frozen, freeze-dried, sterilized by ethylene oxide, and irradiated. These investigators found significantly lower maximum stress values and elastic moduli for irradiated fascia lata and lower values for fresh-frozen than for freeze-dried specimens [15]. A recent study by Paulos et al. addressed the same topic, but also included testing of Achilles and patellar tendons. Irradiated specimens had the lowest values for ultimate stress, ultimate strain, and modulus of elasticity. The Achilles tendon, which showed significantly lower ultimate stress and modulus of elasticity, also had the highest ultimate strain when compared with patellar tendon and fascia lata. All parameters were normalized using lengths and cross-sectional areas [24].

STRENGTH DURING INCORPORATION

The above studies have all addressed the mechanical properties of the grafts at the time of implantation. Equally important, however, is the in vivo strength of the grafts during the period of necrosis, revascularization, and replacement. Several studies have included mechanical testing of animal tendons after implantation. The animal data on mature allograft strengths are quite variable. Webster and Werner, [38, 39] who used freeze-dried dog-paw flexor tendons as intra-articular anterior cruciate ligament (ACL) grafts, found that by eight months the tendon grafts were repopulated by host cells, with some areas of presumed remaining donor collagen occupying up to one third of the cross-sectional area of the tendon. Mechanical testing showed only 29 per cent normal load to failure and a 15 per cent increase in strain to failure. Histology sectioning showed a very close junction of the tendon graft in the bone tunnel.

In 1984, Shino et al. [30] published an elaborate study using fresh-frozen patellar-tendon allograft ACLs in dogs. Microangiography demonstrated early revascularization at three weeks, most of the new blood vessels coming from the infrapatellar fat pad. Knee vascularity appeared to reach its peak at 6 weeks, subsiding to near normal vascularity at 30 weeks. Histology showed a sequence of peripheral cellular invasion with central necrosis at 6 weeks, followed by slow maturation to longitudinally arranged bundles with normal cellularity at 52 weeks. The mature specimens had a columnar appearance of fibrocartilage at their bony insertions. Evidence of rejection or progression of necrosis was absent in all specimens. This study included a group of autogenous central patellar tendons for comparison. Mechanical testing at 30 weeks showed 30 per cent mean maximum load to failure for the autografts and 28 per cent for the allografts. Another group of allografts that were twice as wide and allowed to mature to 52 weeks were also tested, demonstrating only a significant increase in the strain to failure.

Curtis et al. [11] used a somewhat different technique of canine intra-articular ACL grafting with freeze-dried, rolled fascia lata. Their findings paralleled Shino's observations on the sequence of vascularization in the extra-articular portion of the allografts. Mechanical testing at 24 weeks showed a maximum load to failure at 67 per cent of control values. They felt that revascularization required synovialization first in the intra-articular region of the graft. The more rapid revascularization of the extra-articular portion of the graft was attributed to well vascularized, neighboring tissue.

Nikalaou et al. [21] proposed using the anterior cruciate ligament itself as a bone–ligament–bone allograft. Their elaborate canine study included microangiograms, histology, and mechanical testing of grafts as late as 78 weeks after implantation. But the seemingly high load to failure (89 per cent of control) observed by these investigators must be interpreted cautiously since the absolute value of the control ACL was surprisingly low.

No data on implanted soft-tissue allograft strength is available for human beings. The final strength of any successful allograft ligament would depend on how well tension was maintained during revascularization. The process of replacement and revascularization appears to depend upon synovialization of the graft across the exposed surface followed by revascularization from the outside in. This sequence suggests that the rate of incorporation of the graft depends upon the surface area of the exposed allograft. Synovial-fluid transport is also important in normal ACL nutrition [28]. Theoretically then, there should be advantages to a graft composed by grouping several round flexor tendons, as compared with a larger single graft with the same cross-sectional area. A greater distance from the peripheral fibrovascular invasion to the core of the collagen graft may retard completeness of incorporation, and numerous small tendons should revascularize more quickly. One problem with this multiple tendon approach is that adequate fixation of each unit may be less likely.

Several animal studies have found a persistent central core of necrosis in both autografts and allografts [38]. These areas have been assumed to be nonincorporated donor collagen. Heiple et al. addressed this issue using ^{14}C-labeled collagen in flexor tendon transplants and found a significant residual of donor collagen even after two years [17]. Whether reincorporation of larger grafts is ever complete is not known. The low metabolic rate of ligamentous tissue may be, in part, responsible for incomplete incorporation. Whatever the reason for persistent large portions of unaltered donor graft, they could lead to failure and fragmentation due to mechanical wear.

Several histologic studies of animal-tendon allografts and autografts show a very similar sequence of events [2, 3, 8, 9, 11, 21, 30]. The grafts demonstrated necrosis, followed by revascularization from host tissues, and ultimately conversion to collagen with cellularity that appeared very similar to normal tendon. These events were consistent, regardless of the method of preservation. But, the process of healing was prolonged in allografts as compared with autografts [8, 10, 11, 18].

PROCUREMENT AND PROCESSING

Any allograft program must rely heavily on a well-run tissue bank. Criteria for donors has been outlined quite well by the American Association of Tissue Banks. They recommend excluding any potential donor with bacterial infection, viral illness, cancer, rheumatoid arthritis, metabolic bone diseases, toxic drug reactions, death from unknown causes, any jaundice, hepatitis, Acquired Immune Deficiency Syndrome (AIDS) or treatment on a respirator for more than 48 hours. Any extremity with an open wound for more than 12 hours should be excluded. Donors are tested for HTLV-III and hepatitis [13]. One major concern is the AIDS virus, since HTLV-III serum testing may not be positive until six to twelve months after initial contamination. This is a problem that has not been solved and applies to all types of tissues and transplants.

Ideally, tissues should be harvested in an operating room using strictly sterile techniques. The alternative is to harvest nonsterilely and then secondarily sterilize during the preservation steps. Using the first approach, each specimen should be cultured separately during harvest, and again when opened for use. Fresh, sterile tissue is individually wrapped in three layers of sterile wraps and carefully labelled. Specimens may then be deep frozen and freeze-dried. Deep freezing should be below $-70°C$ for at least two weeks. Tissues processed in this manner have the least possible number of problems, with bacterial contamination as the major concern.

The processing of nonsterilely harvested specimens adds a number of steps, with each step possibly altering or damaging the graft. Nonsterile tissues may be processed by freeze drying (lyophilization) and ethylene oxide sterilization [36]. While ethylene oxide has been shown to penetrate cortical bone to a depth of 1 cm, only minimal information is available concerning the effectiveness of ethylene oxide sterilization of ligamentous tissues. Prolo and Oklund did find a lack of chemical residues in thin specimens of fascia lata and dura after adequate aeration [28]. No data is available on possible chemical residues in thicker segments of dense collagenous tissue. Of special concern is the dense, necrotic core of tendon allografts that can measure up to 15 mm in diameter. If ethylene oxide is used, to be effective it must be done while the tissue is moist, i.e., prior to lyophilization [28]. Irradiation has been used in the past, but considerable strength was lost at the doses used [6, 24]. Irradiation was also shown be less effective than freezing with regard to limiting the grafts' immunogenicity [20].

SELECTION OF GRAFTS

The most commonly used allograft for ACL reconstruction is the bone–tendon–bone patellar tendon. This preparation offers the advantages of bony fixation in tunnels and the possibility of preserving the bone–tendon junction. Fascia lata has been used intra-articularly, but fixation in the bone tunnel may not be reliable due to the layering of the fascia, which results in a soft-tissue junction with the host. Achilles tendons can provide a very large piece of sturdy-appearing tissue, but on testing they are weaker per unit area than others [23]. One reason for this weakness is that collagen fibers in the Achilles tendon are not in linear continuity along the entire tendon. Rather, they are arranged in short bundles and layers similar to fish scales.

At least one investigator has added steps to processing by thoroughly washing each graft free of surface cells and marrow elements. These efforts are aimed at reducing the immunogenic load of remaining cellular elements and any toxic chemical residues. Operative time at implantation can be lessened if the grafts are also presized during processing [18, 32].

EXPERIENCE WITH HUMAN ACL GRAFTS

There are only anecdotal reports on human ACL allografts. Shino's procedure for ACL grafting consists of intra-articular deep frozen grafts combined with medial or lateral extra-articular reconstruction. The grafts were of mixed types, including Achilles tendon, tibialis anterior tendon, and groupings of several flexor tendons. Instrumented laxity testing was done and showed remarkably good results. In a recent report on ACL allograft reconstruction with at least two years of follow-up, Shino found that 30 of 31 patients were functioning well in strenuous athletic activities. This optimistic report must be interpreted with caution. It is significantly limited by the fact that only 37 per cent of the patients receiving grafts were included in the study [31]. Hence, no conclusions can be made based on these data.

Our experience over the past five years includes over 200 cases of intra-articular and extra-articular soft-tissue allografts. The majority of tissues were freeze-dried, ethylene oxide sterilized, patellar tendon–bone preparations. Several problems have been identified and are currently under intense study. On initial review, there appears to be two forms of freeze-dried (ethylene oxide sterilized) allograft failure: (1) an acute synovial reaction manifested by swelling and pain approximately 5 to 18 months from the time of surgery, and (2) a late, gradual failure manifested from 9 to 24 months, which appears to be a failure of incorporation of the graft. The first mode of failure, which occurs in approximately 15 per cent of patients, is

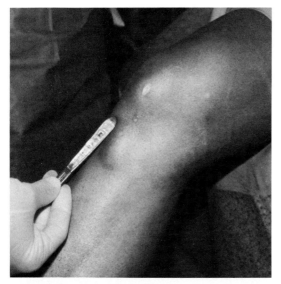

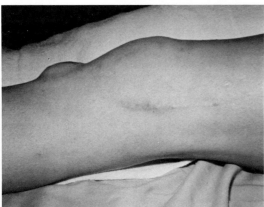

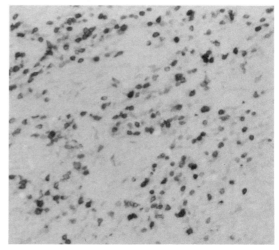

Figure 26–2. T-cell lymphocytes in "explanted" graft tissue—immunoperoxidase staining of T-cell surface antigen marker. (Photo courtesy of Dr. William Lanzer.)

Figure 26–1. Tibial bubbles—A ganglionlike cyst that can form at the tibial attachment sites of ACL allografts. These may occasionally form direct fistulae to the knee joint.

graft tissue. Ethylene glycol and ethylene chlorhydrin are known residues that are formed when ethylene oxide is exposed to water or chlorine, respectively [28]. The reaction to ethylene glycol may be responsible for the foreign-body-type response. Further investigation on these residues is currently under way. If our hypothesis proves true, then this form of failure can be avoided by using sterilely harvested tissues.

manifested by an intense reaction either intra-articularly or at attachment sites (Fig. 26–1). Histocompatibility studies in these patients are being performed, and early results reveal T-cell proliferation in the synovial tissue (Fig. 26–2). Large foreign-body giant cells are also present, bearing witness to an intense foreign-body or toxic reaction (Fig. 26–3). Whether foreign-body reaction or antigenic rejection is the main cause of failure is unknown at this time, but both probably have a role. Our present hypothesis is that with thicker allograft tissues, it is possible that ethylene oxide residues remain in the core of the tissue and if abrasion of the graft occurs (prior to incorporation and replacement), a form of foreign-body reaction is elicited from these residues. We have assayed ethylene oxide levels in freeze-dried allografts. These samples showed very low levels of ethylene oxide but had high levels of ethylene glycol residues in the

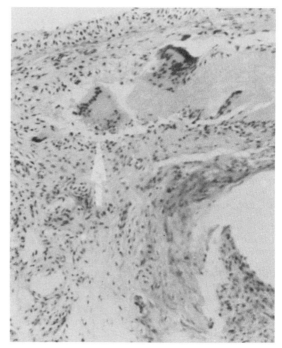

Figure 26–3. Large foreign-body-type giant cells found in the "explanted" graft seen in Figure 26–2. Hematoxylin and eosin stain. (Photo courtesy of Dr. William Lanzer.)

The second form of failure, an ultimate lack of incorporation, manifests itself 9 to 24 months after implantation as an increase in laxity unassociated with gains in motion, thereby eliminating nonisometric placement as the cause. Arthroscopy in these cases reveals an "empty sock" of synovial tissue with no reaction or scarification present. A variation on this kind of failure is also seen as increased compliance of the knee restraints to low- and high-force instrumented testing. The same phenomenon is seen with autografts, but to a lesser extent. Again, whether the use of sterilely harvested rather than secondarily sterilized tissues will prevent this second form of failure is unknown. It is also possible that this second form of failure is only a less reactive phase of the first form.

We feel that the potential advantages of avoiding tissue harvest from patients by using allograft tissues is currently outweighed by a higher failure rate. The reduction of morbidity is slight, and rehabilitation time is unchanged. We currently consider the use of allograft tissues, freeze dried or fresh frozen, as investigational, and reserve its use for patients in whom autografts are not available. We also recommend that ethylene oxide sterilized tissues not be used until more is learned about their behavior and better controls on tissue procurement, sterilization, and distribution are established.

REFERENCES

1. Andreeff L. A comparative experimental study on transplant of autogenous and homogenous tendon tissues. Acta Orthop Scand 1967; 38:35.
2. Arnoczky SP, Tarvin GB, Marshall JL. Anterior cruciate ligament replacement using patellar tendon: an evaluation of graft revascularization in the dog. J Bone Joint Surg (Am) 1982; 64:217–224.
3. Arnoczky SP, Warren RF, Ashlock MA. Replacement of the anterior cruciate ligament using a patellar tendon allograft: an experimental study. J Bone Joint Surg (Am) 1986; 68:376–385.
4. Bos GD, Goldberg VM, Powell AE, et al. The effect of histocompatibility matching on canine frozen bone allografts. J Bone Joint Surg (Am) 1983; 65:89–96.
5. Bright RW, Green WT. Freeze-dried fascia lata allografts: a review of 47 cases. J Pediatr Orthop 1981; Vol. 1: 12–22.
6. Bright RW, Smarsh JD, Gambill VM. Sterilization of human bone by irradiation. In: Friedlaender GE, Mankin HJ, Sell KW, eds. Osteochondral Allografts, biology, banking and clinical applications. Boston: Little, Brown, 1982:223–225.
7. Bunnell S. Surgery of the hand, I. Philadelphia: JB Lippincott, 1944:293–294.
8. Cameron PR, Conrad RN, et al. Freeze-dried composite tendon allografts: an experimental study. Plastic Reconstr Surg 1971; 47:39.
9. Chiroff RT. Experimental replacement of the anterior cruciate ligament. J Bone Joint Surg (Am) 1975; 5:1124.
10. Cordrey LJ, McCorkel H. A comparative study of fresh autogenous and preserved homogenous tendon grafts in rabbits. J Bone Joint Surg (Br) 1963; 45:182–195.
11. Curtis R, DeLee J, Drez D. Reconstruction of the anterior cruciate ligament with freeze-dried fascia lata allografts in dogs. Am J Sports Med 1985; 13:408.
12. Friedlaender GE. Guidelines for banking osteochondral allografts. In: Friedlaender GE, Mankin HJ, Sell KW, eds. Osteochondral allografts, biology, banking and clinical applications. Boston: Little, Brown, 1982:178–180.
13. Friedlaender GE, Strong DM, Sell KW. Studies on the antigenicity of bone. I. Freeze-dried and deep-frozen: bone allografts in rabbits. J Bone Joint Surg (Am) 1976; 58:854–858.
14. Gallie WE, LeMesurier AB. A clinical and experimental study of the free transplantation of fascia and tendon. J Bone Joint Surg 1922; 4:600–612.
15. Gibbons MJ, Butler DL, Noyes FR, et al. The inherent mechanical properties of allograft fascia lata. Proceedings of 1986 European Society of Knee Surgery and Arthroscopy 1986 (unpublished).
16. Graham WC, Smith DA, McGuire MP. The use of frozen stored tendons for grafting: an experimental study. J Bone Joint Surg (Am) 1955; 37:624.
17. Heiple KG, Nash CL, Klein L. A study of C-14 labeled collagen of rat homograft tendon. J Bone Joint Surg (Am) 1967; 49:1109–1118.
18. Liu T. Transplantation of preserved composite tendon allografts. J Bone Joint Surg (Am) 1975; 57:65.
19. Matthews LS, Ellis D. Viscoelastic properties of cat tendon: effects of time after death and preservation by freezing. J Biomechanics 1968; 1:65–71.
20. Minami A, Ishii S, Ogino T. Effect of the immunological antigenicity of the allogeneic tendinosus tendon grafting. Hand 1982; 14(2):111–119.
21. Nikalaou PK, Glisson AV, Seaber FH. Mechanical properties of cryopreserved anterior cruciate ligaments. Trans Orthop Res Soc 1986; 12:80.
22. Noyes FR, Butler DL, Grood ES, et al. Biomechanical analysis of human ligament grafts used in knee-ligament repairs and reconstructions. J Bone Joint Surg (Am) 1984; 66:344–352.
23. Oikawa T, Gothoda E, Austin FC, et al. Temperature-dependent alteration in immunogenicity of tumor-associated transplantation antigen monitored via paraformaldehyde fixation. Cancer Res 1979; 39:3519–3523.
24. Paulos LE, France EP, Rosenberg TD, et al. Comparative material properties of allograft tissues for ligament replacement: effects of type, age, sterilization and preservation. Presented to the Orthopedic Research Society, San Francisco, January 19, 1987.
25. Peacock EE, Madden JW. Human composite flexor tendon allografts. Clin Orthop 1967; 166:624–629.
26. Peacock EE, Petty J. Antigenicity of tendon. J Surg Gynecol Obstet 1960; 110:187–192.
27. Potenza AD, Melone C. Evaluation of freeze-dried flexor tendon grafts in the dog. J Hand Surg 1978; 3:157–162.
28. Prolo DJ, Oklund SA. Sterilization of bone by chemicals. In: Friedlaender GE, Mankin HJ, Sell KW, eds. Osteochondral allografts, biology, banking, and clinical applications. Boston: Little, Brown, 1982:233–238.
29. Renzoni SA, Amiel D, Harwood FL, Akeson WH. Synovial nutrition of knee ligaments. Trans Orthop Res Soc 1984; 10:277.
30. Shino K, Kawasaki T, Hirose H, et al. Replacement of the anterior cruciate ligament by an allogeneic tendon graft:

an experimental study in the dog. J Bone Joint Surg (Br) 1984; 66:672–681.

31. Shino K, Kimura T, Hirose H, et al. Reconstruction of the anterior cruciate ligament by allogeneic tendon graft. J Bone Joint Surg (Br) 1986; 68:739–746.

32. Simon TM, Jackson DW. Anterior cruciate ligament allografts. In: Jackson DW, Drez D, eds. The anterior cruciate deficient knee. St Louis: CV Mosby, 1987:211–225.

33. Stevenson S, Hohn RB, Templeton JW. Effects of tissue antigen matching on the healing of fresh cancellous bone allografts in dogs. Am J Vet Res 1983; 44(2):201–206.

34. Thomas ED, Gresham RB. Comparative tensile strength study of fresh, frozen, and freeze-dried human fascia lata. Surg Forum 1963; 14:442.

35. Tomford WW. Cryopreservation of articular cartilage, In: Friedlaender GE, Mankin HJ, Sell KW, eds. Osteochon-

dral allografts, biology, banking, and clinical applications. Boston: Little, Brown, 1982:215–218.

36. *Idem*. Sterility control in bone backing. In: Friedlaender GE, Mankin HJ, Sell KW, eds. Osteochondral allografts, biology, banking, and clinical applications. Boston: Little, Brown, 1982:219–221.

37. Urist MR, Mikulski A, Lietze A. Solubilized and insolubilized bone morphogenetic protein. Proc Natl Acad Sci USA 1979; 76:1828.

38. Webster DA, Werner FW. Freeze-dried flexor tendons in anterior cruciate ligament reconstruction. Clin Orthop 1983; 181:238–243.

39. *Idem*. Mechanical and functional properties of implanted freeze-dried flexor tendons. Clin Orthop 1983; 180:301–309.

27

ALLOGRAFT ANTERIOR CRUCIATE LIGAMENT RECONSTRUCTION: AN ARTHROSCOPICALLY GUIDED TECHNIQUE

THOMAS D. ROSENBERG, M.D.
LONNIE E. PAULOS, M.D.
RICHARD D. PARKER, M.D.

Arthroscopically guided anterior cruciate (ACL) reconstruction using allografts is a relatively new procedure. It employs virtually the same concepts as the autograft technique, but autogenous tendon harvest about the knee is unnecessary. Although this would appear to be a distinct advantage, allograft tissue for ACL reconstruction is still experimental, and its efficacy will be determined only by long-term follow-up. In the past five years, we have performed allograft ACL reconstructions in selected cases using fascia lata, bone–patellar tendon–bone, and Achilles tendon. Others have used ACL, posterior cruciate ligament (PCL), and quadriceps tendon–bone (Fig. 27–1). At present, the bone–patellar tendon–bone allograft is generally preferred because of its strength, macrostructure, and associated bone blocks; hence, its technique of insertion will be described.

PREPARATION

Preparation is critical to the success of any surgical procedure, and this is especially true of arthroscopically guided ACL reconstruction using patellar-tendon allografts. One overlooked step can mean the difference between a smoothly performed procedure and one fraught with difficulty.

Arthroscopically guided allograft ACL reconstruction is currently performed as an inpatient surgical procedure. The patient is admitted on the day of surgery and discharged on the third or fourth postoperative day.

Anesthesia

The surgery can be performed under regional or general anesthesia. General anesthesia is preferred, since it allows complete muscle relaxation and precludes tourniquet pain. The surgeon can concentrate on the efficiency of his operative task without being preoccupied with a conscious patient. Regional anesthesia requires a block to the D_5 level to ensure absence of tourniquet pain.

Examination

After induction of the chosen anesthesia, the leg to be operated on is examined in routine fashion and compared to the well leg. The grade of the Lachman and pivot-shift tests are noted, as well as any associated laxity patterns.

193

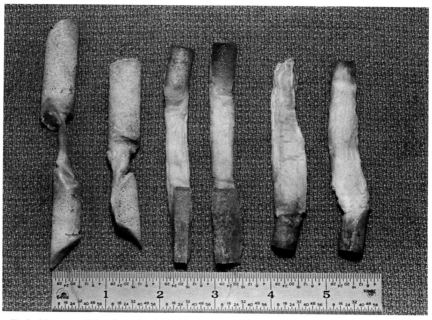

Figure 27–1. Typical harvest of six allografts obtainable from one knee. From left to right, ACL, PCL, two of bone–patellar tendon–bone, and two of quadriceps tendon–bone. (Simon TM, Jackson DW [10].)

Positioning

We have found the presence of a trained surgical assistant and the use of a thigh-holding device essential. The thigh-holding device is placed 10 to 12 in. above the joint line. This placement provides a generous proximal sterile field. If meniscal surgery is deemed necessary, the device facilitates opening of the lateral or medial compartments and ensures safe passage of instruments without articular injury. The surgical assistant should be able to interpret the images appearing on the video monitor in order to position the limb properly and to apply stress to it.

A thigh tourniquet is usually employed and is inflated between 350 and 400 mm Hg after exsanguinating the leg with an Esmarch bandage. Generally, the tourniquet is inflated for no longer than 120 minutes.

After the patient's affected leg has been placed in a thigh-holding device and the tourniquet is in place, the patient's contralateral or well leg is placed in a well-leg support. This support externally rotates, abducts, and mildly flexes the well leg allowing the surgeon more room about the injured knee to operate (Fig. 27–2). When medial meniscal repair or medial side ligamentous repair or reconstruction is necessary, space for maneuvering is especially helpful. The well-leg support also ensures flattening of the lumbar lordosis and prevents femoral nerve traction, a possibility if the

well leg is dangled off the end of the operating table for a long period of time.

After the patient's legs are positioned, the operative leg is prepped with a 2 per cent iodine solution or a povidone iodine gel scrub and solution in order to prepare the leg for surgery. The leg is draped in a routine sterile technique to ensure a watertight seal both proximally and distally. Prior to inflation of the tourniquet, the patient receives 1 gm of a broad-spectrum cephalosporin intravenously as a form of antibiotic prophylaxis.

DIAGNOSTIC AND OPERATIVE ARTHROSCOPY

Diagnostic and operative arthroscopy using a 25-degree, 5-mm arthroscope is performed through the standard anteromedial and anterolateral portals. Through these portals, the knee can be systematically evaluated in order to diagnose and treat any associated pathology. Accessory suprapatellar, posteromedial, posterolateral portals are employed if necessary. Initially, the patellofemoral articulation is evaluated, and care is taken to note any signs of associated patellar dislocation, chondrosis, or malalignment. Evaluation of the medial and lateral cartilage spaces reveals the presence of associated meniscal tears. If a meniscal

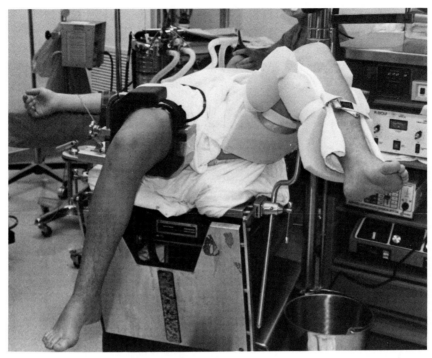

Figure 27–2. Thigh holder is secured around the tourniquet. The contralateral leg is secured in a well-leg support, which externally rotates, abducts, and mildly flexes the well leg.

tear is peripheral and deemed reparable, it is repaired arthroscopically [9]. If it is irreparable, a partial arthroscopic meniscectomy is performed. Small stable tears are simply documented. The articular surface of the femoral condyles and the tibial plateaus are also evaluated. The degree (grade 1, 2, 3, or 4) of chondrosis is documented and, if appropriate, debridement of these areas is performed. Next, the intercondylar notch is evaluated, and the status of the PCL as well as the shape and size of the intercondylar notch are noted.

Preparation of the Intercondylar Notch

The ACL reconstruction begins with assessment of the notch. In chronic cases where osteophytes have developed and in acute cases with a narrow or so-called A-frame notch, a notchplasty should be performed. Superior and lateral expansion of the intercondylar notch should be undertaken in these cases to prevent graft impingement and to improve exposure of the femoral anatomic attachment site (FAAS). The dimensions of the intercondylar notch must be considered relative to the dimensions of the graft. Excess removal of the bone and cartilage should be avoided in order to minimize the exposed length of the biologic substitute. Since nonanatomical graft placement on the tibia may require additional expansion of the notch, it should be avoided.

Exposure of the notch may be facilitated by selective debridement of the ACL remnants and synovium. Viable synovium and ACL tissues that do not interfere with exposure are preserved as a vascular bed for allograft tissue incorporation. Care is taken to avoid injury to the PCL and its synovium. Anteriorly, the notch is approached with the knee flexed 30 to 45 degrees. The posterior outlet may be reached with knee flexed 90 degrees. Routinely, 3 to 5 mm of cartilage and bone are removed using a one-quarter inch curved osteotome or gouge inserted through the anteromedial portal, while viewing through the anterolateral portal. Osteochondral fragments are torn free and removed with a Schlesinger clamp. Final contouring is achieved using a motorized abrader (Fig. 27–3). The lateral extent of the notchplasty slightly exposes the posterior horn of the lateral meniscus, and the superior notchplasty clearly avoids impingement of the proposed tibial attachment site in full extension. As the notchplasty progresses posteriorly, the "posterior dropoff" or "over-the-top" point is identified with a probe, and a small curette is used to mark the FAAS. This site is chosen 2 to 3 mm anterior and distal to the over-the-

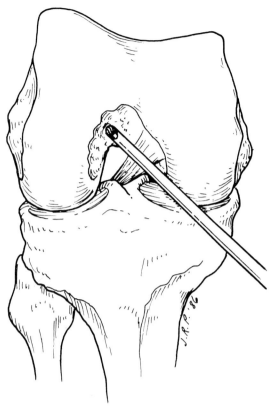

Figure 27–3. Superior and lateral expansion of the intercondylar notch reduces risk of allograft impingement. Final contouring is achieved with a motorized abrader.

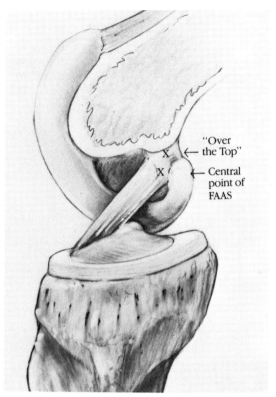

Figure 27–4. Femoral anatomic attachment site (FAAS) is 2 to 3 mm anterior and distal to the "over-the-top" point. (Rosenberg TD [6].)

top point (Fig. 27–4). The femoral ACL stump usually confirms the proper site.

Femoral Tunnel

After completion of the notchplasty and marking of the FAAS, the arthroscope is removed from the knee, and a lateral longitudinal incision is made over the distal femur superficial to the iliotibial band. The iliotibial band is incised at its anterior border, and a limited lateral release (remaining extrasynovially) is performed, allowing the iliotibial band to drop posteriorly. The vastus lateralis is bluntly elevated from the iliotibial band and intermuscular septum. The vastus lateralis is retracted anteriorly, and the midlateral metaphyseal cortex of the femur is exposed. A finger is inserted posteriorly along the distal fibers of the intermuscular septum toward the intercondylar notch, developing this plane.

Current technique employs a rear-entry guide, which enters the joint posteriorly and firmly affixes to the femur at the FAAS [7]. A curved passer is used through the anterolateral portal piercing the posterior capsule at the over-the-top position. The rear-entry guide is then attached and

pulled into the intercondylar notch (Fig. 27–5). Under arthroscopic visualization, the tip of the guide is directed into the hole previously used to mark the FAAS (Fig. 27–6). A K-wire is directed through the "bullet" and guide to this point. This position of the wire can be evaluated arthroscopic-

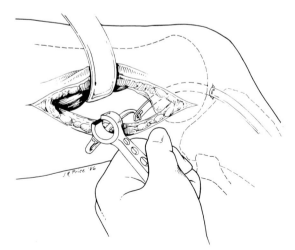

Figure 27–5. Curved passer inserted through the anterolateral portal draws the rear-entry guide into position.

ally with a probe. The guide is removed, and the appropriate cannulated drill bit (usually 10 to 11 mm) reams the femoral tunnel. The apertures are chamfered or curetted to avoid graft abrasion and then plugged. This wound is then irrigated with triple antibiotic solution and packed with an antibiotic-soaked sponge.

Tibial Tunnel

With the arthroscope in the anterolateral portal, the tibial anatomic attachment site (TAAS) is studied. A 2- to 3-cm vertical incision is made medial

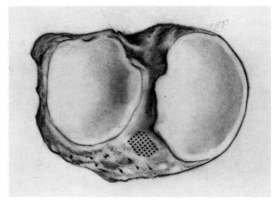

Figure 27–7. Tibial anatomic attachment site (TAAS) is located on the anterolateral slope of the medial intercondylar eminence using the residual ACL stump as a reference. (Rosenberg TD [6].)

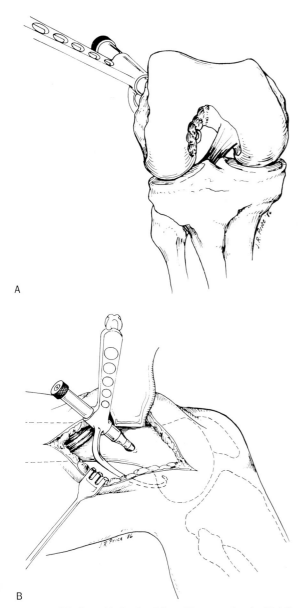

A

B

Figure 27–6. With the tip of the guide engaged at the FAAS (a), the "bullet" slides into the pilot hole and the guide is locked in place (b).

to the tibial tubercle, 3 cm distal to the joint line. The periosteum is incised and elevated medially 1 to 1.5 cm. An aiming device is placed through the anteromedial portal and impaled at the TAAS. Using the residual ACL stump as a reference, this site is identified on the anterolateral slope of the medial intercondylar eminence (Fig. 27–7). In chronic cases, where exact placement is difficult to ascertain, one must refer to the lateral margin of the notch and the posterior cruciate ligament as well. If placement remains unclear, it is better to err slightly anteriorly and medially. This will have negligible effects on isometricity but may require additional expansion of the notch. A K-wire is inserted to the selected site through the guide (Fig. 27–8), followed by a cannulated reamer corresponding to the size of the substitute (usually 10 to 11 mm). The apertures are also selectively chamfered to prevent graft abrasion, and afterward plugged. The arthroscope is then removed from the knee.

ALLOGRAFT PREPARATION

The bone–patellar tendon–bone allograft has been procured and processed under aseptic conditions and preserved by either deep freezing (−80°C; fresh frozen) or by lyophilization (freeze drying). The donor has been screened for malignancy, neurologic disorders, active infectious diseases, sepsis, and diseases of unknown etiology. In addition, the donor blood sample has proved negative for hepatitis B surface antigen and for HTLV-III. With fresh-frozen grafts, cultures of each graft are taken at the time of harvest. If any culture is positive, all grafts from a specific donor are discarded. Lyophilized grafts, sterilized using

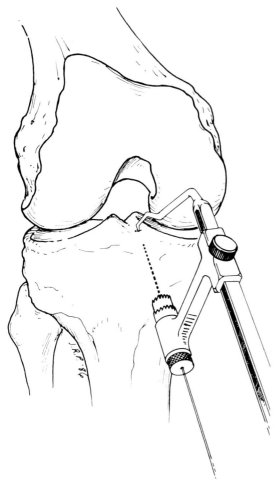

Figure 27–8. Tibial aimer is inserted through the anteromedial portal, and a K-wire is inserted.

ethylene oxide, are unaccepptable due to the presence of ETO (ethylene oxide) residues in the graft which can impede biological incorporation.

Rehydration of a sterilely harvested or irradiated lyophilized allograft is performed 24 hours before insertion [10]. Two hundred fifty milliliters of sterile triple-antibiotic solution consisting of normal saline, bacitracin (500 mg per liter), gentamicin (80 mg per liter), and neomycin (500 mg per liter) are used to rehydrate the allograft. This allows for its complete rehydration and also facilitates its easy removal from the storage bottle. The allograft is removed from the storage bottle under sterile conditions and placed in a basin filled with triple antibiotic solution. Fresh-frozen allografts are thawed in triple-antibiotic solution at room temperature for one hour before the insertion. The graft is then examined, and excess tissue is trimmed. Since most grafts have been previously sized to 11 mm (Fig. 27–9), an 11-mm presizing tube is used to confirm the size of the allograft. Normally, the lengths of the bone plugs are trimmed to approximately 3 cm, making insertion easier, yet allowing for sufficient fixation and bony incorporation. Transverse holes are made in both bone plugs with a 0.062-K-wire, and No. 2 Ethibond sutures are placed through these holes in order to pull the graft into position. The graft is then immersed in triple-antibiotic solution.

GRAFT PLACEMENT

The arthroscope is once again inserted through the anterolateral portal. A doubled 18-gauge wire helps pull the graft into place, usually from distal to proximal position. A probe aids in the deflection

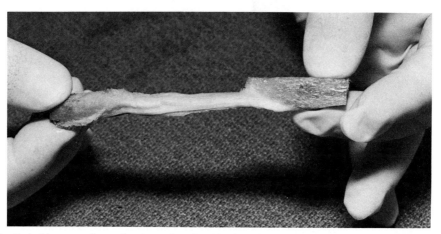

Figure 27–9. Typical bone–patellar tendon–bone allograft, which has been presized to 11 mm. (Simon TM, Jackson DW [10].)

of the bone plug as it enters the femoral tunnel. The graft is positioned such that the bone–tendon junction is flush, if possible, with the opening of the femoral tunnel in the intercondylar notch. The proximal end is fixed by an interference screw technique as described by Lambert [3]. Usually, a 30-mm No. 6.5 cancellous screw is employed. After proximal fixation, the knee is placed through a range of motion to observe excursion and to confirm the absence of impingement within the notch. With anatomic placement, there should be no more than 2 mm of excursion. With the knee flexed 20 degrees and with 10 to 20 lb of tension on the graft, the tibial portion of the allograft is secured by similar interference screw fixation (Fig. 27–10). Final assessment of the intercondylar notch is done. Absence of graft impingement and appropriate graft tension are confirmed. If graft impingement is present, careful additional notchplasty is performed in the appropriate area. If abnormal graft tension is present, the tibial interference screw is removed and the tension adjusted.

If grade II or III anterolateral rotary laxity is present on examination under anesthesia, we perform an extra-articular ACL reconstruction. Either a modified Andrews or iliotibial-band tenodesis (with screw and toothed-washer fixation) is used and performed through the lateral exposure previously described. Krackow's region serves as the fixation point for the iliotibial band in both methods [2]. If grade II or III anteromedial rotary laxity is present as demonstrated by the external-rotation pivot-shift test, then a posterior oblique ligament (POL) reefing is performed [5]. If associated valgus laxity at 30 degrees is also present, then the medial collateral ligament is repaired, recessed proximally, or advanced distally and anteriorly prior to POL reefing [5].

WOUND CLOSURE

The femoral and tibial wounds are irrigated with copious amounts of triple-antibiotic solution. The tourniquet is deflated, and the thigh-holding device is loosened. Hemostasis is achieved using electrocauter with special attention to the lateral femoral wound. After proximal lateral hemovac drainage has been established, the femoral wound is closed in anatomical fashion. Closure of the tibial wound is performed in a layered fashion, first by trimming the exposed allograft bone and then covering the screw and tunnel with the previously elevated periosteum. A sterile dressing is applied to the wounds, and a postoperative rehabilitation brace is applied and locked at 45 degrees of flexion, while the patient is still anesthetized. The patient is then transferred to the recovery room.

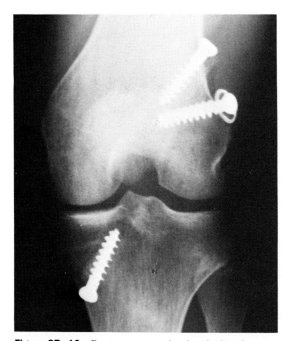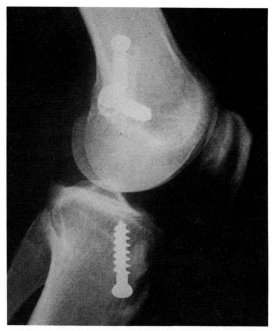

Figure 27–10. Roentgenograms showing the interference screw fixation of allograft bone–patellar tendon–bone to femur and tibia. Note the near straight alignment of the tunnels on anteroposterior (a) and lateral (b) views. Also note the 6.5 mm cancellous screw and toothed washed used in the tenodesis of the iliotibial band in Krackow's region.

SALT LAKE KNEE & SPORTS MEDICINE KNEE REHABILITATION FORM
LONNIE PAULOS, M.D.

Patient: _____ Date: _____

Surgical Procedure: <u>Arthroscopic ACL Reconstruction (Allograft) With Andrews Procedure</u>

Physical Therapist: _____ Post Op Week (POW): _____

PHASE I—IMMOBILITY
☒ Immobility ends on ____1____ POW: Locked flexion angle ___45___ °   ☒ Unlock for ROM exercises only
Leave unlocked after ___3___ POW

PHASE II—MOTION
Begin Passive Range of Motion on _____1_____ POW; Begin Active Range of Motion on ____3____ POW
☒ Passive ROM from __40__ ° to __70__ flexion; Increase ___5___ ° extension and __10__ ° flexion per week beginning on _3_ POW
☒ Active ROM from __40__ ° to __70__ flexion; Increase ___5___ ° extension and __10__ ° flexion per week beginning on _6_ POW
Other _____

PHASE III—PROGRESSIVE WEIGHT BEARING
Begin weight bearing on ___6___ POW: Start with ___25___ % body weight; Increase ___25___ % per week
☒ Keep on one crutch (75%) until notified;   ☒ Use functional brace on ___8___ POW

PHASE IV—ISOMETRIC
☒ Isometrics   ☒ Spectrum isometrics   ☒ Straight leg raises   ☒ Patella glides and tilts   ☐ Tens
☒ Neuromuscular Stimulation: ☒ Hamstrings ☒ Quadriceps ☐ Frequency ___2___/day; Duration ___2___ hrs/session
☐ Other _____

PHASE V—ISOTONIC
☒ Start concentric PRE on ___6___ POW   Start eccentric PRE on ___4___ POW; Body position: ☐ (**Sitting)—Prone
☐ Knee Extension PRE: Increase to ___none___ lbs.; from _____ ° to _____ ° flexion until _____ POW; then advance
    PRN; No limits on weight from _____ ° lbs; from _____ ° to _____ ° flexion
☒ Knee Flexion PRE: Increase to _no limit_ lbs.; from __20__ ° to __100__ ° flexion until ___16___ POW; then advance
    PRN; No limits on weight from _____ ° to _____ ° flexion.
☒ Leg Press PRE; Increase to ___75___ lbs; from __10__ ° to __40__ ° flexion until ___12___ POW.
No limit on weight from __40__ ° to __100__ ° flexion
☒ Must wear brace during PRES

PHASE VI—ISOKINETIC
Start on ___24___ POW; Pad placement: (**High)—Low tibia; Body position: (Sitting)—Prone
☐ Patellar restraining brace   ☐ Burn outs   ☒ High speed only   ☒ Must wear brace
☐ ROM restriction: High speed performance from _____ ° to _____ ° flexion; Low speed from _____ ° to _____ ° flexion

PHASE VII—ENDURANCE
Start cycling on ___8___ POW
☒ Stationary only   ☒ Adjust seat: High—(**Low)   ☐ Patellar Restraint   ☒ Outdoor biking on ___12___ POW
Start swimming on ___4___ POW   ☐ Functional brace
     Bent
☒ ~~Straight leg kicks only~~   ☐ Pool jogging   ☐ Unlimited
☒ Stationary track   ☒ Rowing

PHASE VIII—RUNNING
Beginning progressive running on ___36___ POW (If no swelling or pain and 75% strength)
☒ Stretch cords   ☒ Trampoline   ☐ Functional brace   ☐ Level ground only   ☒ Pogo stick
Progressive sprints on ___40___ POW: Progressive cutting on ___44___ POW; Progressive jumping on ___48___ POW
☐ Other _____

PHASE IX—SPORTS
Begin sports participation on ___48___ POW
☐ Skills drills only   ☒ Functional brace   ☐ Sports restrictions: _____
☐ Other: _____

Figure 27–11. Salt Lake Knee and Sports Medicine Knee Rehabilitation Form for the rehabilitation of an arthroscopically guided ACL reconstruction using allograft (bone–patellar tendon–bone) with an Andrew's augmentation.

REHABILITATION

Rehabilitation of the knee stabilized by an allograft ACL reconstruction is very similar to an autograft. It is the authors' opinion that a rehabilitation prescription must be individualized based on the patient and the associated ligamentous injury patterns. A "cookbook" approach should not be used. Nevertheless, a generalized approach can be used as a guideline. We have, therefore, included a Salt Lake Knee and Sports Medicine Knee Rehabilitation Form as an example of our rehabilitation for a knee stabilized with an allograft (bone–patellar tendon–bone) ACL reconstruction and an extra-articular (Andrew's) augmentation (Fig. 27–11).

REFERENCES

1. Jackson DW, Reiman PR. Principles of arthroscopic anterior cruciate reconstruction. In: Jackson DW, Drez D, eds. The anterior cruciate deficient knee. St Louis: CV Mosby, 1987.
2. Krackow KA, Brooks RL. Optimization of knee ligament position for lateral extraarticular reconstruction. Am J Sports Med 1983; 11(5):293–302.
3. Lambert KL. Vascularized patellar tendon graft with rigid internal fixation for anterior cruciate ligament insufficiency. Clin Orthop 1983; 172:85–89.
4. Moyer RA, Betz RR, Iaquinto J, et al. Arthroscopic anterior cruciate reconstruction using the semitendinosis and gracilis tendons: preliminary report. Contemp Orthop 1986; 12(1):17–23.
5. Paulos LE, Rosenberg TD, Parker RD. The external rotation pivot shift test: anatomy, biomechanics, significance, and surgical corrections. Techniques Orthop 1987; 2(1).
6. Rosenberg TD. Arthroscopic technique for anterior cruciate ligament surgery, technical bulletin. Norwood, Mass.: Acufex Microsurgical, 1984.
7. Rosenberg TD, Abbot PJ. Technique for rear entry ACL guide, technical bulletin. Norwood, Mass.: Acufex Microsurgical, 1986.
8. Rosenberg TD, Paulos LE, Abbot PJ. Arthroscopic cruciate repair and reconstruction: an overview and description of technique. In: Feagin JA, ed. The crucial ligament. New York: Churchill Livingstone (in press).
9. Rosenberg TD, Paulos LE, Parker RD. Arthroscopy of the knee. In: Chapman MW, Coward DB, eds. Operative orthopaedics. Philadelphia: JB Lippincott (in press).
10. Simon TM, Jackson DW. Anterior cruciate ligament allografts. In: Jackson DW, Drez D, eds. The anterior cruciate deficient knee. St Louis: CV Mosby, 1987.

28

FDA REGULATION OF PROSTHETIC LIGAMENT DEVICES

JANET G. FERL, M.S.
KAREN L. GOLDENTHAL, M.D.
NIRMAL K. MISHRA, D.V.M., PH.D.

HISTORY OF MEDICAL-DEVICE REGULATION

President Theodore Roosevelt signed into law the first Food and Drug Act in 1906. The Act defined misbranded and adulterated foods and drugs and included provisions for seizure of these products. The Bureau of Chemistry, U.S. Department of Agriculture enforced the Act until 1927, at which time the Food, Drug, and Insecticide Administration was formed. The agency was renamed the Food and Drug Administration (FDA) in 1931. In 1940, FDA was transferred from the Department of Agriculture to the Federal Security Agency, which today is called the Department of Health and Human Services.

Enforcement of the 1906 Act was difficult due to the government's inability to inspect manufacturing plants and to establish standards of purity under the law. In 1938, after the death of over 100 people from a toxic "Elixer of Sulfanilamide" containing diethylene glycol, the new Federal Food, Drug, and Cosmetic Act was signed by President Franklin D. Roosevelt. The new law authorized factory inspections. It established regulations for drug manufacturers by requiring that they provide scientific proof that their products could be used safely, and by no longer requiring proof of fraud to stop the misbranding of drugs. It also al-

lowed cosmetics and therapeutic devices to be regulated for the first time and made it unlawful to sell medical devices that were dangerous or marketed with false claims. In 1969, after a search of the literature revealed 751 deaths and over 9000 injuries directly related to medical devices in a 10-year period, the Cooper Committee was appointed to study the problems associated with regulating devices under existing laws and to recommend procedures to protect the consumer from unsafe and ineffective devices [1]. The Cooper Committee report was one of the factors that led to the establishment of the Medical Device Amendments of 1976 to the Federal Food, Drug, and Cosmetic Act. These amendments identify three classes of devices based on the degree of regulatory control required to ensure device safety and effectiveness. They authorize FDA to require manufacturers of devices used in supporting or sustaining human life to provide scientific proof that such a device is both safe and effective for its intended use, prior to marketing. Furthermore, the amendments define the legal role of advisory panels of non-FDA experts. The use of panels to classify devices and to review evidence of device safety and effectiveness is unique among FDA programs.

In 1982, the Center for Devices and Radiological Health (CDRH) was created. This became one of five centers included within FDA (the others

202

being the Center for Food Safety and Applied Nutrition, the Center for Drugs and Biologics, the Center for Veterinary Medicine, and the Center for Toxicological Research). Within CDRH, the Division of Surgical and Rehabilitation Devices (DSRD) has the responsibility of reviewing applications for the marketing of prosthetic-ligament devices. This division currently responds to applications concerning general and plastic surgery devices such as sutures, surgical lasers, collagen products, etc.; orthopedic devices such as artificial joints, bone cements, bone growth stimulators, ligaments, etc.; and physical medicine devices such as wheelchairs, muscle stimulators, diathermy devices, etc. The advisory panels of non-FDA experts associated with the division are the General and Plastic Surgery Devices Panel and the Orthopedic and Rehabilitation Devices Panel. The Orthopedic and Rehabilitation Devices Panel, which reviews applications concerning prosthetic ligament devices, consists of seven voting members, two nonvoting members representing consumer and industry interests, and six to seven expert clinical and scientific consultants. To help ensure fairness and objectivity, the background of each panel member and consultant is extensively scrutinized for conflicts of interest.

THE APPROVAL PROCESS

The 1938 Act as amended in 1976 is the basic law governing medical devices. It is intended to ensure that devices are safe and effective for their intended use and that labeling and packaging is truthful, informative, and not deceptive. It prohibits the distribution within or importation into the United States of adulterated or misbranded devices or any device that is required to be approved by FDA if approval has not already been given. It requires manufacturers and/or importers to provide certain reports and to allow inspection of regulated activities. The Act is enforced for all devices distributed in the United States and imported devices, but not exports. Exported products must meet the specifications and laws of the importing country and contain proper labeling.

The Act requires that all medical devices marketed prior to the 1976 Amendments (pre-amendment devices) be classified into one of three categories, based on the recommendation of the appropriate advisory panel, so that adequate controls will be required reasonably to ensure the safety and effectiveness of each device. Class I devices are subject to general controls only, including the registration of manufacturers, recordkeeping regulations, labeling regulations, and the

Good Manufacturing Practice (GMP) regulation. General controls apply also to Class II and Class III devices. Class II devices are subject to performance standards to be established by FDA because general controls alone are not sufficient to ensure device safety and effectiveness. Generally, Class III devices are those represented to be life supporting or life sustaining, those implanted in the human body, and those presenting potential unreasonable risk of illness or injury. New Class III devices are required to have approved Premarket Approval Applications (PMAs) prior to marketing because there is insufficient information to establish that performance standards and general controls will provide reasonable assurance of safety and effectiveness.

Manufacturers are required to notify FDA 90 days before marketing a device. Premarket notification submissions are referred to as 510(k)s, which is the section of the Act that requires premarket notification. During the 90-day period, FDA determines whether or not the device is substantially equivalent to a pre-amendment device. If the device is found to be substantially equivalent, it is classified the same as the pre-amendment device and is subject to the appropriate controls. If the device is not substantially equivalent, it is considered a new device and is automatically classified as a Class III device required to have approval prior to marketing.

Device manufacturers may apply for an Investigational Device Exemption (IDE). The IDE allows exemptions from certain requirements of the Act so that the manufacturer may investigate the safety and effectiveness of the device in regulated clinical trials in the United States. In order to obtain IDE approval, the manufacturer must supply data obtained through literature and laboratory or animal studies that demonstrate that the device is reasonably safe and effective for use on human subjects during carefully controlled trials. The application must also contain the design for clinical trials and an analysis of risk to the patient. The manufacturer must identify investigators and the Investigational Review Boards (IRBs) that will monitor the investigation.

At the completion of an IDE, or at any time when a manufacturer has sufficient data to provide scientific proof of the safety and effectiveness of the new device, the manufacturer may submit a PMA in order to obtain FDA approval to market the device. Every approval process involves a review by FDA scientific staff of the preclinical studies, investigational methods, clinical data, and labeling. An advisory panel of experts provides FDA with recommendations based on their knowledge of the field and their review of the PMA.

FDA will then make a final decision to either approve or disapprove the PMA. If approved, the manufacturer may market the device within the United States with the specific labeling approved by FDA. Any change in the device design, intended use, or labeling requires further FDA approval [10].

HISTORY OF PROSTHETIC LIGAMENT DEVICE REGULATION

Prior to 1976 the only prosthetic knee ligament device marketed in the United States was the Richards Polyflex System. The system consisted of an ultra-high-molecular-weight polyethylene ligament and stainless steel tubes for fixation with bone screws and polymethyl methacrylate cement.

The clinical experience with the device was discussed at a meeting of the Orthopedic and Rehabilitation Devices Panel on April 15, 1977 [2]. A motion was made to ban the device because of evidence of adverse effects. However, the final decision was to recommend that the sponsor collect additional data. At this early date, it became apparent that there was a great lack of knowledge about the use of prosthetic ligament devices. Emmett Lunceford, M.D., Chairman of the Panel, stated that the repair of cruciate ligaments is a very difficult type of operative procedure; and, he was unaware of any procedure that was really effective in correcting the knee malfunction.

Edward Grood, Ph.D., and Frank Noyes, M.D., presented results of mechanical testing of human ligaments and of the Polyflex System at a Panel meeting on July 15, 1977 [3]. Dr. Noyes stated that ''The use of a ligament in a young population means that in all likelihood the ligament will be subjected to high *in vivo* forces due simply to the activity status of this younger population. For this reason, it is our opinion that safety margins should be very wide. Also, any ligament implant should have extensive laboratory tests and animal studies and then careful clinical trials to prove clinical efficacy.'' They concluded that the safety margin of the Polyflex System is minimal and that a combination of repetitive high forces close to or beyond the elastic limit, on bent polyethylene meant a high long-term failure rate.

Although the overall failure rate for the Polyflex System implanted in patients up to that time was never established, a 17 per cent device breakage rate was determined for 114 patients. On November 15, 1977, Richards voluntarily ceased commercial distribution of the device and further attempts to classify the device with the assistance of the Panel also ceased [4]. Presently, these devices

are considered Class III devices and are required to have PMA approval prior to marketing in the United States.

By the early 1980s several manufacturers had developed prosthetic ligament devices and had investigated their use in laboratory and animal studies. After extensive review of preclinical data and study design, FDA approved IDEs for these devices and clinical trials began.

FDA recognized and supported the need for prosthetic ligament devices but also recognized the difficulty in designing and evaluating these devices, as predicted by Drs. Lunceford, Grood, and Noyes. In 1983, FDA staff members met with representatives from the Society of Sports Medicine, where it was decided that an open advisory Panel meeting was necessary. Therefore FDA gathered experts in the field and on November 8, 1983, a Panel meeting was held solely for the discussion of research and regulation of prosthetic ligament devices [5]. Comments were made by William C. Allen, M.D., Chairman of the Panel; James Funk, M.D., Chairman of the American Academy of Orthopedic Surgeons Knee Committee; Frank Noyes, M.D., Chairman of the American Orthopedic Society of Sports Medicine Research Committee; and Clinton Miller, Ph.D., Chairman of the Department of Biometry, Medical University of South Carolina. Eight investigators presented information about research being conducted on prosthetic ligament devices.

The Panel discussed questions that should be raised in evaluating data on safety and effectiveness. With respect to safety, Kurt Niemann, M.D., Panel consultant, stated that this is a broad category, which includes not only biocompatibility but device breakage and the fate of particles released from the device. Dr. Funk also mentioned the importance of demonstrating that particles released from the device are not going to be antigens or irritants that will cause arthritis in the future.

Regarding the criteria and evaluations used for determining device effectiveness, Dr. Funk stated that more detail should be added to the subjective examination, such as data on range of motion and swelling. Dr. Noyes discussed three categories of evaluations: the subjective evaluations such as pain, swelling, and giving way; the functional evaluations such as return to work and activities of daily living; and the objective evaluations such as measurement of knee laxity. Most Panel members discussed the need for uniform measurements and reporting, which would allow comparisons to be made of the effectiveness of different devices.

The Panel also discussed design of clinical trials. Dr. Miller discussed the need for a rationale for admission of patients and a clinical design that accounts for the variability of patients. Randall Lewis, M.D., Panel member, introduced the idea that patient selection must be based on the device indications. For example, acute and chronic patients should be investigated separately, with appropriate controls, rather than questioning whether or not a device can be used for the acute injury once it has been approved for another condition. William Woods, M.D., investigator, in responding to the question of patient-selection criteria, stated his opinion that at that time the synthetic devices were to be used for the worst knees, when there was no other option for effective treatment. In general, the Panel agreed that 2-year follow-up was necessary to establish device safety and effectiveness, but no number of patients was agreed upon. The standardization of clinical design was recognized as being restrictive, potentially causing new and better analysis methods to be unrecognized. This concern brought to light the need for controls.

Mr. Eldon Frisch summarized on behalf of the Orthopedic Surgical Manufacturers Association. The responsibility of FDA is to protect the public from an unsafe or ineffective device and also to make reasonable requirements of the manufacturer so that, eventually, the device can be made available to fill a great need.

Since 1983 FDA has received PMAs and has continued to receive new IDEs for prosthetic ligaments. FDA has carefully reviewed all preclinical engineering and biologic data contained in these submissions and has made numerous suggestions to improve proposed studies. On several occasions, FDA scientific staff assisted the sponsor in designing appropriate mechanical and animal testing protocols. Some of these results, which have been reported widely in the literature, formed the basis of multicenter clinical trials for new prosthetic devices. As of November, 1986, FDA has authorized the implantation of prosthetic knee ligaments in nearly 4000 patients, approximately 3100 of whom had intra-articular procedures. There are continuous technological and medical advances such as new device materials, the use of arthrometers, new subjective evaluations, and improved surgical techniques. Although FDA does not wish to burden manufacturers with advances that were developed after establishment of their investigational protocol, the agency is obliged to evaluate results based on the most current knowledge available in order to ensure that the safety and effectiveness of the device is based on valid scientific evidence. Therefore FDA has worked individually with each manufacturer to require that new IDEs incorporate the most current technology and medical practice, and to attempt to incorporate into ongoing IDEs and PMAs the advances that can be

reasonably applied and that are necessary or important to the evaluation of data. This most critical function of FDA, namely, the evaluation of data and scientific interchange, by law remains confidential in order to protect information contained in a manufacturer's submission. The history of prosthetic ligament device regulation is therefore limited to information presented in open public meetings such as a Panel meeting.

As of November, 1986, PMAs for four prosthetic ligament devices have been reviewed at Panel meetings: the Hexcel Integraft™ Stent, the Stryker® Knee Augmentation Device, the Gore-Tex™ Cruciate Ligament Prosthesis, and the 3M Kennedy LAD™ Ligament Augmentation Device. The Hexcel Integraft stent consists of carbon filaments covered with a resorbable polymer. It is intended to be a scaffolding device that provides temporary mechanical support at the repair site until new tissue assumes the mechanical function of the damaged structure. The Integraft stent was investigated in the repair of anterior cruciate ligaments (ACLs), posterior cruciate ligaments (PCLs), extra-articular knee structures, shoulder rotator cuffs, and ankles. The Hexcel PMA was initially reviewed by the Orthopedic and Rehabilitation Devices Panel on July 11, 1984 [6]. The Panel recommended to FDA that the device was not approvable primarily because of insufficient patient data and also because the data had not been stratified according to implantation site and acute-versus-chronic injuries. The PMA was updated and again reviewed at a Panel meeting on November 26, 1985 [7]. The Panel deferred voting and requested additional information. Supplemental information was provided and the PMA was again reviewed at the June 19, 1986, Panel meeting [8]. The Panel voted, unanimously, to recommend that the PMA again was not approvable. All Panel members expressed concern for the long-term safety of the device. Specifically, they questioned the fate of any carbon particles released from the device. Several Panel members also stated that the data did not support the effectiveness of the device. The consensus was that, for the ACL indication, the use of the device was not better than autogenous reconstruction alone; therefore the risks of the device were believed to outweigh the potential benefits of its use.

The Stryker knee augmentation graft is a composite of four Dacron woven tapes surrounded by a knitted Dacron fabric tubing that is augmented by a small amount of host tissue; it is indicated for repair of the ACL in chronically insufficient knees. The Stryker PMA was also discussed at the June 19, 1986, Panel meeting [8]. Two Panel members voted to recommend that the PMA was approvable for use in salvage patients only. The remaining five Panel members voted to recommend that the PMA was not approvable. The majority concluded that, because only seven salvage patients had 2-year follow-up, there was insufficient evidence to support the safety and effectiveness of the device for this indication. All Panel members expressed concern that preclinical animal studies and mechanical testing were not adequate to predict long-term fate of the device.

The Gore-Tex cruciate ligament prosthesis is fabricated from a continuous filament of expanded polytetrafluoroethylene (PTFE), which is wound and plaited into three bundles of strands. It is indicated for use as a permanent replacement for the ACL in chronically insufficient knees. The Gore-Tex PMA was the third device discussed at the June 19, 1986, Panel meeting [8]. The majority of Panel members voted to recommend that the PMA was approvable, with several conditions. One member voted to recommend that the PMA was not approvable because of insufficient preclinical mechanical testing. The Panel was concerned with the fate of broken strands, evident in arthroscopic examinations of implanted devices, which could eventually result in device rupture. The Panel was also concerned with the fate of PTFE particles released into the joint and the high incidence of effusion. However, it was thought that the extent of an inflammatory response is dependent on the volume of particles released and the sponsor presented data indicating that the volume of released PTFE particles was small. The recommended conditions of approval were that further mechanical tests be conducted, patients be monitored for effusions, the device be used only in salvage patients, and a 5-year postmarket surveillance of PMA patients be performed. Salvage patients were defined as those patients having had at least one failed autogenous intra-articular knee reconstruction. The Panel concurred with the manufacturer that the device labeling should indicate that only specially trained surgeons implant the device. FDA concurred with the Panel's recommendations and the Gore-Tex cruciate ligament prosthesis was approved for marketing in the United States with labeling restricting the indication for use in salvage patients only.

The 3M Kennedy LAD ligament augmentation device is a high-tenacity polypropylene braid, heat-sealed at both ends. It is indicated for augmentation and strengthening of a portion of the quadriceps tendon–prepatellar tissue–central third of the patellar tendon modified by over-the-top femoral fixation to the lateral femoral cortex. The Kennedy LAD PMA was discussed at the October 31, 1986, Panel meeting [9]. The majority of Panel

members voted to recommend that the PMA was approvable, with several conditions. Two Panel members voted to recommend that the PMA was not approvable, based on their concern that the device was actually functioning as a prosthesis rather than as an augmentation device and that the prospective patients required longer follow-up to establish device effectiveness. The remaining three Panel members also expressed concern about the effectiveness of the device. Because the clinical trial was conducted using the Marshall–MacIntosh procedure only, one of the recommendations for conditions of approval was that labeling state that all indications other than augmentation of autogenous tissue used in the Marshall–MacIntosh procedure remain investigational. Further recommendations were that additional mechanical tests be conducted, additional histologic studies be conducted, and a 5-year postmarket surveillance of PMA patients be performed.

GUIDANCE FOR MANUFACTURERS

Throughout recent years FDA has recognized certain criteria on which to base the evaluation of prosthetic knee ligaments. These are to be included in a guidance document for the preparation of IDEs and PMAs for prosthetic knee ligament devices. The intention of the document is to suggest to the manufacturer important preclinical and clinical tests that should be performed to generate data that will reasonably ensure the safety and effectiveness of these devices. The intention is also to establish standards for evaluation that can be used to relate the clinical performance of different devices without being so strict as to limit the creativity of investigators and the discovery of better devices, clinical designs, evaluation techniques, etc.

FDA has gained much of its knowledge from research being conducted by manufacturers investigating prosthetic knee ligament devices. In this sense, the guidance document can be considered a composite of criteria established by different manufacturers. Before being finalized the document will have been reviewed by Panel members, industry, surgeons, and any interested citizen.

As of November, 1986, the following issues have been proposed for comment. FDA has defined two types of intra-articular prosthetic knee ligament devices: devices intended as frank replacements and devices intended to augment natural tissue. Frank replacement type devices include prostheses whose function is not dependent on tissue ingrowth or mechanical support from autogenous structures. The augmentation type devices include a broad category of prostheses with diverse functions: prostheses that act as a scaffold for tissue ingrowth; prostheses that give mechanical support to autogenous reconstruction procedures; prostheses that resorb or degrade with time and are intended to be replaced with ingrown host tissue; and other prostheses whose function is dependent on tissue ingrowth or mechanical support from autogenous structures. Preclinical and clinical studies for these two device types will vary according to differences in materials, intended function, and risk–benefit considerations.

Preclinical tests must include *in vitro* biologic and mechanical tests and *in vivo* animal studies. The purpose of the *in vitro* biologic tests is to establish that the material and processing used to fabricate the device do not present adverse toxicologic effects. Mechanical tests should ensure acceptable strength, stiffness, elongation due to creep, and tensile and bending fatigue life. Device life should be predicted. *In vivo* studies may include several protocols to provide evidence of the histologic, biologic, and immunologic reactions to the device; device integrity; the migration of particles released from the device; the histologic and biologic reaction to particles released from the device; the strength of fixation; and the general integrity of the joint. Depending on the material used to fabricate the device, immunologic potential testing and/or a carcinogenesis bioassay may be necessary to provide evidence of safety. FDA will not approve an IDE for clinical trials to commence without reasonable assurance that the device will be safe when used in human beings and an indication that the device will be effective as established by these preclinical studies.

FDA will not approve an IDE without reasonable assurance that the clinical trial will accrue useful information that will constitute valid scientific evidence of the safety and effectiveness of the device. The clinical protocol should state the purpose of the study, the number of patients, the number of investigators, the study period, patient selection criteria, a detailed description of the surgical procedure, patient evaluation techniques, and success–failure criteria. FDA suggests that a multicenter trial with a minimum of 100 patients with a 2-year follow-up period may provide adequate data. However, sufficient patient numbers and follow-up periods should be used so that clinical results are statistically significant. FDA also suggests that a prospective concurrent control population should be included to provide scientific evidence of the significance of results. Evaluations should include preoperative and postoperative subjective measurements such as pain, giving way, swelling, stiffness, etc.; functional assessments such as function, activity level, etc.; and a physical examination including Lachman, pivot-shift, anterior drawer, arthrometer, thigh circumference, range of motion, effusion, etc., measurements.

Data presented in the PMA should be stratified by anatomical site, by acute-versus-chronic injury, by surgical procedure, by investigator or U.S. versus foreign data, etc., in order to establish the specific indications for which the device is the most effective and in order to demonstrate a lack of investigator–site bias. FDA has defined an acute injury as one that has occurred 3 weeks or less before surgery. A chronic injury is defined as one that has occurred more than 6 months before surgery. Salvage patients are defined as those having had at least one failed autogenous intra-articular knee reconstruction.

PMA data should also include individual patient data and a tabulation of patients lost to follow-up and patients having any complication, device-related or otherwise. Complications include device breakage, infection, synovitis, or instability. These data must be analyzed using accepted success–failure criteria and valid statistical tests. Final conclusions should be based on the benefits and risks of the device for each intended use.

Upon PMA approval, a summary of safety and effectiveness data will be available to the public. The summary contains the above preclinical and clinical information that is the basis for approval. This and all other releasable information can be obtained from the Freedom of Information Staff, FDA, HFW-35, 5600 Fishers Lane, Rockville, MD 20857. The Division of Surgical and Rehabilitation Devices, FDA, HFZ-410, 8757 Georgia Ave., Silver Spring, MD 20910, is also available to answer questions regarding the regulation of prosthetic ligament devices.

REFERENCES

1. Jansenn WF. The U.S. Food and Drug Law: how it came, how it works. Washington, D.C.: Government Printing Office, 1979. (DHHS publication no. (FDA) 79-1054.)
2. Orthopedic and Rehabilitation Devices Panel Meeting, transcripts. Rockville, MD: Dockets Management Branch, Food and Drug Administration, April 15, 1977.
3. Orthopedic and Rehabilitation Devices Panel Meeting, transcripts. Rockville, MD: Dockets Management Branch, Food and Drug Administration, April 15, 1977.
4. Orthopedic and Rehabilitation Devices Panel Meeting, transcripts. Rockville, MD: Dockets Management Branch, Food and Drug Administration, April 15, 1977.
5. Orthopedic and Rehabilitation Devices Panel Meeting, transcripts. Rockville, MD: Dockets Management Branch, Food and Drug Administration, April 15, 1977.

6. Orthopedic and Rehabilitation Devices Panel Meeting, transcripts. Rockville, MD: Dockets Management Branch, Food and Drug Administration, April 15, 1977.
7. Orthopedic and Rehabilitation Devices Panel Meeting, transcripts. Rockville, MD: Dockets Management Branch, Food and Drug Administration, April 15, 1977.
8. Orthopedic and Rehabilitation Devices Panel Meeting, transcripts. Rockville, MD: Dockets Management Branch, Food and Drug Administration, April 15, 1977.
9. Orthopedic and Rehabilitation Devices Panel Meeting, transcripts. Rockville, MD: Dockets Management Branch, Food and Drug Administration, April 15, 1977.
10. U.S. Department of Health and Human Services. Everything you always wanted to know about the medical device amendments . . . and weren't afraid to ask. Washington, D.C.: Government Printing Office, 1984. (DHHS publication no. (FDA) 84-4173.)

29

FUTURE OF PROSTHETIC LIGAMENT RECONSTRUCTION

ROBERT L. LARSON, M.D.

INTRODUCTION

The first requirement for use of synthetic materials about the knee is an understanding of the principles of ligamentous surgery that have been developed over the past 70 years. The kinematics of knee function require proper placement of substituted tissue or material, proper tension, and the proper tensile strength either initially or by development as vascularization and healing occurs. Many variables are associated with anterior cruciate ligament surgery. Evaluation of results are often inconsistent and confusing. However, there does appear to be a learning curve that improves with the use of the synthetic materials. The original investigators of the various materials and devices have developed techniques and instrumentation that have improved the results. Those who follow with the use of the artificial materials must abide by the same techniques and principles in order to achieve like results.

One of the fears of both the manufacturers and the FDA is that once released for general use, these materials or devices might be used inappropriately for less than suggested indications or used indiscriminately. Some may think that for every anterior cruciate ligament injury, 100 per cent satisfactory results will be obtained by the use of an artificial substance. Such is not the case, and if the artificial substances are not used properly and for the right indications, the reputation they acquire may be unjustly bad. Their use may become suspect and the normal progression of indications, improvements, and ultimate benefit may become mired in legal or regulatory obstacles.

As with any product in its developing stages, improvements will occur with use and familiarity with techniques. Present designs and materials will probably change. Present devices may be antiquated in future years as our instrumentation, technical skills, and understanding of synthetic materials and how they are accepted and tolerated over long-term use is evaluated in the human knee joint. As manufacturers develop newer products, we may find that one has a better fixation system, another a better material, and a third may have the best design and configuration. We will then have to choose which device is best for the given situation. There is already research going on making ligaments with more than one axis of tension, which will better mimic the normal anterior cruciate ligament. More-precise methods of placement and stronger fixation, more exact tensioning of the materials as they are inserted, and more exact methods of evaluating preoperative and postoperative laxity to provide better interpretation of the results are improvements to present techniques. Biologic glue has already been used for temporary fixation of materials in bony tunnels. This may lead to repair of menisci and cruciate ligaments in a practical and reasonable arthroscopic manner.

209

PRECAUTIONS

Because synthetic materials do not have the healing potential of living tissue, wear changes are inevitable. Any permanent prosthesis subjected to the stresses of a human knee joint is ultimately going to fail. This is not a reason for not using it. Every car we buy is ultimately going to fail and we know that every once in a while we run across a "lemon." If the prosthesis lasts for a reasonable length of time and if the method of insertion is relatively easy with little morbidity and a short rehabilitation time, its use and replacement as required becomes both justifiable and practical.

Materials that have been used to date show little problems with toxic or immunologic response. The synovitis that has occurred, appears to be a response to the particulate matter produced by fragmentation from erosion and wear. This may produce a mechanical irritation within the joint. Techniques that help to prolong wear and minimize erosion continue to be developed. Radialization of the edges of the bone tunnels, enlarging the intra-articular notch to prevent any impingement of the synthetic or biologic tissue, placement of the bone tunnels to eliminate stress risers from bone contact as the knee is flexed or extended helps prolong the life of the synthetic material.

Until we can precisely reproduce the entirety of the physiologic joint, we may be creating other problems. Our articular cartilage is designed to allow a constant unit load (21 kg/sq cm). Underloading or overloading as well as instantaneous surface velocity change may be factors in creating articular cartilage problems, as suggested in studies of the causes of osteoarthritis. The unyielding characteristics of some of the synthetic materials may so capture the joint that unphysiologic mechanics might produce abnormal articular wear and degeneration.

PRESENT ADVANTAGES

The theoretical advantages of synthetic materials to either augment or replace the anterior cruciate ligament often do not conform to the clinical demands that are required. Time is a demanding test of clinical results. The production of a stable knee for functional use is the immediate benefit. The synthetic materials' enhancement of the tensile strength of biologic tissue, providing a quicker rehabilitation and a more rapid return to activity, is the theoretical gain. A continuous monitoring of results and their comparison with results of previous studies is at present the only method of evaluation. Such comparisons are often fraught with in-

consistencies and inaccuracies because of the variables of types and severity of injury, interpretation of clinical tests, methods of postoperative care and rehabilitation, differences in the type of activity, and improvements in surgical techniques. A prospective, randomized study of treatment and control groups of patients, though ideal, is not, in my opinion, practical or justifiable in a clinical setting. If safety of the device is ensured, the theoretical advantages of an improved technique providing less morbidity, shorter rehabilitation, and quicker return to activity is justification for its use to improve the results of chronic reconstruction of an anterior-cruciate–deficient knee. The efficacy of such techniques can only be determined by long-term evaluation. There is nothing to suggest that results will be any less successful than the present methods of autogenous reconstruction.

The use of a true prosthetic replacement, particularly in the salvage knee or in the patient who requires early mobilization and use, does not require the protection for healing and revascularization as does the augmented autogenous tissue. Their use then becomes self evident and the advantages apparent. The question of longevity of the device and tolerance of the joint to its presence again must be determined by long-term studies.

FUTURE ADVANCEMENTS

The arthroscopic placement of both augmented autogenous tissue and prosthetic devices has been accomplished with relative ease and consistency. The use of autogenous tissue still requires the harvesting of such tissue and a degree of protected mobilization to allow for revascularization, healing, and collagen maturation to ensure the development of proper tensile strength. This increases the morbidity and prolongs recovery. The use of allografts to eliminate the necessity for harvesting an autogenous graft has been used. Such tissue, though providing biologic collagen and the advantages of living tissue, must still be protected during its healing phase, where its tensile strength becomes minimal. The augmentation by synthetic materials to provide early tensile strength and quicker rehabilitation is being investigated in animal studies. Synthetically augmented allografts with high tensile strength, which can be inserted arthroscopically and can be provided with adequate fixation strength to allow early motion and more immediate use, would bestow to the joint the advantages of living tissue within the joint along with immediate joint use as with the use of a true prosthesis.

A problem with knees that have had ligament

injury and resultant laxity is the damage that occurs to the meniscus. Though peripheral repairs are now accepted and produce acceptable results, prolonged protection to allow adequate healing is still felt to be required. Relatively few damaged menisci, particularly with a chronic ligamentous laxity, are repairable. Preservation of as much meniscal tissue as possible is the goal, since loss of the meniscus enhances joint deterioration. Hopefully, we will produce a more acceptable solution to this enigma in the future.

More widespread use of artificial materials to augment tissue or to provide a prosthetic substitution for ligamentous tissue about the knee is, in my opinion, bound to occur. The arthroscopic insertion of such tissue avoids capsular incisions and allows shorter incisions at fixation sites, which preserves proprioceptive sensation around the knee and decreases the reflex inhibition that incisions into the quadriceps mechanism sometimes produce.

The problem of anterior cruciate disruption was first recognized some 130 years ago. We are still searching for the "elegant solution." At the present time, there is no "ideal ligament replacement" [1]. The original ligament, which withstood the stresses of use until its first failure, has not yielded its position of superiority to any biologic or synthetic replacement presently in use.

REFERENCE

1. Larson RL. Overview of synthetic ligaments. In: Feagin JA, ed. The crucial ligaments. Philadelphia: JB Lippincott (in press).

INDEX

Note: Page numbers in *italics* indicate illustrations. Page numbers followed by t indicate tables.

Abrader, 175, *177*, 195, *196*
Abrasion
  with allograft, 190, 195, *196,* 199
  with Gore-Tex ligament, 159, *195,* 175, *176,* 178, *178*
  with ProCol bioprosthesis, 98, 99, 108–109, 111, 113–114, 116
Absorption. *See* Degradation *and* Ingrowth
Achilles tendon, as allograft, 180, 181, 181t, 182, 182t, 183, 183t, 187, 189
Activities of daily living. *See* Function
Allograft, 186–201, *194,* 198. *See also* Kennedy LAD *and* ProCol bioprosthesis
  biomechanics of, 180–185, 181t, 182t, *183,* 183t, 184t
  and types of proestheses, 34, 35
Anatomy of the knee, 3–6. *See also* Biomechanics
Anchoring. *See* Attachment
Anesthesia, with arthroscopic insertion of allograft, 193
Anterior cruciate ligament (ACL)
  anatomy and kinematics of, 4–5
  reconstruction, history of, 1–2
Anterior displacement. *See also* Load-deformation curve
  with Gore-Tex ligament, 142–144, *146*
  with Marshall/Macintosh reconstruction, 75, 76, *76,* 77
  with ProCol bioprosthesis, 106, 106t, 107, 107t
Anterior drawer test, 10, 14
  with Gore-Tex ligament, 160, *161*
  with Intergraft, 57
  with Leeds-Keio ligament, 137
  with ProCol bioprosthesis, 96, 97, 102, 106, 107
Antibiotics
  with allograft procedure, 194
  with arthroscopic Gore-Tex insertion, 169
Antigen. *See* Immunologic response
Arthrofibrosis, with polypropylene braid, 85
Arthrometer. *See also* K-T 1000 device
  in instrumented testing, 12–13, 14
Arthroscope. *See also* K-T 1000 device
  with allograft, 191, 193–201, *195, 196, 197, 198, 199*
  future of, 210
  with Gore-Tex ligament, 159, 165–179, *167,* 169t, *170, 171, 172, 173, 175, 176, 177, 178*
  with Intergraft, 59–64, *60, 61, 62, 63, 64*
  with Leeds-Keio ligament, 137–138, *138*
  with ProCol bioprosthesis, 112–117, *114, 115, 116*

Athletics. *See also* Injuries, Load, *and* Strength
  with allograft, 189, *200*
  with Intergraft, 55–56, *56*
  with Leeds-Keio ligament, 136
  with ProCol bioprosthesis, 106, 107
  with prosthetic materials, 36, 39
Attachment, 35. *See also* Attachment site, Flexion, *and* Surgical technique
  of allograft, 198–199, *198, 199*
  with biograft, 65–67
  with Gore-Tex ligament, 140, 142, 146, 158–159, 162, 170, *171, 176,* 177–179
  of Kennedy LAD, 67–68, 73
  of Leeds-Keio ligament, 119–122, *121,* 133–136, *135, 136*
  with ProCol bioprosthesis, *110,* 113–115
  with soft tissue, 45–47, 48–50, 52, 59, 83
Attachment site, 5–6, *5, 6,* 34, 35
  Bone. *See* Bone as attachment site
  for Intergraft, 45–47, 48–49, 54, 59, 61
  isometry of, 18–19
  for Leeds-Keio ligament, 119–120, *120*
  and maximum absolute value of strain (MAS), 104–105
  for ProCol bioprosthesis, 104–105, 109–110
Augmentation, synthetic, 65–70. *See also* Ingrowth, Ligament augmentation device (LAD), Scaffold, *and* Stent
  with autogenous graft, 65–78, 79, 82–88, *86, 87, 88*
  biomechanics of, 65–67
  FDA review of, 206–207
  with Kennedy LAD, 67–78, 206
  with polpropylene braid, 79–88
Autogenous graft, 22–27
  for augmentation, 65–78, 79, 82–88, *86, 87, 88*
  degradation of, 79, 81, 82
  with Integraft, 59–61
  and types of prosthesis, 34, 35

Biologic graft. *See* Allograft, Autogenous graft, ProCol bioprosthesis, and Xenograft, bovine
Biomechanics
  of allografts, 180–185

Biomechanics *(Continued)*
of augmentation, 65–67
of Gore-Tex prosthesis, 140–148
of the knee, 3–9
of ProCol bioprosthesis, 83–93
Bioprosthesis. *See* Allograft, Autogenous graft, Ligament
augmentation device (LAD), *and* ProCol
bioprosthesis
Bone, for allograft, 186, 189, 193–199, *194, 198*
Bone as attachment site
with allograft, 189, 195–197, *196, 197,* 198–199, *198,*
199
with carbon fiber stent, 49, 50
with Intergraft, 61, 62
with Kennedy LAD, 73
with Leeds-Keio ligament, 119–125, 133–136, *135, 136*
with polypropylene braid, 80, *80,* 83, 84, 85
with ProCol bioprosthesis, 98, 99, 102–104
Bone plug, *103, 125, 127,* 132, 133. *See also* Bone as
attachment site *and* Leeds-Keio ligament
extractor, 123, *123, 124,* 134
introducer, 123, *125, 126,* 134
in laboratory animals, 126, 127
Bovine collagen, 48. *See also* ProCol bioprosthesis
Breakage, LAD. *See also* Failure
with Marshall/Macintosh reconstruction, 74
Burmester curve, 6

Carbon fibers
in Intergraft, 41–64
in ligament reconstruction, 41–50, *49,* 52–55, 59–64
in ligament reinforcement, 39–40
as prosthetic material, 31, 35
Cellular response. *See* Immunologic response
Center for Devices and Radiological Health, (CDRH), 202–
203
Chamfering devices, 172, 173, 179
Cobalt irradiation. *See* Sterilization of autograft
Collagen. *See also* Ingrowth *and* Xenograft, bovine
with ProCol bioprosthesis, 91–92, 95, 96, 97t, 110
with synthetic augmentation, 79, 82
in tissues, 49t
Collagen ingrowth. *See also* Ingrowth
with polymer-coated carbon fiber, 48, 49, 50, 52
with ProCol bioprosthesis, 109, *110,* 111
Compliance, of ACL, 35
Complications. *See also* Creep, Effusion, Infection, Pain,
and Synovitis
with Gore-Tex ligament, 162, *162,* 162t, 165, 169, 169t
with Intergraft, 57
with Leeds-Keio ligament, 138
with Marshall/Macintosh reconstruction, 74, 74t
with ProCol bioprosthesis, 97–98, 107–108
Creep, 6t. *See also* Complications
of augmentation material, 67, 75
with Gore-Tex Prosthesis, 140, 142, *144,* 146, 147, *147*
with Marshall/Macintosh reconstruction, 70
with ProCol bioprosthesis, 90–91, 93

Dacron as prosthetic material, 30, 31, 32, 35, 205–206. *See
also* Leeds-Keio ligament
Deformation, 6t, *7. See also* Load-deformation curve *and*
Load failure
and graft tensioning, 20–21

Degradation
of autogenous grafts, 79, 81, 82
of carbon-fiber implants, 41–42, 52, 53
within synovium, 44–45
Devices. *See* Instrumented Knee Testing *and* Prostheses
Division of Surgical and Rehabilitation Devices (DSRD),
203
Drill hole
for Gore-Tex ligament, *158*
for Intergraft, 61, *61*
Drilling
for Gore-Tex arthroscopic insertion, 170, *172*
for Intergraft, 62, *62,* 63, *64*
with ProCol bioprosthesis, 113–114, *114*
Dye, as diagnostic tool, 2

Effusion. *See also* Complications *and* Particulate debris
with Gore-Tex ligament, 162, 163, 169
with Marshall/Macintosh reconstruction, 74, 75, 77, 77t
with Intergraft, 57
with ProCol bioprosthesis, 96, 106, 107
Elasticity. *See also* Elongation *and* Visoelasticity
with ProCol bioprosthesis, 92, 93
Elongation. *See also* Elasticity *and* Length
with Gore-Tex ligament, 143, *145,* 147, *147,* 154–155
with ProCol bioprosthesis, 93, 101–102, 108
Ethylene oxide (ETO). *See also* Sterilization, of allograft
in allograft, 190, *190,* 191
Evaluation. *See also* Complications
of biologic augmentation of LAD, 69–70
of Intergraft, 41–50
of Marshall/Macintosh reconstruction, 76–77
Exercise. *See* Athletics, Function, *and* Rehabilitation
Extension *See also* Flexion *and* Function
and biomechanics of the knee, 7–8
and kinematics of the knee, 3–6
Extensometer, 91
Extra-articular procedure. *See also* Surgical technique
with allograft, 189, 199
with Gore-Tex ligament, 165, *172*
with Leeds-Keio ligament, 133, 134, 136, 138–139
with ProCol bioprosthesis, 101–102, *102,* 104, 110, 111

Failure. *See also* Load failure
of allograft, 189–191
of Gore-Tex ligament, 162–163, 169, 169t
of Marshall/Macintosh reconstruction, 74
Fascia lata as allograft, 190, 181, 181t, 182, 182t, 183,
183, 183t, 187, 189
Fastener. *See* Attachment *and* Surgical technique
Fatigue. *See also* Load-deformation curve *and* Load failure
of augmentation material, 67
Fatigue testing. *See also* Load *and* Testing
of Leeds-Keio ligament, 129–130, 130t
Femoral anatomic attachment site (FAAS), 195, 196, *196.
See also* Bone as attachment site
Femoral condyles, and kinematics of the knee, 3–4, 5
Femoral-tibial joint, kinematics of, 3–4
Fibers, 4–5. *See also* Carbon fiber
Fibroblasts, with polymer-coated carbon fiber, 43, *44,* 48,
52
Fixation. *See* Attachment
Flexion. *See also* Function, Hyper flexion, Laxity, Length
pattern, *and* Range of motion
and biomechanics of the knee, 7–8

with Gore-Tex ligament, 140, 141, 143, 146, 154
and graft isometry, 19, 104, 136
and kinematics of the knee, 3–6
with Leeds-Keio ligament, 136
and patient needs, 118–119
Food and Drug Administration (FDA), 202–208 and ProCol
bioprosthesis, 111
Foot rotation, with Gore-Tex ligament, 151–152, *152*
Four-bar linkage, crossed, *5, 18,*
Freeze drying of allograft, 180, 181–182, 181t, 189, 191,
197–198
effects of 183, *183,* 183t, 184, 184t, 186, 187
Fresh freezing of allograft, 180, 181–182, 181t, 182t, 183t,
186, 187, 189, 191, 197–198
effects of, 184, 184t
Function, 35. *See also* Laxity *and* Range of Motion
with Gore-Tex ligament, 150–153, 161–162, *161, 162,*
165–169, *166, 167, 168*
with Intergraft, 55, *56*
with Leeds-Keio ligament, 136–138
with Marshall/Macintosh reconstruction, 75–76, 77t
with ProCol bioprosthesis, 96t, 106–107, 105, 109, *109*

Genucom knee-analysis system, 14–15
Giving-way symptoms, with Gore-Tex ligament, 150, 150t,
161, *161,* 165, *168*
Gore-Tex ligament, 32, 35–36, 37–38
biomechanics and tensioning of, 140–148
clinical and laboratory studies of, 149–155
FDA review of, 205, 206
properties of, 7t
US experience with, 156–164
Glutaraldehyde, with bovine xenograft, 96, 101
Graft. *See also* Allograft, Attachment, Attachment site,
Autogenous graft, *and* Xenograft, bovine
biologic, for augmentation, 65–78. *See also* Ligament
augmentation device (LAD)
Graft isometry, 17–20
with Leeds-Keio ligament, 135–136
Graft rejection. *See* Failure
Grips, mechanical, 89–90, 90–91, 92
Guide pin, 113, *113,* 114, *157, 170, 172, 174*

Harvesting
for allograft, 188–189, *194*
for Intergraft, 61, *61*
Healing. *See* Ingrowth, Recollagenization, *and* Remodeling
Histocompatibility. *See* Immunologic response
Histology, of Leeds-Keio ligament, 137–138, *138*
Host reponse. *See* Immunologic response
Hydraulic clinical testing device, 12
with ProCol Bioprosthesis, 91, 92
Hydron, as prosthetic material, 30
Hyperflexion, with Marshall/Macintosh reconstruction, 74

Iliotibial band
as ACL graft, 23–24, 59–61
with Intergraft, 54–55, 59–61
with ProCol bioprosthesis, 105
Immobilization. *See* Rehabilitation
Immunologic response
with allograft, 186–187, 190, *190*

with bovine xenograft, 96, 101, 109, 116
with polylactic acid, 42, 43
Impingement. *See* Abrasion
Incision. *See also* Surgical technique
for Gore-Tex arthroscopy, *171, 173, 174*
Indications
for Gore-Tex ligament, 141, 156
for Leeds-Keio ligament, 118, 133
for prosthetic ACL reconstruction, 38
Infection. *See also* Complications *and* Synovitis
with Gore-Tex ligament, 162, 169
with Intergraft, 57
with Marshall/Macintosh reconstruction, 74
with ProCol bioprosthesis, 97, 98, 107–108
Inflammatory response
with polymer-coated carbon fiber, 44–45, 52
with polypropylene braid, 80, 82
with ProCol bioprosthesis, 108–109, 111
Ingrowth. *See also* Augmentation, synthetic; Collagen;
Recollagenization; Remodeling; Scaffold; *and*
Stent
with bovine xenograft, 109, *110,* 111,
with Gore-Tex ligament, 156–157
with polymer-coated carbon fiber, 45–50, *49, 52*
Injuries. *See also* Athletics *and* Complications
and Gore-Tex ligament, 160, *160*
and indications for prostheses, 36, 38
and Intergraft, 54, 55
and laxity, *13*
and Leeds-Keio ligament, 118–119, 133
and Marshall/Macintosh reconstruction, 74
and ProCol bioprosthesis, 97–98, 108
Insertion site. *See* Attachment site
Instability. *See* Stability
with Gore-Tex prosthesis, 144, 162–163, 165, 169t
with Intergraft, 57
with Leeds-Keio ligament, 137, *137*
overview of, 1–2, 7–8
with ProCol bioprosthesis, 96, 97, 101–102, 106–107
with prostheses, 38
testing of, 10, 96
Instrumentation. *See also* Surgical technique *and* Testing
for Intergraft, 53, 60–64, *53, 60, 61, 62, 63, 64*
for Leeds-Keio ligament, 122–125, *123, 134*
for ProCol bioprosthesis, 114, 115, *114, 115, 116*
Instrumented knee testing, 10–16, 149–150, *150, 151–153.*
See also Testing
Intercondylar notch
with allograft, 195–196, *196,* 199
with Gore-Tex ligament, 157, *157,* 158, 170, *170,* 178
with ProCol bioprosthesis, 98, 99, 103–104, *103*
Intergraft
clinical testing of, 53
FDA review of, 205
preclinical studies of, 41–51, 53
properties of, 7t
reconstruction with, 52–64, *60, 61, 62, 63, 64*
Intra-articular procedure. *See also* Surgical technique
with allograft, 186, 189–190
with Gore-Tex ligament, 165, *172, 173, 175, 177*
with Leeds-Keio ligament, 133–135, *134,* 136, 138–139
with polypropylene braid, 79, 82–88, *83, 84, 85, 86, 87,*
88
with ProCol bioprosthesis, 103–105, *103, 110*
Investigational Device Exemption (IDE), 203, 205, 206,
207
Isometry, graft, 17–21
with Leeds-Keio ligament, 135–136

James–Larson knee-rating forms, 150
Jerk test, with Leeds-Keio ligament, 137
Joint disease, degenerative, 36, 38

Kennedy LAD
  FDA review of, 205, 206
  Marshall/Macintosh reconstruction with 71–78
  modifications of, 83–88
  studies of, 67–70
Kinematics of the knee, 3–6
KT-1000 device, 13–14, *14*
  in Marshall/Macintosh reconstruction, 72, 73, 75
  in ProCol bioprosthesis, 106, 107, 107t
K-wire, 197, *198*

Laboratory setting, for testing, 10
Lachman test
  with allograft, 193
  with Gore-Tex ligament, 141–142, *141, 143,* 146, *147,*
    152, 153, 161, *161,* 165, *166*
  with Intergraft, 56–57
  with Leeds-Keio ligament, 137
  with Marshall/Macintosh reconstruction, 75
  with polypropylene braid, 86, 88
  with ProCol bioprosthesis, 96, 97, 106
LAD. *See* Ligament augmentation device (LAD)
Laxity. *See also* Function *and* Range of Motion
  with allograft, 193
  with Gore-Tex prosthesis, 142–143, *143,* 144–147, *144,*
    147, 151–153, *151, 152, 153,* 154–155, 154t, 177,
    179
  with Intergraft, *47,* 47–48, 50, 57
  with Marshall/Macintosh reconstruction, 72, 73–74, 77
  with ProCol bioprosthesis, 93
  and prosthetic reconstruction, 35
  testing of, 10, 11–16, 149–150, *150*
Leeds-Keio ligament, 31–32, 35, *122, 133*
  biomechanics of, 118–131
  properties of, 7t, 35
  reconstruction with 132–139
Length. *See also* Elongation *and* Length patterns and
    placement sites, 120, 120t, 121, 121t
Length patterns, 104
  and maximum absolute value of strain, *104*
  with tibial and femoral graft sites, 18
Ligament
  for allograft, 186, 187
  augmentation. *See* Augmentation, Synthetic, *and*
    Ligament augmentation device
  reinforcement with carbon fiber, 39–40. *See also*
    Intergraft, Scaffold, *and* Stent
Ligament augmentation device (LAD), 30–31, 35, 36–37,
    66
  Kennedy, 67–78, 83–88, 205, 206
  properties of, 7t
Load. *See also* Load-deformation curve *and* Load failure
  with biologic graft, 65–67, 68–69
  with Gore-Tex prosthesis, 142–144, 145–147, *147*
  with graft tensioning, 20–21, 74
  with Leeds-Keio ligament, 119, 127–128
Load-deformation curve, 6t, *7. See also* Deformation *and*
    Load failure
  and Gore-Tex ligament, 146
  and Leeds-Keio ligament, 128
  for normal knee, *12*
  and ProCol bioprosthesis, 90, 91, 92

Load displacement. *See* Load-deformation curve *and* Load
    failure
Load failure. *See* Load-deformation curve
  with allograft, 188
  with LAD, 67, *68*
  with polypropylene braid, *34*
  with ProCol bioprosthesis, 89–90, 91, 92, 93, 115–116
Longevity, of prostheses, 35, 36
Lyophilization. *See* Freeze drying
Lysholm score, with ProCol bioprosthesis, 107, 107t

Marshall/Macintosh reconstruction, with Kennedy LAD, 71–
    78, 206
Maximum absolute value of strain (MAS), *104,* 104–105,
    105
Mechanical devices. *See also* Instrumentation
  and testing for laxity, 11–14
Medmetric KT-100, 13–14, *14*
Medmetric Tension/Isometer (TI), 19–20, 21, *21*
Meniscus
  as ACL graft, 26–27
  with Marshall/Macintosh reconstruction, 73, 73t
Metachromasia, of articular cartilage of the knee, 45, *46*
Musculature, and success of prosthesis, 38

Notchplasty. *See* Intercondylar notch

Orientation of graft, 18t, *21. See also* attachment
  of Gore-Tex ligament, 154
Orthopedic and Rehabilitation Devices Panel, 203
Osteophyte, with Gore-Tex ligament, 178, *178*

Pain
  in clinical trials of Intergraft, 55, *56*
  with Gore-Tex ligament, 161, *162,* 163, 169
  with Marshall/Macintosh reconstruction, 74
Particulate debris. *See also* Complications, Effusion,
    Infection, *and* Synovitis
  with Intergraft, 46
  with Kennedy LAD, 77, 77t
  with ProCol bioprosthesis, 99, 111, 116
Patellar tendon
  as ACL graft, 23, 25–26, 67–69
  for allograft, 180, 181, 181t, 182, 182t, 183, *183,* 185,
    187, 189, 193–199, *194, 198, 199*
  and augmentation with polypropylene braid, 85, 86, 88
  with Intergraft, 55, 61, *61*
Pes tendon, as ACL graft, 24–25
Pin
  guide, 113, *113, 114, 157, 170, 172, 174*
  Steinman, 62, 177
Pivot shift test
  with allograft, 193
  with Gore-Tex prosthesis, 141, 142, *142,* 150–151, 152–
    153, *153,* 160–161, *161,* 165, *167*
  with Intergraft, 57
  with Marshall/Macintosh reconstruction, 74, 75, 76, *76,*
    77
  with polypropylene braid augmentation, 86, 88
  with ProCol bioprosthesis, 96, 97, 101, 106
Placement. *See* Attachment *and* Attachment site

Plug
    bone. *See* Bone plug
    silicone, *173*
Polycaprolactone. *See also* Intergraft
    as carbon-fiber coating, 42–43, 52, 53
Polyester, as ACL prosthetic material, 30, 31
Polyethylene, as ACL prosthetic material, 30
Polyflex System, 30, 204
Polyglycolic acid, as ACL prosthetic material, 31
Polylactic acid (PLA). *See also* Intergraft
    with ACL prosthetic material, 31
    as carbon-fiber coating, 42–43, 52, 53
    fastener with Intergraft, 63, 64
Polymer coating. *See also* Intergraft
    of carbon-fiber stent, 41–43, 52
Polypropylene braid, 72–88, *81, 82, 83, 85, 86, 87*
    as ACL prosthetic material, 30–31, 35, 36–37
    FDA regulation of, 205, 206
    in Marshall/Macintosh reconstruction, 77
Polytetrafluoroethylene (PTPE). *See also* Gore-Tex ligament
    as ACL prosthetic material, 23, 140, 206
Positioning. *See also* Surgical technique
    for allograft, 194
Posterior cruciate ligament, 4–5
Postoperative results. *See* Complications, Function, *and* Rehabilitation
Preconditioning, of Gore-Tex ligament, 146, 154, 178–179
Preload, with Gore-Tex ligament, 143, 144, 145, *145*
Premarket Approval Application (PMA), 203–204, 205, 206, 207
    for ProCol bioprosthesis, 111
Prepatellar periosteum, in augmentation with polypropylene braid, 83, 85, 86
Prepatellar retinaculum, in Marshall/Macintosh reconstruction, 71, 73
Preservation of allograft, 180–181, 181t, 182, 182t, 183–184, *183*, 184t, 186, 187
Procedures. *See also* Surgical technique
    overview of, 1–2
ProCol bioprosthesis. *See also* Xenograft, bovine
    arthroscopic reconstruction with, 112–117
    biomechanics of, 89–94
    clinical experience with, 101–111
    in open ACL reconstruction, 95–100
Proplast, 29–30, 35
Proprioception, 34
Prostheses. *See also* Allograft, Autogenous graft, Ligament augmentation device (LAD), *and* Xenograft, bovine
    future of, 209–211
    FDA regulation of, 203, 208
    Gore-Tex, 140–179
    history of, 1, 29–33
    indications for, 34–38
    ProCol, 89–117
    results with, in laboratory animals, 79–82

Quadriceps tendon
    in Marshall/Macintosh reconstruction, 71, 73
    in polypropylene braid augmentation, 83, 86

Range of motion. *See also* Function, Laxity, *and* Rehabilitation
    with brace, 88, 96
    with crossed four-bar linkage, 5
    with Gore-Tex prosthesis, 141, 160, 161, 177

    with graft isometry, 17, 18, 19
    with graft tensioning, 21
    with Leeds-Keio ligament, 136, 137, 173t
    with polypropylene braid, 88
    with ProCol bioprosthesis, 96, 98, 104, 115
Recollagenization. *See also* Collagen *and* Ingrowth
    with synthetic augmentation, 78, 82
Regulation, FDA, of prosthetic ligament devices, 202–208
Rehabilitation. *See also* Function *and* Range of Motion
    with allograft, *200, 201*
    considerations in, 1–2
    with Gore-Tex ligament, 156, 159–160
    with Intergraft, 64
    with Leeds-Keio ligament, 137
    with ProCol bioprosthesis, 106, 111
Rehydration of allograft, 198
Reinforcement. *See* Augmentation *and* Ligament augmentation device (LAD)
Rejection, graft. *See* Failure
Remodeling. *See also* Ingrowth, Recollagenization, Scaffold, *and* Stent
    with biologic graft, 65, 70, 71, 98
    with ProCol bioprosthesis, 98, 108, 115
Remote sensors, in laxity testing, 11, 14–15
Retensioning, in Marshall/Macintosh reconstruction, 74, 75t
Revascularization. *See* Vascular supply
Rongeur, for Gore-Tex arthroscopic insertion, 174–175, *175*
Rotation, testing for, 11

Scaffold, 35. *See also* Augmentation, synthetic; Ingrowth; *and* Stent
    with Leeds-Keio ligament, 118–119, 132–133
Screws
    with Gore-Tex ligament, 177, *178*
    revisions of, 162, 169
Semitendinosus tendon, *80, 81*
    as allograft, 181
Soft tissue
    as allograft, 186, 187, 189
    attachment, 45–47, 48–50, 52, 59, 83
    with Gore-Tex prosthesis, 144
Sports. *See* Athletics
Spring theory, and augmentation, 66
Stability. *See also* Instability
    with Gore-Tex ligament, 177
    of Intergraft, 47–48, 55, 56, 57
    of ProCol bioprosthesis, 96–98, *98*, 101–102, 106t, 106–107, 108, *108*, 111
Stabilizer, *113*
Staining. *See* Metachromasia
Steinmann pin, 62, 177
Stent, 35. *See also* Augmentation, synthetic; Ingrowth; Intergraft: *and* Scaffold
    for augmentation, 67
Sterilization
    of allograft, 180, 181–182, 184, 184t, 189, 190, 198
    with Leeds-Keio ligament, 129, 130
Stiffness, 6t
    of allograft, 180, 181
    with Gore-Tex ligament, 143–144, 151–153, *152*
    with Kennedy LAD, 67, *68*
    with LAD, *66*
    with Leeds-Keio ligament, 119, 129
    testing of, 149–150, *150*. *See also* Instrumented knee testing

Strain, 6t, *7*
  of allograft, 180, 182, 182t, 183, *183,* 183t, 184, 184t
  with Gore-Tex ligament, 143
  with Leeds-Keio ligament, 129, 136
  maximum absolute value of, 104–105
  and ProCol bioprosthesis, 90, 93
  and tests of motion, 17
Strength. *See also* Load, Load-deformation curve, *and* Load failure
  of allograft, 180–181, 182, 182t, 183, *183,* 183t, 184, 184t, 187–188
  of Intergraft, 41, 42, 46, 47, 50, 54
  of intra-articular autograft, 79, 81
  with Kennedy LAD, 67, 68, 71, 77
  of Leeds-Keio ligament, 119, 129–130
  with Marshall/Macintosh reconstruction, 71, 77
  with ProCol bioprosthesis, 90–91, 92, 93, 116–117
  relative, of graft material, 23t
  testing of, 89, 90
  ultimate. *See* Ultimate strength
Stress, 6t, *7*
  with ProCol bioprosthesis, 90, 93
Stress radiograph, *11*
Stress-strain curve, 6t
  with ProCol bioprosthesis, 83
Stretch. *See* Elongation
Stover hook, with Gore-Tex ligament, *158,* 159
Stryker, properties of, 7t
Stryker ® Knee Augmentation Device, FDA review of, 205–206
Stryker Meadox ligament graft, 32, 35
Stryker knee-laxity tester, 14, *15*
Surgical technique. *See also* Attachment
  with allograft, 193–200, *195, 196, 197, 198, 199*
  with arthroscopy, 59–64, *60, 61, 62, 63, 64,* 73, 165–179, *170, 171, 172, 173, 174, 175, 176, 177, 178,* 193–199, *195, 196, 197, 198, 199*
  for autogenous reconstruction, 23–27
  with Gore-Tex ligament, 144–145, 146, 157–159, *157, 158, 159,* 169–179, *170, 171, 172, 173, 174, 175, 176, 177, 178*
  for Intergraft, 54–55, 59–64
  with Leeds-Keio ligament, 120–125, 133–135, *134, 135,* 138–139
  for ligament reinforcement with carbon fiber, 39–40, 54–55
  with Marshall/Macintosh reconstruction, 73
  with Medmetric Tension/Isometer, 19–20
  for polypropylene braid augmentation, 85–88
  for ProCol bioprosthesis, 101, 102–105, 111, 112–117
Suturing. *See·also* Surgical technique
  with allograft, 199
  with arthroscopic Gore-Tex insertion, 177
  with Kennedy LAD, 68–69, *69*
  with polypropylene braid, 87
  with ProCol bioprosthesis, 114–115
Swelling, with Gore-Tex ligament, 161, *162*
Synovitis. *See also* Infection *and* Synovium
  with Intergraft, 44–45, 57
  with Marshall/Macintosh reconstruction, 77, 77t
  with ProCol bioprosthesis, 99, 107–108, 111, 116, *116,*177
Synovium. *See also* Synovitis
  with allograft, 188, 191, 195
  and bovine xenograft, 99, 107–108, 110, 111, *116, 117*
  carbon debris in, 44–45, *45*
  in laboratory animals, 80, *80*

Talc, and synovitis, 44–45, *46*
Tape, umbilical, with arthroscopic Gore-Tex insertion, 174, 175, *175, 176*

Teflon (tetrafluorethylene). *See also* Proplast
  as prosthetic material, 35
Tendon. *See also* Achilles tendon, as allograft; Patellar tendon; Pes tendon; Quadriceps tendon; *and* Semitendinosus tendon
  as allograft, 186, 187, 188, 189
Tensile strength, 35. *See also* Strength *and* Tensioning
Tensile test curve, with ProCol bioprosthesis, *93*
Tensioning, *20,* 20–21
  of Gore-Tex ligament, 140–148
  in Marshall/Macintosh reconstruction, 71, 73–74, 75t
Tensionmeter, in Marshall/Macintosh reconstruction, 73
Tension/Isometer, Medmetric, 19–20
Testing. *See also* Lachman test, Laxity, *and* Pivot shift test
  of allograft, 188, 191
  of augmentation with polypropylene braid, 85
  comparisons of, 89, 90
  FDA guidelines for, 207
  of Gore-Tex ligament, 149–150, *150,* 151–153
  hydraulic devices for, 12, 91, 92
  instrumented, 10–16, 149–150, *150,* 151–153.
  of Intergraft, 43–49, 53, 55–57
  laboratory setting for, 10
  of Leeds-Keio ligament, 125, 129–130, 130t, 137, 137t
  with Marshall/Macintosh reconstruction, 75–76
  of ProCol bioprosthesis, 90–92, 96–97
Thawing, of allograft, 198
Thigh holder
  with allograft, 194, *195*
  with ProCol bioprosthesis, *113, 114*
Tibial aimer, 197, *198*
Tibial anatomic attachment site (TAAS), 197 *197. See also* Bone as attachment site
Tibial-femoral displacement. *See* Laxity
Tibial plateaus, 4
Tissue banking, for allograft, 188–189, 191
Transplantation, types of, 186. *See also* Allograft
Tube, for Intergraft, 60, *60,* 62, *63*
Tunnel, 109, *110*
  femoral, 102, 103, *103,* 114, *114, 115,* 196–197, *196, 197*
  for Leeds-Keio ligament insertion, *128,* 134–135, *135*
  tibial, 102, *103,* 114, *114,* 115, *115, 128,* 197, *197*

UCLA apparatus, 11–13, *13,* 149–150, *150*
Ultimate strength, 6t
  of allograft, 181, 182, 182t, 183, *183* 183t, 184, 184t
  in rabbit graft, *6*

Vascular supply
  of allograft, 188
  of graft, 23, 26
  with Leeds-Keio ligament, 138
Vector ® system, 170, *171, 174*
Velocity vector, *4*
Visoelasticity, 6t, *7,* 34

Weaving, of carbon fiber, 61, *61*

Xenograft, bovine, 31, 35, 36, 89–117
  with carbon fiber, 48
  immunologic response with, 96, 101, 109, 116
Xenograft, Pro-Tek, 36
Xeontech, properties of, 7t